Clinical Parasitology

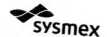

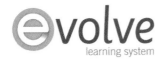 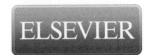
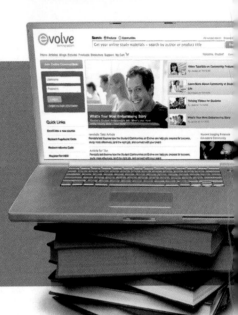

Clinical Parasitology

A PRACTICAL APPROACH

Second Edition

Elizabeth A. Gockel-Blessing (formerly Zeibig), PhD, MLS(ASCP)^{CM}

Interim Associate Dean for Student and Academic Affairs
Program Director, Master of Science in Health Sciences
Associate Professor, Department of Clinical Laboratory Science
Doisy College for Health Sciences
Saint Louis University
St. Louis, Missouri

ELSEVIER
SAUNDERS

3251 Riverport Lane
St. Louis, Missouri 63043

CLINICAL PARASITOLOGY: A PRACTICAL APPROACH   ISBN: 978-1-4160-6044-4
Copyright © 2013, 1997 by Saunders, an imprint of Elsevier Inc.

No part of this publication may be reproduced or transmitted in any form or by any means, electronic
or mechanical, including photocopying, recording, or any information storage and retrieval system,
without permission in writing from the publisher. Details on how to seek permission, further
information about the Publisher's permissions policies and our arrangements with organizations such
as the Copyright Clearance Center and the Copyright Licensing Agency, can be found at our website:
www.elsevier.com/permissions.

This book and the individual contributions contained in it are protected under copyright by the
Publisher (other than as may be noted herein).

Notices

Knowledge and best practice in this field are constantly changing. As new research and experience
broaden our understanding, changes in research methods, professional practices, or medical
treatment may become necessary.

Practitioners and researchers must always rely on their own experience and knowledge in
evaluating and using any information, methods, compounds, or experiments described herein. In
using such information or methods they should be mindful of their own safety and the safety of
others, including parties for whom they have a professional responsibility.

With respect to any drug or pharmaceutical products identified, readers are advised to check
the most current information provided (i) on procedures featured or (ii) by the manufacturer of
each product to be administered, to verify the recommended dose or formula, the method and
duration of administration, and contraindications. It is the responsibility of practitioners, relying
on their own experience and knowledge of their patients, to make diagnoses, to determine dosages
and the best treatment for each individual patient, and to take all appropriate safety precautions.

To the fullest extent of the law, neither the Publisher nor the authors, contributors, or editors,
assume any liability for any injury and/or damage to persons or property as a matter of products
liability, negligence or otherwise, or from any use or operation of any methods, products,
instructions, or ideas contained in the material herein.

Publishing Director: Andrew Allen
Content Manager: Ellen Wurm-Cutter
Publishing Services Manager: Julie Eddy
Senior Project Manager: Marquita Parker
Design Manager: Teresa McBryan

Printed in the United States of America

Last digit is the print number: 9   8   7   6   5   4   3

**Working together to grow
libraries in developing countries**

www.elsevier.com | www.bookaid.org | www.sabre.org

ELSEVIER   BOOK AID International   Sabre Foundation

For Bob

Charity E. Accurso, PhD, MT(ASCP)
Assistant Professor
Medical Laboratory Science Program
University of Cincinnati
Cincinnati, Ohio

Hassan A. Aziz, PhD, MLS(ASCP)^{CM}
Director and Associate Professor
Biomedical Sciences
Qatar University
Doha, Qatar

Lynda A. Britton, PhD, MLS(ASCP)^{CM} SM
Program Director and Professor
Program in Clinical Laboratory Sciences
Department of Clinical Sciences
School of Allied Health Professions
LSU Health Sciences Center
Shreveport, Louisiana

Janice M. Conway-Klaassen, PhD,
MT(ASCP)SM
Director, Clinical Laboratory Science
University of Minnesota
Minneapolis, Minnesota

Jill Dennis, EdD, MLS(ASCP)^{CM}
Associate Dean of Academic Operations
Assistant Professor of Medical Laboratory
Science
Thomas University
Thomasville, Georgia

Linda J. Graeter, PhD, MT(ASCP)
Associate Professor
Medical Laboratory Science Program
University of Cincinnati
Cincinnati, Ohio

Michelle Mantooth, MSc, MLS(ASCP)^{CM},
CG(ASCP)^{CM}
MLT Instructor
Trident Technical College
Charleston, South Carolina

Lauren Roberts, MS, MT(ASCP)
Microbiology Laboratory
St. Joseph's Hospital and Medical Center
Phoenix, Arizona

John P. Seabolt, EdD, MT(ASCP)SM
Senior Academic Coordinator
Department of Biology
University of Kentucky
Lexington, Kentucky

Teresa A. Taff, MA, MT(ASCP)SM
Laboratory Manager and Program Director
School of Clinical Laboratory Science
Mercy Hospital St. Louis
St. Louis, Missouri

TEST BANK WRITER

Janice M. Conway-Klaassen, PhD,
MT(ASCP)SM
Director, Clinical Laboratory Science
University of Minnesota
Minneapolis, Minnesota

Thomas Betsy, DC
Professor
Bergen Community College
Paramus, New Jersey
Adjunct Professor
Felician College
Lodi, New Jersey
Adjunct Professor
SUNY Rockland Community College
Suffern, New York

Dorothy M. Boisvert, EdD, MT(ASCP)
Professor
Department of Biology/Chemistry
Fitchburg State College
Fitchburg, Massachusetts

Donna M. Duberg, MA, MS, MT(ASCP)SM
Vice-Chair, Assistant Professor
Clinical Laboratory Science Department
Doisy College of Health Sciences
Saint Louis University
St. Louis, Missouri

Alese M. Furnald, BS, MLS(ASCP)[CM]
Clinical Laboratory Scientist and
 Microbiologist
Harry S. Truman Memorial Veterans Hospital
Columbia, Missouri

Lynne Hamilton, PhD, MT(ASCP)
Assistant Professor
Clinical Laboratory Science Program
School of Allied Health Sciences
Texas Tech University Health Sciences Center
Lubbock, Texas

Katherine M. Hopper, MS, MT
Vanderbilt University Medical Center
Nashville, Tennessee

Amy R. Kapanka, MS, MT(ASCP)SC
MLT Program Director
Hawkeye Community College
Waterloo, Iowa

Perthena Latchaw, MS, MLS(ASCP)[CM]
MLT Program Director
Seminole State College
Seminole, Oklahoma

Laura A. Mayer
Office Assistant
Doisy College of Health Sciences
Office of the Dean
Saint Louis University
St. Louis, Missouri

Paula C. Mister, MS, MT, SM(ASCP)
Educational Coordinator and Clinical
 Microbiology Instructor
Medical Microbiology
Johns Hopkins Hospital
Instructor, Biology Department
Community Colleges of Baltimore County
Pathogenic Microbiology Laboratory
 Instructor
Stevenson University
Baltimore, Maryland

Cynthia Parsons, MS, MT(ASCP)
Program Director, Medical Laboratory
 Technology
Northeast Texas Community College
Mt. Pleasant, Texas

Lauren Roberts, MS, MT(ASCP)
Microbiology Laboratory
St. Joseph's Hospital and Medical Center
Phoenix, Arizona

Anne T. Rodgers, PhD, MT(ASCP)
Retired Professor of Medical Technology
Hendersonville, North Carolina

Wendy Warren Sweatt, MT(ASCP), MS, CLS
Clinical Coordinator
Center for Professional, Career, and Technical
  Education
Jefferson State Community College
Birmingham, Alabama

Teresa A. Taff, MA, MT(ASCP)SM
Laboratory Manager and Program Director
School of Clinical Laboratory Science
Mercy Hospital St. Louis
St. Louis, Missouri

Valerie A. Watson, MS
Department of Microbiology, Immunology &
  Cell Biology
West Virginia University
Morgantown, West Virginia

Linda Layne Williford Pifer, PhD, SM(ASCP),
  GS(ABB)
Professor, Department of Clinical Laboratory
  Sciences
University of Tennessee Health Science Center
Memphis, Tennessee

Michele B. Zitzmann, MHS, MLS(ASCP)
Associate Professor
Department of Clinical Laboratory Sciences
Louisiana State University Health Sciences
  Center
New Orleans, Louisiana

Parasitology is an important component of clinical laboratory medicine. The results obtained through specimen examination for parasites, provide invaluable information regarding the diagnosis and treatment of human disease. Tracking the epidemiology of such organisms as well as establishing prevention mechanisms may be accomplished with the assistance of this information.

Although numerous advances in technology have been developed during recent years, the traditional technique of manually processing and examining the samples both macroscopically and microscopically still occurs in select clinical settings. It is critical that well-educated and highly trained individuals perform these procedures as well as read and interpret the results. Thus, the goal of this second edition is to provide such information for students preparing for a career in laboratory medicine, for learners in related disciplines, which include parasitology, and for clinical practitioners.

This "learner friendly" text is designed to assist learners in both the didactic and laboratory components associated with human clinical parasitology. Students using this book will have the opportunity to develop the skills necessary to become proficient entry-level practitioners. Currently practicing clinicians may also find this book of use as both a reference at the bench and as a mechanism for these individuals to review and sharpen their skills. In alignment with Elsevier standards, the term laboratory technicians is used throughout the book when referring to practicing laboratorians. The term in this context does not refer to a specific level of practitioner but rather to all practitioners.

In order to accomplish the aforementioned goal, the primary focus of this text is two-fold. First is that assurance that proper diagnostic laboratory techniques are employed when conducting parasitology testing. The major adjustments/new features designed to address this component of the two-fold focus are as follows.

The location of this chapter has been moved from the last chapter in the book to the second chapter of the book right after the introduction discussion. An *updated*, where appropriate, laboratory diagnosis section is incorporated under the discussion of each parasite. Second is that of accurate organism identification, which is paramount to successful parasitology. To enhance proper organism identification, full-color photomicrographs are now embedded within the corresponding parasite discussions. Full-color detailed line drawings, many of which are enlarged to show detail, with structures labelled, where appropriate and updated "Typical Characteristics at a Glance" tables have been added. Periodic references to other chapters, without being redundant, are strategically placed in the text to assist the reader in quickly finding additional information.

Several parasites deemed appropriate, primarily in the Arthropod Chapter (Chapter 13) have been added to this second edition. Under the individual parasite descriptions concise information is incorporated regarding life cycle notes, epidemiology, clinical symptomatology, treatment, prevention and control, and notes of interest and new trends, where appropriate.

Features such as side-by-side comparison drawings and an entire chapter dedicated to common artifacts and confusers (Chapter 12) that were placed into the first edition are also included in this edition with revisions for clarity made as appropriate. The introduction to each chapter is now known as a feature called "Focusing In," whereas the summary of each chapter constitutes the section entitled "Looking Back." A series of chapter review questions and a case study with questions for consideration comprise the section at the end of appropriate chapters entitled "Test Your Knowledge."

This second edition contains several additional features worthy of mentioning that pertain to the book in general, to specific chapters, and/or to individual parasite discussions. Learning objectives have been updated as appropriate for each chapter. A list of key terms is embedded within each set of appropriate chapter objectives. Each term is then bolded and defined in the chapter where it first appears. A comprehensive alphabetized glossary is located at the back of the book. The common disease/condition name(s) associated with each pathogenic parasite appears below the pronunciation for quick and easy reference.

This text provides a way of enhancing problem solving skills through the use of case studies, each identified as "Case Study: Under the Microscope," as these abilities are critical to the practice of laboratory and primary care medicine. Each appropriate chapter begins with a case study based on the chapter content that follows and contains questions for consideration. A second case study complete with patient history and symptomatology, pertinent laboratory findings, drawings of the organism(s) present and a series of questions appears at the end of each appropriate chapter. Periodic self-assessment questions, each of which is entitled "Test Your Knowledge" and a set of review questions have been incorporated into each chapter. Answers for both the chapter "Quick Quiz" and review questions are located in the appendices located in the back of the book.

A new addition to this second edition is an Evolve website. This Evolve site provides free material for both students and instructors. Instructors have access to a test bank, PowerPoint slides, and an electronic image collection featuring all the images from the book. Students have access to interactive quizzes which test them on the content from individual chapters.

Every attempt has been made to ensure that this text is as accurate and as up-to-date as possible. As with every field of study, disagreements and discrepancies exist about particular facts. Parasitology is no exception. In select instances where this was encountered, notations were made in the text. It is important to point out here that in all such occurrences appropriate decisions on how to remedy these situations for the purpose of this book were reached primarily by considering views from content experts and my personal clinical experience.

This text was written to serve as a concise and practical guide to clinical parasitology. It is not intended to be exhaustive in nature. It is my sincere hope that users of this text will find it to be a positive learning experience as well as enjoyable and helpful. I welcome comments and suggestions from students, educators and practitioners. After all, this text has been designed with you in mind.

Elizabeth A. Gockel-Blessing (formerly Zeibig)

ACKNOWLEDGMENTS

First and foremost, I would like to thank all of the individuals who helped in the preparing of the first and second edition manuscript for publication. Their roles in this project ranged from typists and photographers, proofreaders, editors, and content consultants. I would like to extend a special thanks to each chapter contributor who took time out of his/her busy schedule to review the first edition chapters, revise and update content as appropriate and incorporate the new features into this second edition. The dedication, support, and enthusiasm of all of these individuals were instrumental in producing both editions of this text. I apologize in advance for those I may have inadvertently omitted.

PROJECT CONSULTANTS

Peggy A. Edwards, MA, MT(ASCP)
Assistant Dean of Student and Academic Affairs, Retired
Department of Clinical Laboratory Science
Saint Louis University
St. Louis, MO

Michael P. Grady, Ph.D.
Professor of Education
Saint Louis University
St. Louis, MO

James A. Taylor, Ed.D.
Director, School of Allied Health Sciences
Northeast Louisiana University
Monroe, LA

Eugene C. Wienke, M.D.
Pathologist/Microbiology Laboratory Director, Retired
Deaconess Health Systems
St. Louis, MO

PROJECT ASSISTANTS

Steve Fobian
Peg Gerrity, Illustrator
Ryan Gile
Terry Jo Gile
Shirley Gockel
Bill Matthews
Kelly Rhodes
Gail Ruhling
The late David Zeibig

I would like to extend thanks to Deaconess Health Systems for supplying select samples that were used to obtain photographs as well as the required equipment necessary to take all of the text photography.

STUDENT ASSISTANTS

A sincere thank you to the Saint Louis University Department of Clinical Laboratory Science classes of 1994 and 1995 for their encouragement, support, and help. These students, listed below, were helpful in many ways, including looking up organism pronunciations and creating representative parasite drawings upon which those in this text are based. In addition, information from several of their research projects was incorporated into the manuscript and is cited in the reference section.

Beatrice Bernhart
Theresa Blattner
Karen Casey
Toni Depue
John Drury
David Fulmer
Deidra Hughes
Tricia Konrad
Luann Linsalata
Laura Murat
Bharat Patel
Tracy Pitzer
Dawn Randles
Jennifer Shelley
Munsok So
Claro Yu

SPECIAL THANK-YOUS

To my colleagues in the Saint Louis University Department of Clinical Laboratory Science over the years of undending support throughout the development and revision process associated with both editions of this book.

The late Ann Boggiano
Hillary Daniel
Donna Duberg
Peggy Edwards, Retired
Uthay Ezekiel
Mona Hebert
Rita Heuertz
Linda Hoechst
Kathy Humphrey
Tim Randolph
Sharon Smith
Carol Sykora
Mary Lou Vehige, Retired

Special thanks to following individuals who each in their own way contributed to one or both editions of this book:

- To my late grandmother Grace W. Hull, who spent countless hours teaching me, during my formative years, the skills necessary to effectively write sentences, paragraphs and papers.
- To my medical technology instructor Avril Bernsen, who gave me the opportunity to study Medical Technology (now known as Clinical Laboratory Science) under her direction.
- To Dr. Michael Grady who served as my advisor and mentor during graduate school and served as an outside reviewer for the first edition chapters in this book.
- To my mother, Shirley Gockel, and brother and sister-in-law, Fred and Juanita Gockel, for their unending encouragement and support.
- To my husband, Bob Blessing who provided unending love and support during the editing and production stages of this second edition. Thanks to him for taking care of numerous tasks and in doing so opened up valuable time blocks for me to work on this project.

Last, but by no means least, thanks to the entire staff at Elsevier. Special thanks to Selma Kaszczuk and Rachael Kelly for their support and patience during the preparation of the first edition and to Ellen Wurm-Cutter and Marquita Parker for guidance and assistance during the second edition process.

CONTENTS

CHAPTER 1
INTRODUCTION   1

CHAPTER 2
SPECIMEN COLLECTION AND
PROCESSING   14

CHAPTER 3
THE AMEBAS   41

Entamoeba histolytica   45
Entamoeba hartmanni   51
Entamoeba coli   53
Entamoeba polecki   56
Endolimax nana   58
Iodamoeba bütschlii   60
Entamoeba gingivalis   63
Naegleria fowleri   65
Acanthamoeba species   68

CHAPTER 4
THE FLAGELLATES   77

Giardia intestinalis   80
Chilomastix mesnili   86
Dientamoeba fragilis   88
Trichomonas hominis   91
Enteromonas hominis   92
Retortamonas intestinalis   94
Trichomonas tenax   96
Trichomonas vaginalis   97

CHAPTER 5
THE HEMOFLAGELLATES   104

Leishmania braziliensis complex   111
Leishmania donovani complex   113
Leishmania mexicana complex   116
Leishmania tropica complex   117
Trypanosoma brucei gambiense   120
Trypanosoma brucei rhodesiense   121
Trypanosoma cruzi   123
Trypanosoma rangeli   125

CHAPTER 6
SELECT SPOROZOA: PLASMODIUM AND
BABESIA   129

Plasmodium vivax   136
Plasmodium ovale   141
Plasmodium malariae   143
Plasmodium falciparum   147
Plasmodium knowlesi   151
Babesia microti   154
Babesia divergens   154

CHAPTER 7
MISCELLANEOUS PROTOZOA   159

Balantidium coli   162
Isospora belli   165
Sarcocystis species   168
Cryptosporidium parvum   170
Blastocystis hominis   172
Cyclospora cayetanensis   174
Microsporidia   176
Toxoplasma gondii   177
Pneumocystis jiroveci (Pneumocystis
carinii)   182

CHAPTER 8
THE NEMATODES   188

Enterobius vermicularis   192
Trichuris trichiura   195
Ascaris lumbricoides   197
Necator americanus   202
Ancylostoma duodenale   202
Strongyloides stercoralis   207
Trichinella spiralis   210
Dracunculus medinensis   213

CHAPTER 9
THE FILARIAE   222

Wuchereria bancrofti   225
Brugia malayi   227
Loa loa   229
Onchocerca volvulus   231
Mansonella ozzardi   233
Mansonella perstans   235

CHAPTER 10
THE CESTODES   239

Taenia saginata   242
Taenia solium   242
Hymenolepis diminuta   247
Hymenolepis nana   249
Dipylidium caninum   251
Diphyllobothrium latum   253
Echinococcus granulosus   256

CHAPTER 11
THE TREMATODES   265

Fasciolopsis buski   269
Fasciola hepatica   269
Clonorchis sinensis   271
Heterophyes heterophyes   273
Metagonimus yokogawai   273
Paragonimus westermani   275
Schistosoma mansoni   277
Schistosoma japonicum   277
Schistosoma haematobium   277

CHAPTER 12
ARTIFACTS AND CONFUSERS   286

CHAPTER 13
THE ARTHROPODS   297

Ticks   301
Mites   303

Spiders   305
Scorpions   307
Fleas   308
Flies   310
Lice   312
Mosquitoes   314
Bugs   316

APPENDIX A
GLOSSARY   323

APPENDIX B
ANSWERS TO CASE STUDIES UNDER
THE MICROSCOPE   333

APPENDIX C
ANSWERS TO QUICK QUIZ
QUESTIONS   339

APPENDIX D
ANSWERS TO TEST YOUR KNOWLEDGE
REVIEW QUESTIONS   343

APPENDIX E
BIBLIOGRAPHY   352

INDEX   355

Introduction

Elizabeth Zeibig

WHAT'S AHEAD

Focusing In
Historical Perspective
Epidemiology
Parasite-Host Relationships
Parasitic Life Cycles

Disease Processes and
   Symptoms
Treatment
Prevention and
   Control

Specimen Processing and
   Laboratory Diagnosis
Parasite Nomenclature and
   Classification
Looking Back

LEARNING OBJECTIVES

On completion of this chapter, the successful learner will:

1-1. Define each of the following key terms and phrases:

Accidental or incidental host (*pl.,* hosts)
Animalia
Arthropod (*pl.,* arthropods)
Artifact (*pl.,* artifacts)
Carrier (*pl.,* carriers)
Commensal
Commensalism
Confuser (*pl.,* confusers)
Definitive host
Diagnostic stage (*pl.,* stages)
Disease
Ectoparasite
Elephantiasis
Endoparasite
Epidemiology
Facultative parasite
Helminth (*pl.,* helminthes or helminths)
Host (*pl.,* hosts)
Infection
Infective stage
Infestation
Intermediate host (*pl.,* hosts)

Metazoa
Micron (abbreviated as μ or μm; *pl.,* microns)
Mode of transmission (*pl.,* modes of transmission)
Mutualism
Obligatory parasite
O&P
Parasite (*pl.,* parasites)
Parasitic
Parasitic life cycle
Parasitology
Parasitism
Pathogenic
Protozoa
Reservoir host
Symbiosis
Transport host
Vector (*pl.,* vectors)

1-2. Identify and summarize the key discoveries that have contributed to current knowledge about parasites.

1-3. Select the areas in the world in which parasitic infections are endemic and the factors that contribute to their occurrence.

1-4. Identify and describe the main factors that account for the increased prevalence of parasites in nonendemic areas of the world.

1-5. Choose populations of people at risk of contracting a parasitic infection.

1-6. Identify and describe the primary modes of parasitic transmission.

1-7. State the primary function of a host in a parasite-host relationship.

1-8. Explain, in general terms, the parasite-host relationship.

1-9. Give an example of a parasite defense mechanism that serves to protect it from a host's immune system.

1-10. State the two common phases in the parasitic life cycle and the significance of each.

1-11. Identify and describe the key pieces of information that may be extracted from each of the two common phases in the parasitic life cycle.

1-12. List the major body areas that may be affected as the result of a parasitic infection.

1-13. Name the most commonly observed symptoms associated with parasitic infections.

1-14. Cite examples of available treatment therapies to combat parasitic infections.

1-15. Outline possible parasite prevention and control strategies.

1-16. Select the most commonly submitted specimen type for parasitic study.

1-17. Summarize, in general terms, the components of the ova and parasite (O&P) traditional parasite processing technique performed on a variety of samples including stool.

1-18. Give examples of newer parasite recovery techniques.

1-19. State the name of each of the three major groups of the clinically significant parasites.

1-20. Differentiate Protozoa, Metazoa, and Animalia in terms of definition and the members of each group.

1-21. Analyze case studies with information pertinent to this chapter, and:
A. Interpret and explain the information, data and results provided.
B. Define and explain the parasite-associated terms and processes associated with the case.
C. Construct a generic parasite life cycle.
D. Determine possible parasite-associated epidemiology, generic, symptoms and disease processes, treatment, and prevention and control measures.
E. Explain the parasite-related processes going on in the case.
F. Propose subsequent actions to be taken and/or solutions, with justification.
G. Design an informational brochure that contains generic information about all or select aspects of parasites.

CASE STUDY 1-1   UNDER THE MICROSCOPE

Joe, a third-year medical student, presented to his physician complaining of severe diarrhea and abdominal pain and cramping. Patient history revealed that Joe recently returned home after a 3-month medical missionary trip to Haiti. Suspecting that Joe might be suffering from a parasitic infection, his physician ordered a battery of tests, including a stool sample for parasite examination using a traditional O&P technique.

Questions and Issues for Consideration
1. What is a parasite? (Objective 1-21B)

2. Indicate where Joe might have come into contact with parasites and identify the factors that likely contributed to this contact. (Objective 1-21D)

3. Name two other populations that are at risk of contracting parasitic infections. (Objective 1-21D)

4. Name two other symptoms associated with parasitic infections that individuals like Joe may experience. (Objective 1-21D)

5. What are the key components of a traditional O&P examination? (Objective 1-21B)

FOCUSING IN

The purpose of this chapter is to introduce the reader to the study of **parasites**, organisms that live on and obtain their nutrients from another organism, a field known as **parasitology**. A brief historical perspective of this field is followed by an introduction to epidemiology, the factors that contribute to the frequency and distribution of parasites, parasite-host relationships, and parasitic life cycles, defined as an examination of the route a parasite follows throughout its life. An introduction to disease processes and symptoms, treatment, and prevention and control associated with parasites are presented. Specifics of these topics are discussed on an individual parasite basis, as appropriate. Identification of the three major groups of clinically significant parasites follows a section that provides general information regarding specimen processing and laboratory diagnosis of parasites, covered in more detail in Chapter 2.

HISTORICAL PERSPECTIVE

The documentation of parasite existence by the ancient Persians, Egyptians, and Greeks dates back to prehistoric times. Just as the people of that era were primitive, relatively speaking, so too were parasites. Although underdeveloped areas still exist, humans have progressed through the years into an age of civilization. Parasites have evolved as well.

A number of discoveries over the years has contributed to our current knowledge of parasitology. For example, as increased awareness that parasites were becoming a problem and the realization that they were responsible for invasion in the body (**infection**), invasion on the body (**infestation**), and **disease**, defined as a process with characteristic symptoms, emerged, determining an effective means of healing infected persons became a priority. As more information was discovered regarding parasitic life cycles, especially the fact that transport carriers known as **vectors** were frequently responsible for transmission, parasite control and elimination also became

important. Advances in other areas of medical and biologic science, coupled with the discovery of useful tools, such as microscopes, not only expanded our knowledge of parasites and their makeup, but also their relationships with **hosts**—that is, plants, animals, and humans known to harbor parasites.

Today, parasitologists and clinicians have a wealth of parasite knowledge from which to draw. The escalation of disease caused by the presence of parasites (a concept known as **parasitic**) because of global travel tends to result in higher parasite recovery rates. The increased number and diversity of these organisms may allow practitioners to gain high levels of expertise in parasite identification and treatment.

Enhanced preservation of specimens now allows parasites that otherwise might have been destroyed to remain viable. A number of advances in parasitology, particularly in the area of parasite laboratory diagnosis, promise to be exciting. Measures are also now in place that are designed to protect the practitioner when handling samples for parasite study.

Quick Quiz! 1-1

Which of the following are key discoveries that contributed to current knowledge about parasites? (Objective 1-2)
A. Consistent status quo preservation of samples
B. Techniques that indicate only the presence or absence of parasites
C. Modifications of traditional parasite identification techniques
D. Decrease in parasite incidence because of global travel

EPIDEMIOLOGY

Even though treatment, prevention, and control measures are available, parasitic infections still occur and thus it is important to study and monitor their trends, a field known as **epidemiology**. Although they are distributed worldwide, most parasitic infections are found in underdeveloped tropical and subtropical countries such as Haiti, Guatemala, and Myanmar (Burma) and countries on the African continent. Increased population density, poor sanitation, marginal water sources, poor public health practices, and environmental changes affecting vector breeding areas account for the prevalence of parasites. The habits and customs of the people living in these regions are also contributing factors.

The increased prevalence of global travel likely accounts for parasitic infections being spread to areas other than where these infections originated. Individuals who travel to endemic areas are at risk of contracting parasitic infections. Refugees, immigrants, and foreign visitors may bring parasites with them when entering a nonendemic area.

Representative additional human populations at risk of contracting a parasitic infection are listed in Box 1-1. Historically, a dramatic increase in parasite infection incidence occurred in the homosexual population but it is now also occurring more in the heterosexual population. More recently, parasitic infections have become more prevalent in underdeveloped countries, regardless of a person's sexual orientation.

The means whereby a parasite gains entry into an unsuspecting host, referred to as **mode of transmission**, vary by specific parasite species and those associated with the parasites covered in this text are summarized in Box 1-2. Consuming contaminated food or water and hand-to-mouth transfer are common ways of transmitting select parasites. Others require an insect (**arthropod**) vector through which a parasite is passed on to an uninfected host, most often via a blood meal (bite). Still others will drill their way into the body via the skin through an unprotected bare foot or when an unsuspecting human is swimming in contaminated water. Sexual transmission, mouth-to-mouth contact through kissing, droplet contamination, and eye contact with infected swimming water also serve as routes for parasite transmission.

Quick Quiz! 1-2

Which of the following people may be at risk for contracting a parasitic infection? (Objective 1-5)
A. A toddler who attends an all-day preschool or day care center
B. A 25-year-old man who lives on his own in an apartment complex
C. A 37-year-old South American refugee
D. More than one of these: _____ (specify)

PARASITE-HOST RELATIONSHIPS

The study of parasite-host relationships is over 100 years old. The main focus of this research has been threefold: (1) recognition of these relationships; (2) search for patterns of the relationships; and (3) development of methodologies to study these patterns. Table 1-1 lists the terms associated with parasite-host relationships, along with their definitions.

There are several types of parasites that may be members of a parasite-host relationship. An

TABLE 1-1	Terms Associated with Parasite-Host Relationships
Parameter	**Definition or Description**
Type of Parasite	
Obligatory parasite	Parasite that cannot survive outside of a host
Facultative parasite	Parasite that is capable of existing independently of a host
Endoparasite	Parasite that is established inside of a host
Ectoparasite	Parasite that is established in or on the exterior surface of a host
Type of Host	
Accidental or incidental host	Host other than the normal one that is harboring a parasite
Definitive host	Host in which the adult sexual phase of parasite development occurs
Intermediate host	Host in which the larval asexual phase of parasite development occurs
Reservoir host	Host harboring parasites that are parasitic for humans and from which humans may become infected
Transport host	Host responsible for transferring a parasite from one location to another
Carrier	Parasite-harboring host that is not exhibiting any clinical symptoms but can infect others
Parasite-Host Relationship Terms	
Symbiosis	Living together; the association of two living organisms, each of a different species
Commensalism	Association of two different species of organisms that is beneficial to one and neutral to the other
Mutualism	Association of two different species of organisms that is beneficial to both
Parasitism	Association of two different species of organisms that is beneficial to one at the other's expense
Commensal	Relating to commensalism; the association between two different organisms in which one benefits and has a neutral effect on the other
Pathogenic	Parasite that has demonstrated the ability to cause disease

organism may be an **obligatory parasite** or a **facultative parasite**. It may be an **endoparasite** or an **ectoparasite**. In the same manner, a number of different hosts may be part of this parasite-host relationship. These include **accidental** or **incidental hosts, definitive hosts, intermediate hosts, reservoir hosts, transport hosts,** and **carriers.**

When a parasite infects a host, **symbiosis** results. The primary function of the host is to carry on the parasite's life cycle. This newly formed relationship may develop into **commensalism, mutualism,** or **parasitism.** Some of these associations exist as **commensal** under certain circumstances and **pathogenic** under others.

Parasites have an amazing capability to adapt to their host surroundings. In addition to a number of morphologic adaptations, parasites are capable of protecting themselves from the host's immune system. Parasites alter their antigenic makeup so that the host will not recognize the modified parasites as foreign, and thus the initiation of an immune response does not occur. A more in-depth study of parasite-host relationships is beyond the scope of this chapter. Where appropriate, further consideration of this topic is discussed on an individual parasite basis.

Quick Quiz! 1-3

The primary function of a host in a parasite-host relationship is to: (Objective 1-7)
A. Carry on the parasite's life cycle.
B. Provide immunologic protection for the host.
C. Carry on the host's life cycle.
D. Provide a food source for the host.

PARASITIC LIFE CYCLES

Although **parasitic life cycles** range from simple to complex, they all have three common components—a mode of transmission, a morphologic form that invades humans, known as the **infective stage,** and one (or more) forms that can be detected via laboratory retrieval methods, known as the **diagnostic stage.** Some parasites require only a definitive host, whereas others also require one or more intermediate hosts.

A parasitic life cycle consists of two common phases (Fig. 1-1). One phase involves the route a parasite follows when in or on the human body. This information provides an understanding of the symptomatology and pathology of the parasite. Insights about the best the method of diagnosis and selection of appropriate antiparasitic medication may also be determined. The other phase, the route a parasite follows independently of the human body, provides crucial information pertinent to epidemiology, prevention, and control.

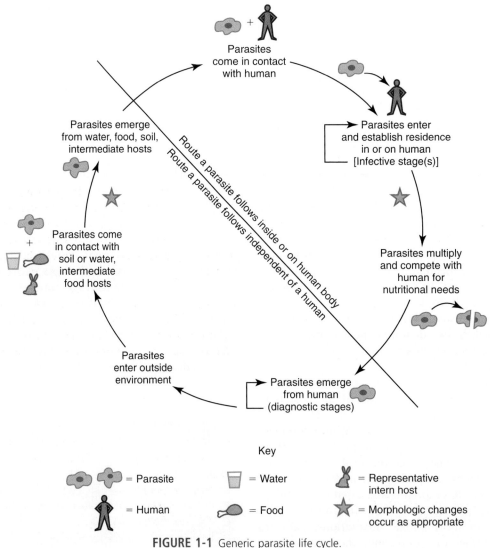

FIGURE 1-1 Generic parasite life cycle.

Quick Quiz! 1-4

Which of the following key pieces of information may be extracted from the portion of a parasite's life cycle that occurs outside the body? (Objective 1-11)
A. Parasitic disease symptoms and disease processes
B. Epidemiology and prevention and control measures
C. Appropriate parasite diagnosis methodologies
D. Selection of appropriate antiparasitic medication

DISEASE PROCESSES AND SYMPTOMS

A parasitic disease may affect the entire body or any of its parts. The major body areas associated with such processes include the following: (1) the gastrointestinal (GI) and urogenital (UG) tracts; (2) blood and tissue; (3) liver, lung, and other major organs; and (4) miscellaneous locations, such as cerebrospinal fluid (CSF), eye, skin, and extremities.

A wide variety of representative symptoms, summarized in Box 1-3, may occur when a parasite infects a human host. Some persons remain asymptomatic, whereas other parasites produce severe symptoms and may result in death. The most commonly observed symptoms include diarrhea, fever, chills, abdominal pain, and abdominal cramping. Other symptoms, such as **elephantiasis** (an enlargement of areas such as the breast, leg, and scrotum caused by a parasite's presence), anemia, vitamin deficiency, bowel obstruction, edema, enlargement of major organs, skin lesions, and blindness, may develop.

 Quick Quiz! 1-5

Which of the following groups of symptoms represents those most commonly observed in parasitic infections? (Objective 1-13)
A. Diarrhea, abdominal cramping, and anemia
B. Enlargement of the spleen, fever, and chills
C. Skin lesions, abdominal pain, and diarrhea
D. Abdominal cramping, abdominal pain, and diarrhea

TREATMENT

There are several options for treating parasitic infections. Examples of such measures are listed in Box 1-4. There are a variety of antiparasitic medications available. Many of these drugs are toxic to the host and care should be exercised when selecting the proper course of treatment. Therapies such as a change in diet, vitamin supplements, fluid replacement, blood transfusion, and bed rest may be indicated solely or in addition to chemotherapy. Treatment for non-pathogenic parasitic infections is usually not indicated.

BOX 1-3	Symptoms Associated with Parasitic Disease Processes

Diarrhea
Fever
Chills
Abdominal pain
Abdominal cramping
Elephantiasis
Anemia
Vitamin deficiency
Bowel obstruction
Edema
Enlargement of major organs
Skin lesions
Blindness

BOX 1-4	Parasite Treatment Options

Antiparasitic medications
Change in diet
Vitamin supplements
Fluid replacement
Blood transfusion
Bed rest

Quick Quiz! 1-6

Which of the following represent examples of available treatment therapies to combat parasitic infections? (Objective 1-14)
A. Regulated exercise plan
B. Change in diet
C. Avoidance of vitamin supplements
D. More than one of these: _____ (specify)

Quick Quiz! 1-7

Which of the following are examples of possible parasite prevention and control measures? (Objective 1-15)
A. Avoiding the use of insecticides
B. Practicing unprotected sex
C. Practicing proper sanitation practices
D. More than one of these: _____ (specify)

PREVENTION AND CONTROL

Prevention and control measures may be taken against every parasite infective to humans. Preventive measures designed to break the transmission cycle are crucial for successful parasite eradication. Examples of such measures are listed in Box 1-5 and include the following: education programs, use of insecticides and other chemicals, protective clothing, protective netting, proper water treatment, good personal hygiene, proper sanitation practices, proper handling and preparation of food, and avoidance of unprotected sexual relations. The vast capital expenditures required to accomplish these measures are not available in many endemic countries in the world. The problem of eradicating parasites is an ongoing process and is a key goal of international health groups such as the World Health Organization (WHO) and Doctors Without Borders (Médecins Sans Frontières [MSF]).

BOX 1-5	Parasite Prevention and Control Strategies

Development and implementation of parasite awareness education programs
Use of insecticides and other chemicals
Use of protective clothing
Use of protective netting
Proper water treatment
Good personal hygiene
Proper sanitation practices
Proper handling, cooking, and protection of food
Avoidance of unprotected sexual relations

SPECIMEN PROCESSING AND LABORATORY DIAGNOSIS

Proper specimen selection and processing are crucial to parasite recovery. There are a variety of acceptable specimen types that may be examined for parasites. Stool is the most commonly submitted sample for such studies. Typical stool analysis consists of performing macroscopic and microscopic techniques on a portion of unpreserved sample when available. A process to remove fecal debris, which often resembles parasitic forms, is performed on a portion of sample after a preservative is added to it. Microscopic analysis of the resultant processed sample follows. This traditional parasite recovery method, often referred to as an **O&P**, in which "O" stands for ova (eggs) and "P" stands for parasites, is still widely used today.

Other specimens, including blood, tissue biopsies, CSF, sputum, urine, and genital material, may also be examined for the presence of parasites. In some cases, the sample is basically processed the same as for stool. Other specimens, such as blood, are traditionally processed differently. For example, a Giemsa stain followed by microscopic examination is the procedure of choice for blood samples submitted for parasite study.

A number of other traditional and new parasite recovery techniques are available. Cellophane tape preparation, a methodology for recovery of pinworm eggs, and the Enterotest (string test) for recovery of several parasites are among the traditional tests. Representative newer methodologies are listed in Box 1-6. Details regarding these various specimen processing techniques are found in Chapter 2, "Specimen Collection and Processing." It is important to note that Chapter 2 was designed to provide representative examples of laboratory methodologies that may be used to recover parasites. In some cases, Chapter 2 contains laboratory methodologies that are not covered in the corresponding individual parasite laboratory diagnosis sections. Similarly, the laboratory diagnosis section of select individual parasites mentions additional possible laboratory techniques that are not specifically identified as being associated with these parasites or are not mentioned at all in Chapter 2. Thus, examination and study of the methods covered in Chapter 2 and those identified in the individual parasite laboratory diagnosis sections are required to understand and appreciate fully the extent of laboratory techniques available.

Careful and thorough microscopic examination of samples for parasites is essential to ensure that accurate patient results are obtained and ultimately reported. Suspicious forms that visually resemble parasites in terms of size and morphology are commonly encountered and are often referred to as **artifacts** and/or **confusers.** For example, the *Entamoeba histolytica* cyst (described in detail in Chapter 3), a single-celled eukaryotic animal known as a **protozoa,** typically measures 12 to 18 **microns** (μm), a measurement defined as one millionth of a meter (10^{-6} m). Similarly, polymorphonuclear leukocytes average 15 μm in size. In addition, the

nuclear structures, although very different on further inspection, may often initially appear almost identical. Plant cells, as another example, resemble the *Ascaris lumbricoides* egg (see Chapter 8 for details), a member of the subkingdom **Metazoa,** which includes multicellular organisms such as parasitic worms. Not only do they share structural similarities, but both may measure in the diameter range of 30 to 50 μm. There are numerous artifacts and confusers (also often referred to as pseudoparasites) that may be present in samples submitted for parasite study. Brief detailed descriptions of a select group of commonly encountered artifacts and confusers are discussed in Chapter 12.

Quick Quiz! 1-8

Which of the following specimen type is most often submitted for parasite study? (Objective 1-16)
A. Blood
B. Sputum
C. Urine
D. Stool

PARASITE NOMENCLATURE AND CLASSIFICATION

The scientific names of parasites are written in italics and consist of two components, genus (*pl.,* genera) and species. An example of a parasite name is *Giardia intestinalis* (covered in detail in Chapter 4), in which *Giardia* is the genus name and *intestinalis* is the species name. When a parasite name first appears in a document, the entire parasite name is written out. Subsequent references to a parasite are often abbreviated by recording only the first letter of the genera name followed by a period, followed by the entire species name. Thus, the abbreviation of our example parasite *Giardia intestinalis* is *G. intestinalis.*

Variations of scientific genus names are used to identify diseases and conditions associated with their presence. The suffix *-iasis* is often used to denote such diseases or conditions. For example, giardiasis refers to the disease or

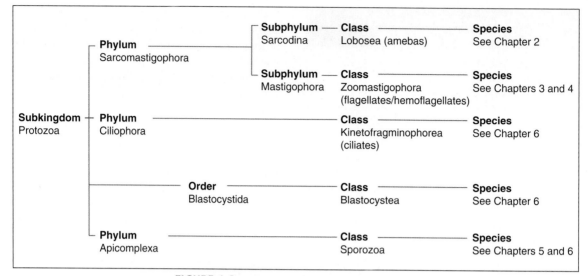

FIGURE 1-2 Parasite classification—the protozoa.

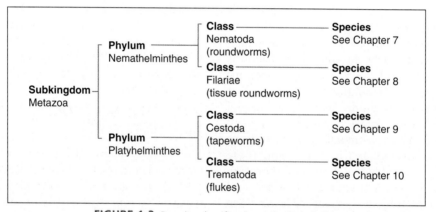

FIGURE 1-3 Parasite classification—the helminths.

condition associated with *Giardia intestinalis*. In some cases, a variation of a scientific genus name may be used to refer to a genus of parasites. Here is an example of this use of a genus name. Chapter 5 of this text discusses two genera of parasites, *Leishmania* and *Trypanosoma*. In general, reference to infections with these two genera is often written as leishmanial infections and trypanosomal infections.

Along with specific parasite name variations, variations of parasite category names are common. An example of this terminology is the

amebas (Chapter 3). When appropriate, reference to the amebas may be written in several ways, such as amebic or ameboid.

There are several different parasite classification systems, ranging from very basic to complex. The system used in this text delineates three major groups of clinically significant parasites:
1. Single-celled parasites—Protozoa (Fig. 1-2)
2. Multicellular worms—Metazoa **helminths** (Fig. 1-3)
3. Arthropods (insects and their allies)—**Animalia** (Fig. 1-4)

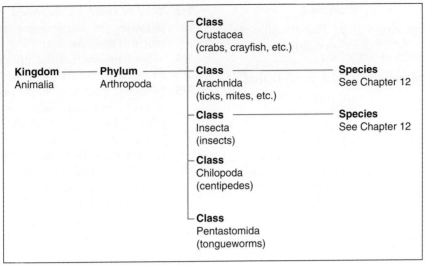

FIGURE 1-4 Parasite classification—the arthropods.

The groups of parasites in each classification table are organized by kingdom and subkingdom, phylum and subphylum, and class. The individual species are classified in their respective chapters.

 Quick Quiz! 1-9

Which of the following correctly represents the three major groups of clinically significant parasites? (Objective 1-20)

A. Protozoa—worms; Metazoa—single-celled parasites; Arthropods—insects and their allies

B. Protozoa—insects and their allies; Metazoa—worms; Arthropods—single-celled parasites

C. Protozoa—single-celled parasites; Metazoa—worms; Arthropods—insects and their allies

D. Protozoa—single-celled parasites; Metazoa—insects and their allies; Arthropods—worms

LOOKING BACK

Over the years, parasites once considered commensal have evolved to become human pathogens. During this time, we have gained tremendous knowledge of the epidemiology, parasite-host relationships, life cycles, disease processes and symptoms, treatment, and prevention and control

of parasites. In addition, parasites are classified based on their individual characteristics. Traditional as well as new methodologies for parasite identification allow for accurate laboratory diagnosis.

Parasitology is an interesting and exciting field of the clinical laboratory sciences. The continued development of high-tech, highly sensitive parasite test methodologies provides the key to the future of parasitology. Because it is highly unlikely that parasites will totally be eradicated in the near future, competent practitioners educated in the field of parasitology are essential to ensure proper parasite identification.

TEST YOUR KNOWLEDGE!

1-1. Match each of the key terms (column A) with its corresponding definition (column B). (Objective 1-1)

Column A	Column B
___ **A.** Ectoparasite	**1.** The form of a parasite that enters a host
___ **B.** Obligatory parasite	**2.** Two organisms of different species living together

Column A	Column B
___ **C.** Infective stage	**3.** The official units of parasite measurement
___ **D.** Commensalism	**4.** A parasite that cannot survive outside its host
___ **E.** Disease	**5.** An insect that transports a parasite from an infected host to an uninfected host
___ **F.** Microns	**6.** A parasite that lives on the outside surface of its host
___ **G.** Transport host	**7.** Parasite-harboring host that is not affected by its presence but can shed the parasite and infect others
___ **H.** Vector	**8.** A destructive process that has characteristic symptoms
___ **I.** Symbiosis	**9.** Association of two different species of organisms that is beneficial to one but neutral to the other
___ **J.** Carrier	**10.** A host responsible for transferring a parasite from one location to another

1-2. In what parts of the world are parasites endemic, and what factors contribute to their occurrence in these areas? (Objective 1-3)

1-3. Why is there an increased prevalence of parasites in nonendemic areas of the world (Objective 1-4)

1-4. What are some of the primary modes of parasitic transmission? (Objective 1-6)

1-5. Suppose that you have been asked to design a one-page informational flyer on parasite-host relationships. Identify the types of parasites, hosts, and parasite-host relationships that you should include in your flyer. (Objective 1-8)
  A. Types of parasites
  B. Types of hosts
  C. Types of parasite-host relationships
Optional activity: Design the actual flyer and share with classmates. (Objective 1-21)

1-6. Give one example of a parasite defense mechanism that serves to protect it from a host's immune system. (Objective 1-9)

1-7. What are the two common phases of a parasitic life cycle? (Objective 1-10)

1-8. Refer to question 1-7. What key pieces of information may be extracted from each of the two common phases of a parasitic life cycle? (Objective 1-11)

1-9. Which of the following major body areas may be affected as the result of a parasitic infection? (Objective 1-12)
  A. Gastrointestinal tract
  B. Respiratory tract
  C. Blood and tissue
  D. Liver and lung
  E. More than one of these: _____ (specify)

1-10. Which of the following are examples of newer parasite recovery techniques? (Objective 1-18)
  A. Carbohydrate immunoassays
  B. RNA hybridization techniques
  C. PCR
  D. Immunochromatographic techniques
  E. More than one of these: _____ (specify)

1-11. What are the three groups of clinically significant parasites? (Objective 1-19)

1-12. Suppose you are asked to speak to a group of grade school–aged children who are preparing to go on a class picnic. The students are currently learning the basics about parasites in their science class. You have been asked to speak about possible parasite prevention and control strategies for the upcoming class outing. What strategies would you discuss with these students? (Objective 1-21)

1-13. Refer to question 1-12. The session with the students went so well that the teacher would like you to take this project to the next level. Design an informational brochure with these strategies detailed, written at a grade school level. (Objective 1-21)

1-14. Suppose that you and a friend are studying for parasitology class together. Your friend is having great difficulty visualizing the concept of parasite life cycles, including the difference between the two common phases and the information derived from each phase. Your friend has asked you for help. Using Figure 1-1 as a guide, construct your version of a generic parasite life cycle in a format that is easy to read and follow. (Objective 1-21)

2

Specimen Collection and Processing

Lauren Roberts and Elizabeth Zeibig

WHAT'S AHEAD

Focusing In
Stool for Ova and Parasite
  Examination
Stool Screening Methods

Other Intestinal Specimens
Other Specimens and
  Laboratory Techniques
Immunologic Testing

Reporting of Results and
  Quality Control
Looking Back

LEARNING OBJECTIVES

On completion of this chapter and review of its tables and ocular micrometer diagram, the successful learner will:

2-1. Define the following key terms:
   Concentration technique (*pl.*, techniques)
   Concentrated iodine wet preparation
     (*pl.*, preparations)
   Concentrated saline wet preparation
   Concentrated wet preparation
   Direct iodine wet preparation
   Direct saline wet preparation
   Direct wet mount (*pl.*, mounts)
   Direct wet preparation
   Fixative (*pl.*, fixatives)
   Micron (*pl.*, microns; abbreviated μ or μm)
   O&P
   Ocular micrometer
   Ova and parasites
   Permanent stained smear (*pl.*, smears)
   Preparation, prep (*pl.*, preparations;
     abbreviated as preps)
   Unfixed
2-2. Identify and describe the proper collection
   and transport of stool samples for parasitic
   study.

2-3. Identify the procedures included in a
   routine O&P examination.
2-4. Discuss the basic composition, purpose,
   advantages, and disadvantages of each of
   the following preservatives and state which
   laboratory procedures can be performed
   using each type:
   A. Formalin
   B. Polyvinyl alcohol (PVA)
   C. Sodium-acetate formalin (SAF)
   D. Modified PVA
   E. Alternative single-vial systems
2-5. Describe the characteristics of the
   macroscopic examination of stool
   specimens.
2-6. Identify the procedures involved in the
   microscopic examination of stool
   specimens.
2-7. State the purpose and procedure involved
   when calibrating and using an ocular
   micrometer.
2-8. Describe the use of a direct wet
   preparation and state when this procedure
   can be eliminated from an O&P
   examination.

2-9. State the purpose of concentration techniques and, for each technique studied, list the advantages and disadvantages.

2-10. Explain the purpose of a permanent stained smear and summarize the characteristics of the stains presented.

2-11. Describe the use of stool screening methods and provide an example when these methods would be used.

2-12. Explain the purpose of examining intestinal specimens other than stool for parasites.

2-13. Describe the purpose, advantages, and disadvantages of performing the proper techniques for examining specimens other than stool and intestinal samples for the presence of parasites.

2-14. Describe the use of immunologic tests for the diagnosis of parasitic diseases and provide an example when antibody testing might be used.

2-15. Match the specific immunologic tests available with the parasite(s) that they can detect.

2-16. Briefly describe the new techniques that have been developed for parasite study.

2-17. Identify and describe the appropriate information to include in the parasitology test report.

2-18. Identify the appropriate areas to be included in a parasitology quality assurance program.

2-19. Analyze case studies with information pertinent to this chapter and do the following:
A. Interpret and explain the information, data, and results provided.
B. Propose subsequent actions to be taken and/or solutions, with justification.

CASE STUDY 2-1 | **UNDER THE MICROSCOPE**

MP, a 26-year-old man, returned home from a spring ski trip to the Rocky Mountain region and began to experience intestinal unease, with nausea and abdominal fullness. He then developed abdominal cramping and diarrhea, along with hives. MP became concerned when the symptoms continued beyond 1 week, and he presented to his family physician. The physician decided to order laboratory tests to determine the cause and ordered a stool for culture and sensitivity. The results indicated "no *Salmonella, Shigella, E. coli* O:157, or *Campylobacter* isolated." On receiving these results, the physician called the laboratory and inquired about a workup for intestinal parasites.

Questions for Consideration
1. Which tests should the laboratory technician recommend to detect the presence of parasites? (Objective 2-19B)
2. Describe the proper collection and transport of stool samples for intestinal parasites. (Objective 2-2)
3. List the procedures that would be included in the routine O&P examination. (Objective 2-3)
4. Suppose that the laboratory technician suggests that a stool screen be performed initially and, if the results are negative, then a complete O&P is indicated. Explain this recommendation. (Objective 2-11)

FOCUSING IN

As noted in Chapter 1, parasitic diseases continue to be a significant threat throughout the world. Although they appear to be more prevalent in underdeveloped tropical and subtropical countries, parasites do occur in developed areas, such as the United States. These diseases are usually brought about by climate conditions desirable for parasitic survival as well as poor sanitation and personal hygiene practices of the inhabitants. Certain populations are more at risk of contracting parasitic infections, including foreign visitors and those traveling and emigrating to other countries.

In areas in which parasitic infections are not considered a major cause of human disease, it can be difficult for health care professionals to recognize that these agents may be a cause of the patient's clinical condition. However, with the increased number of populations at risk for contracting parasitic infections, it is critical for clinicians to obtain knowledge of the clinical manifestations of parasitic diseases and understand the appropriate laboratory test(s) to order. Furthermore, laboratory technicians must have an understanding of these diseases to guide the physician in selecting the appropriate tests. Because the diagnosis of these diseases can be challenging and is not always straightforward, it is imperative that strong communication exist between the physician and clinical laboratory.

This chapter is designed to introduce readers to representative testing methods available for the diagnosis of parasitic infections. Parasites that may be determined using these testing methods are identified. These lists are not intended to be exhaustive in nature. By design, appropriate testing methods are mentioned in the specific parasite laboratory diagnosis sections, which may or may not be noted in this chapter.

Successful laboratory identification of parasites requires the knowledge and practice of laboratory testing in the preanalytic, analytic, and postanalytic steps. For example, in the preanalytic phase, a specimen received in the laboratory that is compromised because of improper collection, labeling, or transport should be rejected and a new specimen requested. Similarly, laboratory techniques performed in the analytic phase of testing of these samples should be completed with care to ensure that accurate results are obtained. Interpretation and reporting of results obtained, completed in the postanalytic phase of testing, should be accurately reported in a timely manner.

Specific topics addressed in this chapter include the following: specimen collection and handling guidelines for stool and intestinal specimens; other specimen types, including tissue, blood, and body fluids; immunologic testing; future methods; and the reporting of results and quality control associated with parasite studies. A concise but comprehensive discussion of each topic follows. This chapter contains terminology that is detailed in other chapters in this text. Reference to the appropriate chapter is made where each appropriate term first appears.

STOOL FOR OVA AND PARASITE EXAMINATION

Without a doubt, the most common procedure performed in the area of parasitology is the examination of a stool specimen for **ova and parasites** (abbreviated as **O&P**), where ova refers to the egg stage of select parasites and parasites encompasses the other morphologic forms that may be present. There are two general components associated with this routine parasitology procedure macroscopic and microscopic examination. The microscopic examination consists of three possible components, each of which is detailed in the sections that follow a discussion of collection, transport, and fixatives for preservation. As in all areas of laboratory testing, the quality of the results is dependent on the appropriate collection of the specimen.

Collection and Transport

Morphologic forms of protozoa and helminths may be detected from a properly collected and prepared stool specimen. When present, the protozoan forms known as trophozoites and cysts (discussed in more detail in Chapter 3) may be recovered from these samples. Helminth stages, such as eggs, larvae, proglottids, and adult worms, may also be found. Definitions of these helminth-related morphologic forms are detailed in the corresponding parasite chapters of this text (Chapters 8 to 11).

Because parasites are often shed (i.e., enter and subsequently passed in the stool) intermittently, they may not appear in a stool specimen on a daily basis; therefore, multiple specimens are recommended for adequate detection. The typical stool collection protocol consists of three specimens, one specimen collected every other day or a total of three collected in 10 days. One exception is in the diagnosis of amebiasis (Chapter 3), in which up to six specimens in 14 days is acceptable.

Certain medications and substances may interfere with the detection of parasites. Stool samples from patients whose therapy includes barium, bismuth, or mineral oil should be collected prior to therapy or not until 5 to 7 days after the completion of therapy. If the samples are taken during the course of therapy, these interfering substances may mask possible parasites during examination. Collection of specimens from patients who have taken antibiotics or antimalarial medications should be delayed for 2 weeks following therapy.

Stool specimens should be collected in a clean, watertight container with a tight-fitting lid. The acceptable amount of stool required for parasite study is 2 to 5 g, often referred to as the size of a walnut. Urine should not be allowed to contaminate the stool specimen because it has been known to destroy some parasites. Stool should not be retrieved from toilet bowl water because free-living protozoa and nematodes may be confused with human parasites. In addition, water may destroy select parasites, such as schistosome (Chapter 12) eggs and amebic trophozoites. Toilet paper in the stool specimen may mask parasites or make examination of the sample difficult.

The specimen container should be labeled with the patient's name and identification number, the physician's name, and the date and time of sample collection. Some form of requisition, paper or computer-based, should accompany the specimen indicating the test(s) requested. Other information, such as suspected diagnosis, travel history, and clinical findings, is helpful, but may not be provided. The specimen should be placed into a zip lock plastic bag for transport to the laboratory. The paperwork accompanying the specimen should be separated from the specimen container.

When handling all specimens, gloves and a protective coat should be worn at all times. Biohazard hoods should also be used in laboratories, when present. Universal precautions, as outlined by the Occupational Safety and Health Administration (OSHA) for handling blood and body fluids, should be exhibited and enforced at all times.

Another important consideration in testing fecal specimens for parasites is the time frame from sample collection to receipt and examination in the laboratory. To demonstrate the motility of protozoan trophozoites, a fresh specimen is required. The trophozoite stage is sensitive to environmental changes and, on release from the body, disintegrates rapidly. Other parasite stages (e.g., protozoan cysts, helminth eggs and larvae) are not as sensitive and can survive for longer periods outside the host. Because trophozoites are usually found in liquid stool, it is recommended that liquid specimens be examined within 30 minutes of passage. In keeping with stool consistency, semiformed specimens may yield a mixture of protozoan cysts and trophozoites and should be evaluated within 1 hour of passage. Formed stool specimens are not likely to contain trophozoites; therefore, they can be held for 24 hours following collection. If these guidelines cannot be met, the specimen should be placed into a preservative. The specimen can be preserved by placing it directly into a fixative at the time it is collected or on receipt in the laboratory (see next section).

Quick Quiz! 2-1

How many stool samples should be collected when following the typical O&P collection protocol? (Objective 2-3)

A. 1

B. 2

C. 3

D. 4

Fixatives for Preservation

A freshly collected stool sample, which is immediately submitted to the laboratory, is the ideal specimen for parasitic examination. When this is not possible, the sample must be preserved to maintain its integrity. **Fixatives** are substances that preserve the morphology of protozoa and prevent further development of certain helminth eggs and larvae. Several preservatives are available commercially (see later). The ratio of fixative to stool is important for the successful recovery of parasites and, whatever fixative is used, the recommended ratio is three parts fixative to one part stool. Commercial kits may contain one or more vials, each containing an appropriate preservative. These kits usually contain vials with fill lines marked to indicate the appropriate sample volume. It is also important that the specimen be mixed well with the preservative to achieve thorough fixation. Because the patient is often responsible for collection of the specimen and transfer to the fixative vials, it is imperative that he or she be given detailed and complete instructions. The specimen must be fixed in the preservative for at least 30 minutes before processing begins.

The choice of fixative(s) for O&P use depends on the preference of the laboratory performing the test. Because the laboratory ideally should have the ability to perform all steps of the O&P test, appropriate fixatives should be on hand to accomplish these steps. Some fixatives are limited to use in certain O&P laboratory procedures. Thus, the laboratory technician must be familiar with and understand the uses and limitations of each fixative. Table 2-1 provides an overview of the procedures that can be performed using specific fixatives. Some laboratories prefer to use a two-vial fixative system; others use a single-vial system. In addition, if other tests are ordered, such as a fecal immunoassay, the laboratory must ensure that the fixative is compatible for use with these techniques. Finally, some fixatives contain mercury and disposal regulations for these compounds could affect the laboratory's decision of which fixatives to use in their testing protocols. A description of representative fixatives used in O&P testing follows.

Formalin. Formalin has been used for many years as an all-purpose fixative for the recovery of protozoa and helminths. Two concentrations of formalin are commonly used; a 5% concentration ideally preserves protozoan cysts and a 10% concentration preserves helminth eggs and larvae. Formalin may be routinely used for direct examinations and concentration procedures, but not for permanent smears.

There are advantages and disadvantages to using formalin as a fixative. There are three primary advantages for the use of formalin: (1) it is easy to prepare; (2) it preserves specimens for up to several years; and (3) it has a long shelf life. One of the biggest disadvantages of formalin is that it does not preserve parasite morphology adequately for permanent smears. Other disadvantages include the fact that trophozoites usually cannot be recovered and morphologic details of cysts and eggs may fade with time.

It is important to note that because the use of formalin is considered a potential health hazard, OSHA has developed formalin handling regulations for laboratories. Monitoring of vapors, use of protective clothing, and a comprehensive,

TABLE 2-1	Stool Preservatives and Applicable Laboratory Procedures		
Preservative	**Concentration**	**Permanent Stain**	**Antigen Tests**
10% formalin	+	−	+
SAF	+	+ (iron hematoxylin)	+
PVA	±	+ (trichrome or iron hematoxylin)	−
Modified PVA (zinc)	±	+ (trichrome or iron hematoxylin)	±
Single-vial system	+	+ (trichrome or iron hematoxylin)	±

written chemical hygiene plan (CHP) are required under these OSHA regulations. Such measures should be in place in all laboratories.

Polyvinyl Alcohol. Polyvinyl alcohol (PVA) is comprised of a plastic powder that acts as an adhesive for the stool specimen when preparing slides for staining. PVA is most often combined with Schaudinn solution, which usually contains zinc sulfate, copper sulfate, or mercuric chloride as a base.

Like formalin, PVA has advantages and disadvantages regarding its use. Trophozoites and cysts of the protozoa, as well as most helminth eggs, may be detected using this fixative. The greatest advantage of this preservative is that it can be used for preparation of a permanent stained smear. PVA-preserved specimens have a long shelf life when stored at room temperature. Although concentration techniques can also be performed from a PVA-preserved specimen, the recovery of certain parasites is not as effective as when formalin is used. Thus, many laboratories choose to use a two-vial system—a formalin vial for the concentration technique and a PVA vial for the stained slide. The biggest disadvantage of the use of PVA is that Schaudinn solution contains mercuric chloride. Because of the potential health problems caused by mercury, strict regulations regarding the use and disposal of PVA have resulted in many laboratories looking for alternatives.

Sodium Acetate Formalin. A viable alternative to the use of PVA and Schaudinn fixative is sodium acetate formalin (SAF). This preservative can be used for performing concentration techniques and permanent stained smears. Some laboratories have adopted this fixative because it only requires a single vial and it is mercury-free. SAF is easy to prepare, has a long shelf life, and can be used for preparing smears for staining with the modified acid-fast stain to detect coccidian oocysts.

SAF also has disadvantages. Because the adhesive properties of SAF are not good, the addition of albumin to the microscope slide may be necessary to ensure adhesion of the specimen to the slide. Furthermore, protozoa morphology from SAF-preserved specimens is not as clear in permanent stains as when mercury-containing preservatives are used. Another limiting factor of SAF is in the choice of permanent stains made from this fixative. Many experts believe that permanent stained smears with iron hematoxylin staining provide better results than staining SAF-preserved material using the Wheatley trichrome stain (both stains are described later in this chapter).

Modified Polyvinyl Alcohol. Other alternatives to mercury-based PVA are the use of substitute compounds containing copper sulfate or zinc sulfate. The advantage of these formulas is that they can be used for concentration methods and permanent stained smears. However, these substitute products do not provide the same quality of preservation for adequate protozoan morphology on a permanent stained slide as the mercury-based fixatives. Therefore, parasite identification will be more difficult. Zinc sulfate fixatives provide better results than copper sulfate reagents. Modified PVA fixatives are more likely to be negatively affected if proper protocol is not followed (e.g., stool-to-fixative ratio, adequate mixing).

Alternative Single-Vial Systems. Several manufacturers have developed alternative nontoxic fixatives. These single-vial fixatives are free of formalin and mercury and can be used for concentration techniques and permanent stained smears. Some of these products can also be used for performing fecal immunoassays. Like the modified PVA fixatives, these products do not provide the same quality of preservation as mercury-based fixatives and organism identification will be more difficult from permanent stained slides.

Quick Quiz! 2-2

What is the purpose of fixatives for the collection of stool samples? (Objective 2-4)
A. Enhance the motility of protozoa.
B. Stain the cytoplasmic inclusions of protozoa.
C. Preserve the morphology of protozoa and prevent further development of helminths.
D. All of the above.

Processing

Once a stool specimen has been received in the laboratory, the analytic phase of laboratory testing, also referred to processing, begins. In this phase, samples are examined from two perspectives, macroscopic and microscopic. A detailed description of each perspective follows.

Macroscopic Examination. Stool specimens submitted for parasitic study should first be examined macroscopically to determine the consistency and color of the sample. The specimen should be screened and examined for the presence of gross abnormalities. To perform this macroscopic examination, the laboratory must receive a fresh, unpreserved stool specimen. Because most laboratories receive fecal specimens already in fixative, this step is often skipped because these macroscopic characteristics cannot be determined. In such situations, a notation of the gross appearance, either on the actual specimen container or on the requisition form, is recommended at the time of specimen collection.

The consistency or degree of moisture in a stool specimen may serve as an indication of the types of potential parasites present. For example, soft or liquid stools may suggest the presence of protozoan trophozoites. Protozoan cysts are more likely to be found in fully formed stools. Helminth eggs and larvae may be found in liquid or formed stools.

The color of a stool is important because it may indicate the condition of the patient, such as whether a patient has recently had a special procedure (e.g., a barium enema) or if the patient is on antibiotic therapy. The range of colors varies, including black to green to clay, and colors in between. The color of normal stool is brown. Unusual colors, such as purple, red, or blue, typically suggest that the patient is on a particular medication.

Gross abnormalities possibly found in stool include adult worms, proglottids, pus, and mucus. First, the surface of the stool should be examined for parasites, such as pinworms (Chapter 8), tapeworm proglottids, and adult worms (Chapter 9). The sample should then be broken up—a wooden applicator stick works nicely for this task—and examined once more for macroscopic parasites, especially adult helminths. Samples containing adult worms may be carefully washed through a wire screen. This process allows for the retrieval and examination of the parasites for identification purposes.

Other macroscopic abnormalities in the specimen may have parasitic indications. For example, blood and/or mucus in loose or liquid stool may suggest the presence of amebic ulcerations in the large intestine. Bright red blood on the surface of a formed stool is usually associated with irritation and bleeding.

A number of possible terms may be used to describe the macroscopic appearance of a stool specimen. A suggested list of possible consistency, color, and gross appearance descriptions is found in Table 2-2.

Quick Quiz! 2-3

Which of the following characteristics is observed during the macroscopic examination of stool specimens? (Objective 2-5)

A. Consistency
B. Color
C. Adult worms
D. All of the above

TABLE 2-2	**Macroscopic Examination of Stool Specimens: Possible Descriptive Terms**		
Consistency Terms	**Possible Colors**	**Gross Appearance Terms**	
Hard	Dark brown	Conspicuously fibrous	
Soft	Black	Fiber scanty to moderate	
Mushy	Brown	Colloidal (homogeneous)	
Loose	Pale brown	Scanty mucus	
Diarrheic	Clay	Much mucus	
Watery, liquid	Yellow	Mucus with scanty blood	
Formed	Red-brown	Other (e.g., blood, barium)	
Semiformed	Green, other		

Microscopic Examination. To detect the presence of parasites in a stool specimen, microscopic examinations are performed. The microscopic examination of stool for ova and parasites involves three distinct procedures, direct wet **preparations** (often, the term *preparations* is abbreviated as **preps**), a concentrated technique resulting in concentrated wet preparations, and a permanently stained smear. All three of these procedures should be performed on a fresh specimen. If the specimen is received in fixative, the direct wet preparation can be eliminated from the O&P procedure; the concentrate and permanent stain techniques are performed. A discussion of each of these procedures follows, and important concepts associated with microscopes as they relate to parasitology analysis are discussed.

Quick Quiz! 2-4

Which of these procedures is involved in the microscopic examination of stool specimens for parasites? (Objective 2-6)
A. Performing a concentration technique
B. Determining specimen consistency
C. Examining sample for gross abnormalities
D. Analyzing sample for color

Microscope Considerations: Ocular Micrometer.

The most important piece of equipment in the parasitology laboratory is the microscope. A microscope with the appropriate features and good optics are critical to the successful detection of parasites. Because size is an important diagnostic feature in parasitology, it is necessary for the microscope to contain a specially designed ocular piece equipped with a measuring scale known as an **ocular micrometer.** Before one begins examining specimens for parasites, the ocular micrometer must be calibrated to ensure accurate measurement.

The diagnostic stages of parasites detected microscopically are measured in units known as **microns** (abbreviated as μ or μm, defined as a unit measuring 0.001 [10^{-3}] millimeter, or 10^{-6} meter). An ocular micrometer is used to

measure objects observed microscopically accurately. The laboratory technician uses size in differentiating parasites from one another and from artifacts. The ocular micrometer is a disk that is inserted into the eyepiece of the microscope. The disk is equipped with a line evenly divided into 50 or 100 units. These units represent different measurements depending on the objectives used. Therefore, it is necessary to calibrate the micrometer to determine how many microns are equivalent to each of these divisions.

Each objective of the microscope is calibrated so that parasites can be measured at any magnification observed. Once the objectives for a given microscope have been calibrated, the ocular containing the disk and these objectives cannot be exchanged with another microscope. Each microscope must be calibrated as a unit. Calibration is usually repeated annually.

The calibration is performed with the use of a stage micrometer containing a calibrated scale divided into 0.01-mm units. The calibration procedure involves aligning the eyepiece and stage scales on the microscope, followed by determining the values of lines superimposed to the right of the zero point with a simple calculation. Figure 2-1 and Procedure 2-1 explain this procedure in detail.

Direct Wet Preparation.

The primary purpose of a **direct wet preparation** (also known as a **direct wet mount**), defined as a slide made by

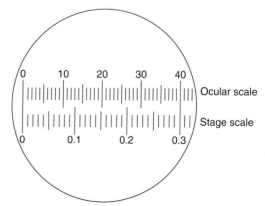

FIGURE 2-1 Calibration of an ocular micrometer.

mixing a small portion of **unfixed** stool (stool with no added preservatives) with saline or iodine and subsequent examination of the resultant mixture under the microscope, is to detect the presence of motile protozoan trophozoites. Trophozoite motility can only be demonstrated in fresh specimens, especially those of a liquid or soft consistency. If the specimen is received in the laboratory in a fixative, this procedure can be eliminated from the O&P assay. Other parasite stages that might be observed in a direct wet preparation include protozoan cysts, oocysts (Chapter 7), helminth eggs, and larvae. Because the diagnostic yield of this procedure is low, most experts agree that technical time is better spent on the concentration procedure and permanent stained smear and recommend only performing the direct wet preparation on fresh specimens.

A **direct saline wet preparation** is made by placing a drop of 0.85% saline on a glass slide (a 3- × 2-inch size is suggested) and mixing with a small portion of **unfixed** stool using a wooden applicator stick or another mixing tool. The resulting slide should be thin enough for newspaper print to be read through the smear. A 22-mm square cover slip is placed on the slide and the preparation is examined microscopically in a systematic fashion. The entire cover glass should be scanned using the low power (10×) objective on the microscope, and the power should only be increased when a suspicious object requires further investigation. The use of oil immersion is not usually recommended on wet preparations unless the cover slip is sealed to the slide. A temporary seal can be prepared using a hot paraffin-petroleum jelly (Vaseline) mixture around the edges of the cover slip. Performing this procedure allows for the ability to observe greater detail using the 100× objective.

A **direct iodine wet preparation** may be made to enhance the detail of protozoan cysts. This type of direct wet preparation is made as described earlier, using a drop of iodine (Lugol's or D'Antoni's formula) in place of saline. A suggested recipe for Lugol's iodine for wet preparation use is given in Procedure 2-2 at the end of this chapter. Because iodine kills any trophozoites present, it is recommended to use direct saline and direct iodine wet preparations on each sample that requires this component of testing. Thus, many laboratories prepare two direct wet preparations side by side on a large microscope slide, one preparation with saline and one with iodine.

Proper adjustment of the microscope is essential to the successful reading and interpreting of wet preparations. For example, the light adjustment of the microscope is critical for the detection of protozoa, which are often translucent and colorless. The light should be reduced using the iris diaphragm to provide contrast between the cellular elements in the specimen. Lowering the condenser is often recommended to lower the light and allow for otherwise transparent structures to be seen. Screening a slide using these adjustments typically takes an experienced laboratory technician approximately 10 minutes.

Quick Quiz! 2-5

The direct wet preparation can be eliminated from the O&P examination if the specimen is received in a fixative. (Objective 2-8)
A. True
B. False

Concentration Methods. The next procedure in an O&P examination is concentration of the fecal specimen. **Concentration techniques** provide the ability to detect small numbers of parasites that might not be detected using direct wet preparations. The purpose of concentration is to aggregate parasites present into a small volume of the sample and to remove as much debris as possible that might hinder the laboratory technician's ability to see any parasites present clearly. Concentration techniques can be performed on fresh or preserved stool specimens. This portion of the O&P examination allows the laboratory technician to detect protozoan cysts, oocysts, helminth eggs, and larvae. Protozoan trophozoites do not usually survive the procedure.

There are two types of concentration methods available, sedimentation and flotation. These techniques use differences in specific gravity and centrifugation to separate the parasites from the fecal debris and increase their recovery. As the name implies, in sedimentation techniques, parasites are concentrated in the sediment of the tube following centrifugation and the sediment is examined microscopically. In flotation techniques, the parasites are less dense than the solutions used and, during centrifugation, they float to the surface. Material from the surface film is examined microscopically. The ideal situation would be to perform both procedures on each specimen, but this approach is not practical; thus, each laboratory must choose which technique to use. Most experts recommend that the sedimentation technique be used, because it is more efficient and easier to perform accurately.

Formalin–Ethyl Acetate Sedimentation Procedure. The most widely used sedimentation technique is the formalin–ethyl acetate sedimentation procedure. The principle of this technique is based on specific gravity. Ethyl acetate is added to a saline-washed formalin-fixed sample and the tube is then centrifuged. Parasites are heavier than the solution and settle in the sediment of the tube, whereas fecal debris is usually lighter and rises to the upper layers of the test tube. The tube is then decanted and the sediment is examined in a wet prep, unstained (i.e., with saline) and with iodine. The advantage of this technique is that it provides good recovery of most parasites and is easy to perform. The disadvantage of this technique is that the preparation contains more fecal debris than a flotation technique and is more challenging to the microscopist. A suggested stepwise procedure for performing the formalin–ethyl acetate concentration technique may be found in Procedure 2-3.

Zinc Sulfate Flotation Technique. The zinc sulfate flotation technique is also based on differences in specific gravity between the sample debris, which in this case is heavy and sinks to the bottom of the test tube, and potential parasites, which are lighter and float toward the top of the tube. In this procedure, zinc sulfate, with a specific gravity of 1.18 to 1.20, is used as the concentrating solution. When the zinc sulfate is added to the specimen and centrifuged, the parasites float to the surface and can be skimmed from the top of the tube. The advantage of this technique is that more fecal debris is removed and it yields a cleaner preparation, making it easier for microscopic examination. The disadvantage of this method is that some helminth eggs are very dense and will not float; therefore, some parasites will be missed. It is recommended that if laboratories perform this technique, they examine saline and iodine preps made from the sediment microscopically, as well as the surface film, so as not to miss any parasites. These **concentrated wet preparations** are referred to as **concentrated saline wet preparations** and **concentrated iodine wet preparations.**

A suggested procedure for performing a modified version of this technique may be found in Procedure 2-4.

Quick Quiz! 2-6

Which of the following parasitic stages is not usually detected after using a concentration technique? (Objective 2-9)

A. Protozoan cysts
B. Protozoan trophozoites
C. Helminth eggs
D. Helminth larvae

Permanent Stains. The final procedure in the O&P examination (Procedure 2-5) is the preparation and examination of a **permanent stained smear,** (defined as a microscope slide that contains a fixed sample that has been allowed to dry and subsequently stained). These slides are considered permanent because after staining, they are typically cover-slipped and sealed, thus allowing them to remain intact long term. This is a critical portion of the O&P examination because it is designed to confirm the presence of protozoa cysts and/or trophozoites. This procedure allows laboratory technicians to observe detailed features of protozoa by staining intracellular organelles. Although some protozoa may be recognized in the direct or concentrated wet preparation, the identification is considered tentative until confirmed with the permanent stained smear. In addition, there are some protozoa that only possess a trophozoite stage and will not be detected in the concentrated wet mount preparation. *Dientamoeba fragilis* (Chapter 4) is one example and, if a permanent stained smear is not performed, this parasite will likely be missed. The permanent stained smear is not the method of choice for the identification of helminth eggs or larvae because these parasites often stain too dark or appear distorted. Helminth eggs or larvae are best detected and identified using a concentration technique.

The sample of choice for such stains is a thinly prepared slide of see-through thickness made from a PVA-preserved sample. Specimens fixed with SAF may also be used, but the choice of stain is limited to iron hematoxylin. The slide should be allowed to air-dry thoroughly before staining. Slides can also be prepared from a fresh stool specimen but must not be allowed to dry and should be immediately placed into a fixative, such as the Shaudinn fixative. On completion of staining, the slides can be sealed with a permanent mounting sealant and can be kept for years, serving as an effective teaching tool. The slides are reviewed under oil immersion (100×); 300 fields are reviewed before the slide can be considered negative. Because the slides being examined are permanently stained, an increased light source is recommended for achieving optimal results. This may be done by adjusting the microscope iris and raising the microscope condenser.

Two common stains used for routine O&P testing include trichrome (Wheatley modification) and iron hematoxylin. Specialized stains are also available for specific groups of parasites. These are not part of the routine O&P examination and must be specifically requested. These specialized stains include the modified acid-fast and modified trichrome stains.

TABLE 2-3	Appearance of Select Protozoan Structures and Background Material on Trichrome Stain
Structure or Material	**Appearance**
Cytoplasm of *Entamoeba histolytica* trophozoites and cysts	Light pink or blue-green
Cytoplasm of *Entamoeba coli* cysts	Purple tint
Nuclear karyosomes	Bright red to red-purple
Degenerated parasites	Light green
Background	Green

Wheatley Trichrome. The most widely used permanent stain is the Wheatley trichrome stain. Laboratory technicians choose this stain because it uses reagents with a relatively long shelf life and the procedure is easy to perform. There are distinct color differences among the cytoplasmic and nuclear structures of select parasitic forms, as well as background material, as noted in Table 2-3. Some technicians find that the distinct color differences between the parasites and background material make this stain easier for review of patient slides. Others think that the contrasting colors are more stressful to their eyes, which is a matter of personal opinion. A suggested procedure for trichrome staining of a slide made from a PVA-fixed specimen may be found in Procedure 2-6.

Iron Hematoxylin. The iron hematoxylin stain may be used instead of the trichrome technique. Historically, this procedure was considered to be time-consuming. However, a shorter technique using this stain, described in Procedure 2-7, is now available. The iron hematoxylin stain reveals excellent morphology of the intestinal protozoa. In some cases, the nuclear detail of these organisms is considered to be stained clearer and sharper than when stained with trichrome. The color variations among specific parasitic structures and background material are not as distinct as with the hematoxylin stain, described in Table 2-4.

TABLE 2-4	Appearance of Select Protozoan Structures and Background Material on Iron Hematoxylin Stain
Structure or Material	**Appearance**
Protozoa cytoplasm	Blue to purple
Protozoa nuclear material	Dark blue to dark purple
Debris and background material	Light blue, sometimes with pink tint

TABLE 2-6	Appearance of Microsporidia on Modified Trichrome Stain
Structure or Material	**Appearance**
Spores of microsporidia	Pink to red with clear interior
Polar tubule	Red horizontal or diagonal bar
Bacteria, yeast, debris	Pink to red
Background	Green

TABLE 2-5	Appearance of Select Protozoan Structures, Yeast, and Background Material on Modified Acid-Fast Stain
Structure or Material	**Appearance**
Oocysts of Cryptosporidium and Isospora	Pink to red
Oocysts of Cyclospora	Variable; clear to pink to red
Yeast	Blue
Background material	Blue or light red

 Quick Quiz! 2-7

The permanent stained smear is critical for detection of helminth eggs and larvae. (Objective 2-10)
A. True
B. False

Specialized Stains. One disadvantage of these stains is that they do not detect oocysts of the coccidian parasites or spores of microsporidia. The modified acid-fast stain, as described in Procedure 2-8, has become an important permanent stain procedure for the detection of the oocysts of *Cryptosporidium*, as well as those of *Isospora* and *Cyclospora* (Chapter 7). Table 2-5 describes the staining characteristics of the modified acid-fast stain. A modified iron hematoxylin stain has been developed that incorporates a carbol fuchsin step; this allows for the detection of acid-fast parasites in addition to the other protozoa normally recovered using the iron hematoxylin stain. This combination stain is being performed in laboratories that use SAF-preserved fecal samples. Although the spores of microsporidia will also stain with the acid-fast technique, their small size (1 to 2 µm) makes it difficult to identify them without the use of special stains. Modifications of the trichrome stain are available to demonstrate these parasites (Table 2-6).

STOOL SCREENING METHODS

The procedures that comprise an O&P examination enable thorough detection of parasites found in stool specimens. These techniques allow detection of a wide variety of parasites but are labor-intensive and require an experienced microscopist. Alternative tests have been developed that are often referred to as rapid methods, or stool-screening methods. These methods can be obtained as kits that contain monoclonal antibody. This commercial antibody is used to detect antigens in patient specimens. Current assays include enzyme immunoassay (EIA), direct fluorescent antibody (DFA), and membrane flow cartridge techniques.

These antigen detection methods are commercially available for specific intestinal protozoa, including *Entamoeba histolytica* (Chapter 3), *Giardia intestinalis* (Chapter 4), and *Cryptosporidium* spp. There are products available for a single parasite antigen as well as products that test for more than one. These tests are highly sensitive and specific and not as technically demanding as the O&P examination, but they only detect one or two pathogens at a time.

The physician must suspect one of these pathogens based on patient history and symptoms to request these tests. For example, in a patient with diarrhea who has returned from a camping trip, tests for *Giardia* and *Cryptosporidium* are indicated. If other parasites are potentially causing the patient's symptoms, a complete O&P examination must be performed. It is recommended that O&P examinations and fecal immunoassays be available in the laboratory test options. Some of the kits require fresh or frozen stool and cannot be done on preserved specimens. This is difficult for many laboratories because they receive their stool specimens in preservative vials. The procedure of the specific kit must be followed carefully for accurate results.

Quick Quiz! 2-8

What is one advantage of the stool screening method? (Objective 2-11)
A. It is highly sensitive and specific.
B. It can detect all parasites.
C. It can be performed on fresh or preserved specimens.
D. It is labor-intensive.

OTHER INTESTINAL SPECIMENS

In certain intestinal parasitic infections, examination of stool specimens may not detect the infectious agent. There are additional procedures that can be performed to reveal the presence of specific parasites. These are often used when the physician suspects a particular parasite and the traditional O&P examination is negative. These procedures include examination of duodenal material, examination of sigmoidoscopy material, and using cellophane tape to detect pinworms (Chapter 8).

Duodenal Material

Parasites that reside in the small intestine may be more difficult to recover in a stool specimen. In these situations, examining material from the duodenal area may yield success. The specimen may be collected by nasogastric intubation or by the enteric capsule test (Enterotest). Parasites that may be observed in this type of specimen include *Giardia intestinalis* trophozoites, *Cryptosporidium* spp., *Isospora belli*, *Strongyloides stercoralis* (Chapter 8), and eggs of *Fasciola hepatica* or *Clonorchis sinensis* (Chapter 11).

Duodenal fluid must be examined promptly because if there are trophozoites present, they will deteriorate rapidly. The material can be examined microscopically as a wet preparation. If the volume of fluid is sufficient (>2 mL), it should be centrifuged and the sediment examined. The material can be mixed with PVA fixative; stained slides can be prepared using trichrome, iron hematoxylin, and/or modified acid-fast stain. The material can also be used to perform antigen tests for *Cryptosporidium* and/or *Giardia*.

The Enterotest is a simpler method for collecting duodenal material without requiring intubation. The patient swallows a gelatin capsule that contains a coiled length of yarn. The capsule dissolves in the stomach and the weighted string is carried to the duodenum. The free end of the string is attached to the patient's neck or cheek with tape. After a 4-hour incubation period, the yarn is pulled back out of the patient. The bile-stained mucous material brought up on the string is then examined microscopically via wet preps and, if necessary, permanent stains.

Sigmoidoscopy Material

Examination of sigmoidoscopy (colon) material is often helpful for detecting *E. histolytica*. Material from ulcers obtained by aspiration or scraping should be examined by direct wet preparations and permanent stains. It is important to realize that if *E. histolytica* is present, the trophozoite stage will often be present and timing is critical because of the fragility of this organism. Coccidian parasites and microsporidia (Chapter 7) may also be recovered from examining material from the sigmoid colon.

Colon biopsy material may also be collected for examination. The specific methods necessary to perform on this biopsy material vary by the organism suspected. For example, samples believed to contain amebae are best processed using surgical pathology methods. A detailed discussion of these techniques is beyond the scope of this chapter.

Cellophane Tape Preparation

The cellophane tape prep is the specimen of choice for the detection of *Enterobius vermicularis* (pinworm) eggs (Chapter 8). Adult female pinworms may also be seen. At night, when the body is at rest, pregnant adult female worms exit the host, typically a child, through the rectum and lay numerous eggs in the perianal region. Therefore, it is important that the specimen be collected in the morning before the patient washes or defecates. In addition to pinworm, there is evidence to support the use of this technique for the recovery of *Taenia* spp. eggs (Chapter 10).

A suggested procedure for the traditional cellophane tape prep test is outlined in Procedure 2-9. Commercial collection kits are also available. It is important to note that the standard protocol for specimens collected daily for the number of negative tests that should be performed to rule out a pinworm infection is five. Laboratory technicians must be knowledgeable regarding collection of this specimen because they may need to explain the procedure to patients, their families, and/or other health care professionals. This is particularly important because, in many cases, parents may need to collect these samples from their children in a home setting. When instructing others, it is also critical to emphasize the importance of exercising proper hygiene and preventive measures during specimen collection to avoid spreading infectious eggs into the environment.

Quick Quiz! 2-9

From which area can the Enterotest be used to collect specimens? (Objective 2-12)

A. Duodenum
B. Sigmoid colon
C. Stomach
D. Perianal area

OTHER SPECIMENS AND LABORATORY TECHNIQUES

Much of this chapter has focused on processing fecal specimens because they are the most common type of specimen evaluated for parasites. There are certain parasites, however, that are not found in the gastrointestinal tract, and therefore the laboratory technician must have knowledge of which specimen must be collected and which techniques need to be applied to detect specific parasites. This section introduces the reader to body sites that may be examined for parasites, as well as specialized laboratory techniques.

Blood

Systemic or blood-borne parasitic infections are diagnosed by demonstrating the diagnostic stage(s) of the responsible parasite(s) in a blood specimen. Parasites that may be recovered in blood include *Leishmania donovani* and *Trypanosoma* spp. (Chapter 5), *Plasmodium* and *Babesia* spp. (Chapter 6), and microfilariae (Chapter 9). The proper collection and handling of blood specimens is essential to obtain adequate smears for examination. There are some parasites (e.g., *Trypanosoma* spp., microfilariae) that can be detected by observing motility in a wet preparation of a fresh blood sample under low- and high-power magnification. Definitive identification, however, requires demonstrating their features in a permanent stained smear. Blood smears can be prepared from fresh whole blood without anticoagulant (fingertip or earlobe) or from venipuncture collection with anticoagulant. There are several standard methods that may be used to identify the blood parasites. A brief description of each follows the discussion of collection.

Collection and Handling. Blood specimens for parasite study must be collected by aseptic technique. Blood from the fingertip or earlobe is obtained by making a puncture at the site. Although these specimens provide the best morphology of the parasites, improper collection or smear preparation can lead to unsatisfactory results. Capillary blood should be free-flowing and not contaminated with the alcohol used to cleanse the puncture site. Blood that is milked from the finger will be diluted with tissue fluids, making it difficult to detect the parasites. Anticoagulants cause some distortion to the staining process and subsequent parasite morphology but most laboratories use venipuncture specimens collected with an anticoagulant. Blood specimens should be collected in tubes containing ethylenediaminetetraacetic acid (EDTA). If malaria is suspected, it is best to prepare smears within 1 hour of collection, because storage of blood for a longer period leads to distortion and possible loss of malarial parasites. Similarly, malarial tests should always be considered immediately because this disease can rapidly progress to life-threatening complications.

The timing of obtaining blood samples varies with the parasite suspected. For example, the malarial forms present in peripheral blood at a given time correlate with the specific phase in the organism's life cycle. In general, the filarial parasites have a certain periodicity, or time at which the microfilariae are most likely to be present in the peripheral blood. Specific details regarding collection time are addressed on an individual basis in the parasite chapters of this text.

Processing. Typical blood sample processing for parasites consists of preparing thick and thin blood smears, staining them using a permanent stain, and examining them microscopically. Blood samples may also be processed by performing the Knott technique, examining buffy coat slides, or setting up and reading cultures. A description of each processing option follows.

Thick and Thin Smears. Once the blood sample has been collected, two types of smears may be made, thick and thin. Thick smears are frequently satisfactory for screening purposes, particularly when malaria is suspected. Thin smears provide the best view of the malarial parasites in red blood cells and are recommended for species identification. It is important to note that dehemoglobinized thick smears typically have a much higher concentration of parasites

than thin smears. Thick smears are primarily used when parasites are few in number or when thin smears are negative. The advantage of the thick smear is increased ability to detect the malarial parasites; the disadvantage is that the red blood cells have been lysed and it is not possible to assess the morphology of parasites that are detected. Suggested procedures for making thick and thin smears are given in Procedures 2-10 and 2-11, respectively.

Permanent Stains. There are two permanent stains commonly used for the detection of blood parasites, Wright's stain, which contains the fixative and stain in one solution, and Giemsa stain, in which the two are separate. Wright's stain typically yields only satisfactory results. Further discussion of Wright's stain may be found in more comprehensive parasitology manuals and in hematology texts. Giemsa stain is thus considered the preferred stain because it allows for the detection of parasite detail necessary for species identification. A suggested procedure for staining thick and thin smears with Giemsa stain is given in Procedure 2-12. A synopsis of the expected blood and tissue parasite colors and of background material seen following Giemsa staining is found in Table 2-7.

TABLE 2-7	Appearance of Select Parasitic Structures and Background Material on Giemsa Stain
Structure or Material	**Appearance**
Leishmania, trypanosome, malaria, and *Babesia* nuclear structures	Red
Cytoplasm	Blue
Schüffner's dots	Red
Filariae	
Nuclei	Blue to purple
Sheath	Clear; may not stain
Background aterial	
Red blood cells	Pale red
White blood cells	Purple
Neutrophilic granules	Pink-purple
Eosinophilic granules	Purple-red

Knott Technique. The Knott technique is designed to concentrate blood specimens suspected of containing low numbers of microfilariae. A simple modified version of this technique consists of combining 1 mL of venipuncture-collected blood with 10 mL of 2% formalin in a centrifuge tube. The mixture should then be thoroughly mixed and spun for 1 minute at 500 × g. Thick slides may be made, dried, and subsequently Giemsa-stained from the resulting sediment.

Buffy Coat Slides. A buffy coat is a layer of white blood cells between the plasma and red blood cells that results from centrifuging whole blood. Buffy coat cells may be extracted from blood specimens, stained with Giemsa stain, and microscopically examined for *Leishmania* and *Trypanosoma*. This may be accomplished by collecting oxalated or citrated blood, placing it in a Wintrobe tube, and spinning it for 30 minutes at 100 × g. The tube should be capped tightly. Centrifuging the tube produces three layers from bottom to top—packed red blood cells, buffy coat, and plasma. The buffy coat may then be extracted using a capillary pipette.

Cultures. Cultures of blood, as well as other associated specimens such as bone marrow and tissue, may be performed. One such culture technique that yields favorable results for the recovery of *Leishmania* spp. and *Trypanosoma cruzi* uses Novy-MacNeal-Nicolle (NNN) medium. The NNN slant is inoculated by the addition of a single drop of collected blood or ground tissue. Penicillin is added to the medium if the specimen originates from a source that may contain bacteria. Periodic examination, every other day, should be conducted by observing the slant under 400× magnification. Negative cultures should be held for 1 month.

Cerebrospinal Fluid and Other Sterile Fluids

Cerebrospinal fluid (CSF) specimens may be collected for the diagnosis of amebic conditions associated with select ameba (Chapter 3) as well as African sleeping sickness (Chapter 5). The CSF must be examined promptly to detect the motility of these parasites. A wet preparation can be prepared to search for the presence of the characteristic morphologic forms of *Naegleria fowleri* and *Acanthamoeba* spp. and the trypomastigote stages of *Trypanosoma* spp. Special stains can also be performed on CSF including Giemsa, trichrome, and modified trichrome stains. If *Naegleria* or *Acanthamoeba* are suspected of being potential pathogens, the specimen can be cultured on non-nutrient agar seeded with *Escherichia coli*. The CSF sediment is inoculated to the medium, sealed, and incubated at 35° C. The plate is then examined for evidence of the amebae feeding on the bacteria. Other pathogens that might be recovered from the central nervous system include *Toxoplasma gondii* and microsporidia (Chapter 7) and *Taenia solium* cysticercus larvae and *Echinococcus* spp. (Chapter 10).

Sterile fluids other than CSF include several specimen types, such as fluid present in cysts, aspirates, peritoneal fluid, pleural fluid, and bronchial washings. Samples submitted for parasitic study should be collected using proper technique and placed in containers equipped with secure lids. The parasites that may be detected, as well as the specific processing techniques necessary to identify them, vary by specimen type. All these samples may be examined using wet preps and/or permanent stains.

Tissue and Biopsy Specimens

Tissue and biopsy specimens are recommended for the recovery of a number of parasites, including intracellular organisms such as *Leishmania* spp. and *T. gondii*. Surgical removal of the specimen followed by the preparation of histologic tissue sections and impression smears is the preferred method for handling these samples. Other parasites that may be detected in these samples include free-living ameba, *Trypanosoma* spp., *Trichinella spiralis* (Chapter 8), and microsporidia. Hepatic abscess material is the specimen of choice for patients suspected of liver abscesses caused by *E. histolytica*. Further discussion of these and of all histologic methods mentioned in this chapter is beyond the scope of this text.

Sputum

Sputum is typically collected and tested from patients suspected of being infected by the lung fluke *Paragonimus westermani* (Chapter 11). Patients with *Strongyloides stercoralis* (Chapter 8) hyperinfection will demonstrate motile larvae in their sputum. Other parasitic infections that may be found in sputum samples include microsporidia, *E. histolytica*, *Entamoeba gingivalis* (Chapter 3), *Ascaris lumbricoides*, and hookworm (Chapter 8). An early-morning specimen is best and should be collected into a wide-mouthed container with a screw cap lid. Saliva should not be mixed with the specimen. The sample may then be examined directly via wet preps and/or concentrated using *N*-acetylcysteine or other appropriate agent. Microscopic examination of the sediment can include wet preps and permanent stains.

Urine and Genital Secretions

Urine is the specimen of choice for the detection of *Schistosoma haematobium* (Chapter 11) eggs and may also yield *Trichomonas vaginalis* trophozoites (Chapter 4). Microfilariae can sometimes be found in the urine of patients with a heavy filarial infection. The specimen should be collected into a clean container with a watertight lid. The sample should be centrifuged on arrival at the laboratory. Microscopic examination of the sediment should reveal the parasites, if they are present.

Vaginal and urethral specimens, as well as prostatic secretions, are typically collected and examined for the presence of *T. vaginalis* trophozoites. These specimens may be collected on a swab or in a collection cup equipped with a lid. Saline wet preparations are the method of choice for demonstrating the motile trophozoites. Prompt examination of these preps is important because it helps ensure the recovery of the delicate organism. Permanent stains may also be used if desired.

Alternative techniques for the diagnosis of *T. vaginalis* include antigen detection methods using latex agglutination and EIA procedures. A commercially available nucleic acid probe is also available. Culture methods are available, including a commercial product that uses a culture pouch. All these methods are highly successful for diagnosing this sexually transmitted parasite.

Eye Specimens

Acanthamoeba keratitis (Chapter 3) is best diagnosed by the collection and examination of corneal scrapings. These scrapings should be placed into an airtight container. It is important that small tissue samples be kept moist with sterile saline. Other specimens that may be tested include a contact lens or contact lens solution. The samples may be processed in several ways. First, it may be cultured on an agar plate seeded with gram-negative bacteria. Examining the culture plate under low dry magnification every day for 1 week should reveal the trophozoites (usually in less than 4 days) and the cysts (in 4 to 5 days). Second, the scrapings may be transferred to glass slides and stained using the calcofluor white stain, followed by microscopic examination using fluorescent microscopy. The *Acanthamoeba* cysts stain apple green. It is important to note that this technique does not stain the trophozoites. Third, the scrapings may be processed using histologic methods.

In addition to *Acanthamoeba*, *T. gondii*, microsporidia, and *Loa loa* (Chapter 9) are also potential eye pathogens. These may be detected with histologic stains and specialized culture methods.

Mouth Scrapings and Nasal Discharge

Mouth scrapings are the sample of choice for the detection of *E. gingivalis* and *Trichomonas tenax* (Chapter 4), whereas nasal discharge specimens are helpful for the recovery of parasites such as *N. fowleri*. Material obtained via mouth scrapings and nasal discharge should be placed in a clean airtight collection container, such as on a swab or in a cup. The material may then be extracted from the swab or transferred from the cup for examination purposes. Wet preps are typically made from mouth scrapings and nasal discharge samples. Permanent stains may also be used if appropriate.

Skin Snips

Useful in the detection of *Onchocerca volvulus* (Chapter 9), skin snips may be made using one of two collection techniques. The objective of both procedures is to obtain skin fluid without bleeding. One of the methods involves making a firm (scleral) punch into skin with a specially designed tool. The other technique uses a razor blade with which a small cut into the skin is made. The resulting material obtained by both techniques may then be placed in approximately 0.2 mL of saline. After a 30-minute incubation period, the sample may be microscopically examined. The jerky movement of the microfilariae should be visible, if present, in the saline because they tend to migrate into the liquid from the skin snip itself.

Culture Methods

Culture methods are not a common means of detecting parasites. There are a few techniques available but they are not usually performed in the routine laboratory. Specialized laboratories and research facilities may offer these services. Parasites that can be isolated with culture include *E. histolytica*, *T. vaginalis*, *Leishmania* spp., *T. cruzi*, and *T. gondii*. The techniques used are beyond the scope of this chapter.

Animal Inoculation and Xenodiagnosis

Appropriate specimens from patients suspected of suffering from *Leishmania* and *Trypanosoma*, as well as *Toxoplasma*, may be tested by means of animal inoculation. Certain parasites have host specificity and require particular animals. Mice, guinea pigs, and hamsters are used. Suitable specimens for animal inoculation vary depending on the parasite suspected; these include blood, lymph node aspirates, CSF, and bone marrow. The specimens should be collected using aseptic technique. Testing takes place in facilities equipped for animal testing.

Xenodiagnosis is a technique used for the diagnosis of Chagas' disease (Chapter 5). An uninfected reduviid bug is allowed to take a blood meal from the patient and the bug's feces is then examined to observe for the presence of *T. cruzi*. This procedure is primarily used in South America and Mexico.

Quick Quiz! 2-10

Thick blood smears for malaria are recommended for species identification. (Objective 2-13)
A. True
B. False

Quick Quiz! 2-11

Giemsa is the preferred stain for the detection of blood parasites. (Objective 2-13)
A. True
B. False

Quick Quiz! 2-12

Which of the following is the specimen of choice to demonstrate intracellular parasites such as *Toxoplasma gondii* and *Leishmania* spp.? (Objective 2-13)
A. Sputum
B. Urine
C. Tissue
D. Genital secretions

IMMUNOLOGIC TESTING

Diagnosis of parasitic diseases is usually dependent on the demonstration of the causative agent in an appropriately collected and processed specimen. Occasionally, however, standard laboratory tests are not sufficient for the diagnosis of a parasite. For example, in some parasitic infections, the diagnostic stage is located deep in the tissues of the host (e.g., toxoplasmosis; see Chapter 7) and it may not be possible to detect its presence or it may be dangerously invasive to attempt it (e.g., echinococcosis; see Chapter 10). In these situations, immunologic assays can be used. Immunologic testing is usually considered as an adjunct or supplement to standard laboratory protocols.

Immunologic tests include methods for antigen and antibody detection. Antigen detection methods are more reliable and a positive test result is indicative of a current infection. Some antigen detection methods for intestinal pathogens were described earlier in the discussion of stool screening methods. These techniques allow for the rapid detection of specific intestinal pathogens. Tests that detect antibody in the patient are more complex and must be interpreted cautiously. The presence of an antibody against a given parasite may not always indicate a current infection, however. Because antibodies remain with a host for many years, a positive test result can occur from a past infection. The detection of an antibody to a given parasite in a patient with no previous exposure prior to travel to an endemic area can be considered a positive result.

There are a wide variety of immunologic tests that have been developed over recent years. These assays are not usually offered by routine laboratories and specimens must be sent out to specialty commercial or reference laboratories that perform them. The Centers for Disease Control and Prevention (CDC) also performs these assays on request. Each laboratory must check with the local public health laboratory to make arrangements for these tests to be performed.

Table 2-8 contains a list of parasitic diseases for which immunologic tests are available and the type of assay used. This table is not intended to be exhaustive in nature, but rather a representation of certain diseases that may be diagnosed

by these tests. The principle of each type of immunoassay is beyond the scope of this text. The reader can refer to an immunology text to review these features.

Nucleic acid tests have also been developed for certain parasites and are primarily performed in a specialized research or reference laboratory. The only commercial molecular test available is for the diagnosis of *T. vaginalis*. Further molecular techniques will become available as manufacturers develop automated systems that can be used by the diagnostic laboratory. Studies designed to incorporate new techniques in the diagnosis of parasitic diseases are performed on a regular basis. There are numerous methods that will no doubt emerge over time and perhaps eventually replace current standard techniques.

 Quick Quiz! 2-13

The detection of an antibody to a given parasite in a patient with no previous exposure prior to travel to an endemic area can be considered a positive result. (Objective 2-14)
A. True
B. False

REPORTING OF RESULTS AND QUALITY CONTROL

Once the analytic phase of testing is completed, the results are interpreted and reported. This is considered the postanalytic phase of laboratory testing. When reporting a positive specimen, the report should state the scientific name (genus and species), along with the stage that is present (e.g., cyst, trophozoite, larvae, eggs, adults). It is also helpful to report the presence of certain cells in the specimen. White blood cells should be reported semiquantitatively—rare, few, moderate, many.

The results of the O&P procedure should include a comment indicating that this procedure does not detect *Cryptosporidium* spp., *Cyclospora cayetanensis*, and microsporidia; it will recover the oocysts of *Isospora belli* (see Chapter 7 for

TABLE 2-8	Immunoassays and Molecular Techniques for Parasitic Diseases		
	Technique		
Disease	**Antigen Test**	**Antibody Test**	**Molecular Test**
African trypanosomiasis		CA, IFA	PCR
Amebiasis	EIA, IFA	EIA, IHA	PCR
Babesiosis		IFA	PCR
Chagas' disease		CF, EIA, IFA	PCR
Cryptosporidiosis	DFA, EIA, IFA, Rapid		PCR
Cysticercosis		EIA, IB	
Echinococcosis		EIA, IB	
Fascioliasis		EIA, IB	
Filariasis	Rapid	EIA	
Giardiasis	DFA, EIA, Rapid		PCR
Leishmaniasis	Rapid	EIA, IFA	PCR
Malaria	Rapid	IFA	PCR
Microsporidiosis	IFA		
Paragonimiasis		EIA, IB	
Schistosomiasis	EIA	EIA, IB	
Strongyloidiasis		EIA	
Toxocariasis		EIA	
Toxoplasmosis		EIA, IFA, LA	PCR
Trichinellosis		BF, EIA	
Trichomoniasis	DFA, LA, Rapid		DNA probe

BF, Bentonite flocculation; *CA,* card agglutination; *CF,* complement fixation; *DFA,* direct fluorescent antibody; *EIA,* enzyme immunoassay; *IB,* immunoblot; *IHA,* indirect hemagglutination; *IFA,* indirect fluorescent antibody; *LA,* latex agglutination; *PCR,* polymerase chain reaction; *Rapid,* immunochromatographic cartridge

details on these parasites). The results of fecal immunoassays should indicate the specific parasite(s) that is (are) tested for in the assay. Communication of this information is an educational tool to help the clinician understand the laboratory test protocols. This will ensure that the most appropriate tests are ordered.

In general, for most parasites, quantitation is not indicated. Situations in which quantitation is important are as follows: *Blastocystis hominis* (Chapter 7), helminth eggs, including *Trichuris trichiura* (Chapter 8), *Clonorchis sinensis* and *Schistosoma* spp. (Chapter 11), and *Plasmodium* and *Babesia* spp. (Chapter 6). Charcot-Leyden crystals (Chapter 12) are also reported when found and can be quantitated.

The quality assurance of parasitology is consistent with the parameters of the microbiology laboratory: procedure manuals must be up to date and readily available; reagents and solutions must be properly labeled; controls must be included in concentration and staining techniques; centrifuges and ocular micrometers must be calibrated; and refrigerator and incubator temperatures must be recorded. Action plans must be documented for anything found to be out of control. The parasitology laboratory must have references available for training and continuing education of personnel. These should include texts and atlases, digital images, and reference specimens (formalin-preserved and -stained slides). The laboratory should participate in an external proficiency test program and should also institute an internal proficiency program to enhance the skills of the laboratory technician.

Quick Quiz! 2-14

Which one of these parasites should be quantitated in the parasitology report? (Objective 2-17)
A. *Giardia intestinalis*
B. *Entamoeba coli*
C. *Trichomonas vaginalis*
D. *Blastocystis hominis*

LOOKING BACK

Accurate detection of parasites requires appropriate specimen collection and processing. This preanalytic phase of the laboratory testing is critical to a successful analysis. Because some parasites will not survive outside the host, it becomes necessary to collect certain specimens into preservatives. The traditional test performed on stool specimens is the O&P examination. This consists of macroscopic and microscopic examinations that include direct wet preparations, concentration technique resulting in concentrated wet preparations, and a permanent stained smear. Stool screening methods are also available for the detection of antigens of certain protozoan parasites. There are situations when other intestinal specimens (e.g., duodenal material, sigmoidoscopy material, cellophane tape preparation) are evaluated for the presence of parasites. Many parasites do not reside in the gastrointestinal tract but in other organs and tissues. Specimens must be collected from the appropriate sites and evaluated accordingly. Finally, there are situations in which it is difficult or impossible to demonstrate the parasite in the laboratory, so immunologic assays are performed to aid in the diagnosis.

The laboratory must complete the diagnostic test by communicating the results effectively and efficiently. This postanalytic process is just as critical as the actual analysis. The physician must understand the report to act appropriately for the patient. All aspects of the parasitology laboratory must follow the quality assurance guidelines necessary for successful testing.

TEST YOUR KNOWLEDGE!

2-1. In the collection and transport of stool specimens for parasites, which parasitic stage is most affected by the length of time from collection to examination? (Objective 2-2)
A. Cysts
B. Trophozoites
C. Oocysts
D. Helminth larvae

2-2. When using preservatives, what is the appropriate ratio of fixative to stool? (Objective 2-4)
A. One part fixative to one part stool
B. Two parts fixative to one part stool
C. Three parts fixative to one part stool
D. Four parts fixative to one part stool

2-3. One of the biggest disadvantages of formalin as a fixative for O&P is that: (Objective 2-4)
A. It cannot be used for concentration procedures.
B. It cannot be used for permanent stained slides.
C. It cannot be used for direct microscopic examinations.
D. It cannot be used for detecting protozoan cysts.

2-4. Which of the preservatives contains mercuric chloride? (Objective 2-4)
A. Formalin
B. SAF
C. PVA
D. Modified PVA

2-5. Trophozoites are found more often in liquid stools rather than formed stools, true or false. (Objective 2-5)

2-6. What is the purpose of using an ocular micrometer? Explain why it must be calibrated. (Objective 2-7)

2-7. A stool specimen is received in the laboratory for an O&P examination in a two-vial system (formalin and PVA). The laboratory technician on duty performs a concentration procedure and prepares a permanent stain slide but decides not to perform a direct wet prep examination. Is this acceptable technique? Why or why not? (Objective 2-8)

2-8. Although the zinc sulfate flotation concentration procedure removes more fecal debris and yields a cleaner microscopic preparation, most laboratories use the sedimentation procedure. Explain why. (Objective 2-9)

2-9. Why is it important to test the specific gravity of the zinc sulfate solution when using this method of concentration? (Objective 2-9)

2-10. Name one parasite that will not be detected if a permanent stained smear is not included in the O&P examination. (Objective 2-10)

2-11. A physician suspects that the patient has a tapeworm and orders a rapid stool screen or direct antigen test. Why is this an inappropriate test request? (Objective 2-11)

2-12. Give an example for which a duodenal aspirate would be tested for parasites. (Objective 2-12)

2-13. Which technique is used to detect the eggs of *Enterobius vermicularis*? (Objective 2-12)
A. Duodenal aspirate
B. Cellophane tape prep
C. Sigmoidoscopy
D. Skin snips

2-14. Describe the techniques used for preparing thick and thin films of blood. What are the advantages and disadvantages of each technique? (Objective 2-13)

2-15. List three parasites that can be recovered using specialized culture methods. (Objective 2-13)

2-16. Match each of the specimen sources (column A) with the corresponding parasite that can be recovered (column B). (Objective 2-13)

Column A	Column B
___ **A.** CSF	1. *Trichomonas vaginalis*
___ **B.** Sputum	2. *Naegleria fowleri*
___ **C.** Muscle tissue	3. *Schistosoma haemotobium*
___ **D.** Urine	4. *Onchocerca volvulus*
___ **E.** Vaginal secretions	5. *Paragonimus westermani*
___ **F.** Skin snips	6. *Trichinella spiralis*

2-17. Describe xenodiagnosis. What parasitic disease is detected with this technique? (Objective 2-13)

2-18. Explain the role of immunologic testing in the diagnosis of parasitic diseases. List examples when antigen and/or antibody tests are used. (Objective 2-14)

2-19. A technologist performs an O&P examination and detects the presence of *Entamoeba coli* cysts. The report that is sent to the physician reads: "*E. coli* detected." Why is this inappropriate reporting and how should it be corrected? (Objective 2-17)

2-20. List the areas in parasitology that need to be part of the quality assurance program. (Objective 2-18)

PROCEDURE 2-1 | **CALIBRATION AND USE OF AN OCULAR MICROMETER**

1. Insert an ocular micrometer disk in the eyepiece of the microscope or replace the ocular eyepiece with one containing an ocular micrometer.
2. Place the stage micrometer on the stage of the microscope.
3. Using the 10× (or lowest) objective, focus in on the stage micrometer and arrange it so that the left edge

of the stage micrometer lines up with the left edge of the ocular micrometer. Successful completion of this step must result in the exact alignment of the zero points of each calibration device—that is, the numbers are superimposed (see Fig. 2-1).
4. Locate a point farthest to the right of the zero points where both devices again superimpose. Each device is

Continued

PROCEDURE 2-1 | **CALIBRATION AND USE OF AN OCULAR MICROMETER—cont'd**

equipped with a numbered scale for easy calculation. Determine the number on each scale where the coinciding line exists. The number of microns (μm) equal to each unit on the ocular micrometer may be calculated by using the following formula:

(No. of stage micrometer units × 1000)/
(no. of ocular micrometer units) = no. of microns

Example 1: Note in Figure 2-1 that the 40th ocular unit aligns up exactly with the 0.3-mm mark on the stage micrometer. Using the formula

(0.3-stage micrometer units × 1000)/(40 ocular units)
= 7.5 μm

We find that at this magnification, each ocular unit is equivalent to 7.5 μm.

5. Repeat this process for each objective and calculate the number of microns equivalent to each ocular unit. This process should be completed on each microscope used for parasite examination a minimum of once annually.

6. To measure a parasite length or width, do the following:
   a. Align the ocular micrometer eyepiece by turning to the parasite so that one end is equivalent to the zero mark.
   b. Count the number of ocular units corresponding to the parasite length or width.
   c. Multiply the number of ocular units obtained by the calculated micron number established for the microscope objective in use to obtain the parasite measurement in microns.

Example 2: Let's assume that the parasite in question is measured using the 10× objective. The organism is 2 ocular units in length. The calibration of the 10× objective, as shown in example 1, revealed that each ocular unit is equivalent to 7.5 μm. Following step 6c,

2 ocular units × 7.5 μm/unit = 15 μm

Therefore, the parasite would measure 15 μm.

NOTE: The number of microns calculated per ocular unit may vary by microscope. Suggested ranges of the micron value per ocular unit by magnification are as follows:
10×: 7.5-10 μm
40×: 2.5-5 μm
100×: 1 μm

PROCEDURE 2-2 | **LUGOL'S IODINE SOLUTION FOR WET PREPARATIONS: SUGGESTED RECIPE**

Materials Needed
Distilled water, 100 mL
Potassium iodide, 10 g
Iodine powdered crystals, 5 g
1. Dissolve the potassium iodide in the distilled water.
2. Slowly add the iodine crystals, shaking the solution gently until they dissolve.

3. Filter the resulting solution.
4. Place the filtered solution, known as the stock solution, into a stoppered container.
5. Dilute the filtered stock solution 1:5 with distilled water, creating a working solution, before use.

NOTE: A new working solution should be diluted from the stock solution every 2 to 3 weeks. When the iodine crystals disappear from the bottom of the bottle, the stock solution is no longer viable and will need to be replaced.
(Data from John DE, Petri WA: Markell and Voge's medical parasitology, ed 9, St. Louis, Saunders, 2006.)

PROCEDURE 2-3 | **FORMALIN–ETHYL ACETATE CONCENTRATION**

1. Strain the specimen through a filter containing a single-layer thickness of gauze into a disposable conical centrifuge tube. The tube should be large enough to hold at least 12 mL of contents.
2. Add saline to the 12-mL mark on the tube and mix well.

3. Centrifuge the tube for 10 minutes at 500 × g (1500 rpm). Decant the supernatant. ≈1 to 1.5 mL of sediment should be left in the tube.
4. If the supernatant in step 3 is cloudy, resuspend the sediment in fresh saline or formalin and repeat steps

---

PROCEDURE 2-3 | FORMALIN–ETHYL ACETATE CONCENTRATION—cont'd

2 and 3. When the supernatant is basically clear, proceed to step 5.

5. Add 9 mL of 10% formalin to the sediment and mix thoroughly.

6. Add 3 mL of ethyl acetate, stopper the tube, and shake the mixture vigorously in an inverted position for at least 30 seconds.

7. Centrifuge the tube for 10 minutes at $500 \times g$ (1500 rpm). Four layers will form in the tube. From top to bottom they are as follows:
   Layer of ethyl acetate
   Plug of specimen debris
   Layer of formalin
   Sediment

8. Remove the stopper and, with an applicator stick, gently rim the plug of debris to loosen it from the sides of the tube. Carefully decant the top three layers.

9. With a cotton-tipped swab, wipe down the sides of the tube, absorbing any remaining ethyl acetate. Excess ethyl acetate may appear as bubbles in the microscopic preparation and can dissolve the plastic in the tube.

10. Make side by side saline and iodine wet preps from the sediment on a large glass slide. These are called concentrated wet preps.

11. Examine each concentrated wet prep under the microscope, as described in text.

NOTE: Specimen should be formalin-fixed for a minimum of 30 minutes prior to beginning this procedure.

PROCEDURE 2-4 | ZINC SULFATE FLOTATION

1. Strain the specimen through a filter containing a single-layer thickness of gauze into a conical centrifuge tube.

2. Fill the tube with saline and centrifuge for 10 minutes at $500 \times g$ (1500 rpm). Decant the supernatant. If the supernate is cloudy, repeat this step for a second wash.

3. Resuspend the sediment with 1-2 mL of zinc sulfate solution. Fill the tube with additional zinc sulfate to within 2-3 mm of the rim. (The zinc sulfate must have a specific gravity of 1.18-1.20.)

4. Centrifuge for 2 minutes at $500 \times g$ (1500 rpm). Allow the centrifuge to come to a complete stop.

5. While the tube is in the centrifuge, remove one or two drops of the top film using a Pasteur pipette or a bent wire loop and place on a slide.

6. Add a cover slip and examine microscopically. Iodine can also be added.

NOTE: Specimen should be formalin-fixed prior to beginning this suggested procedure.

PROCEDURE 2-5 | PREPARING SMEARS FOR PERMANENT STAINING

Fresh Stool

1. Using applicator sticks, spread a thin film of stool on a microscope slide and place immediately into Schaudinn fixative. Allow to fix for 30 minutes to overnight. Prior to staining, the slide must be placed into 70% alcohol to remove fixative.

2. Liquid specimen—add three or four drops of PVA to a slide and mix with several drops of stool. Spread the mixture to allow to dry overnight at room temperature or for 2-3 hours at 35° C.

PVA-Preserved Stool

1. Mix the vial of the PVA-preserved specimen well and pour some of the material onto several layers of paper towels. Let stand for 3 minutes to absorb excess PVA.

2. Using applicator sticks, apply the material to the slide, ensuring that it covers the slide to the edges.

3. Dry the slide overnight at room temperature or for 2-3 hours at 35° C.

SAF-Preserved Stool

1. Mix SAF-preserved specimen well and strain through gauze into a conical centrifuge tube.

2. Centrifuge for 1 minute at $500 \times g$ (1500 rpm) and decant the supernatant.

3. Prepare the slide by adding two drops of albumin to the slide and mixing with one drop of fecal sediment.

4. Allow to dry and place into 70% alcohol to begin the staining procedure.

PROCEDURE 2-6 | WHEATLEY TRICHROME STAIN

1. Label nine glass Coplin staining jars with the jar number and contents, as defined below. It is important that the proper laboratory protocol be followed when labeling the jars.
2. Using the table below as a guide, transfer the slides being stained from one jar to the next following the time lines established below.

3. Following the staining process, seal each slide with a fixative, such as Permount, and let it dry. An alternative to a mounting medium is to let the slide air-dry and, prior to examination, add one drop of immersion oil to the slide. Let the oil sit on the slide for 10-15 minutes and then place a no. 1 cover slip onto the oiled smear.
4. Examine each slide under oil immersion.

Trichrome Stain: Suggested Procedure

	Coplin Jar Number								
	1	2	3	4	5	6	7	8	9
Reagent	Iodine plus 70% ethanol	70% ethanol	70% ethanol	Trichrome stain	90% acidified alcohol	100% ethanol	100% ethanol	Xylene (substitute)	Xylene (substitute)
Purpose	Removes mercuric chloride, hydration	Removes iodine, hydration	Rinse, hydration	Stain	Destain	Halts destaining	Dehydration	Removes debris, dehydration	Removes debris
Time	10 min	5 min	5 min	7 min	5-10 sec	Quick rinse	5 min	10 min	10 min

PROCEDURE 2-7 | IRON HEMATOXYLIN STAIN (TOMPKINS-MILLER METHOD)

Step No.	Reagent	Purpose	Time (min)
1	Iodine + 70% ethanol	Remove fixative	2-5
2	50% ethanol	Rinse	5
3	Running tap water	Rinse	3
4	4% ferric ammonium sulfate	Mordant fixative	5
5	Running tap water	Rinse	1
6	Hematoxylin solution (0.5%)	Stain	2
7	Running tap water	Rinse	1
8	2% phosphotungstic acid	Decolorize	2-5
9	Running tap water	Rinse	10
10	70% ethanol containing a few drops of saturated aqueous lithium carbonate	Dehydrate	3
11	95% ethanol	Dehydrate	5
12	100% alcohol	Dehydrate	5
13	100% alcohol	Dehydrate	5
14	Xylene substitute	Clearing	5
15	Xylene substitute	Clearing	5
16	Mounting fluid (i.e., Permount) (alternative method as described in Procedure 2-6 can be used)	Preserve slides	
17	Microscopically examine slides		

NOTE: Prepare smears as described in Procedure 2-5. SAF-preserved slides begin with step 2.

PROCEDURE 2-8	MODIFIED ACID-FAST STAIN		
Step No.	Reagent	Purpose	Time
1	Kinyoun carbol fuchsin	Stain	5 min
2	50% ethanol	Rinse	Briefly
3	Tap water	Rinse	Thorough
4	1% sulfuric acid	Decolorizer	2 min
5	Tap water	Rinse	1-2 min
6	Methylene blue	Counterstain	1 min
7	Tap water	Rinse	1-2 min
8	Air-dry, examine under oil immersion		

NOTE: This procedure may be used for unpreserved specimens or for samples fixed in formalin. The sample should be smeared on the slide and allowed to air-dry. The slide should be fixed in absolute methanol for 1 minute and allowed to air-dry before proceeding with this procedure.

PROCEDURE 2-9	CELLOPHANE TAPE PREPARATION

1. Fold the end of a 10-cm piece of transparent tape, adhesive side out, over the end of a tongue depressor. It is important not to use frosted tape because it might mask the appearance of the eggs.
2. Press the adhesive side of the tape firmly against the perianal region of the patient. Using a rocking motion, cover as much of the region as possible.
3. Place the tape, adhesive side down, on a clean glass microscope slide. Avoid trapping air bubbles during this step.
4. Microscopically examine the slide under low power. Reduced light is recommended because the eggs will appear colorless, making them difficult to detect under high light intensity.

NOTE: Commercial collection kits are also available for use. Each kit contains a plastic collection paddle. In this procedure, the paddle is used for collection and examination.

PROCEDURE 2-10	PREPARATION OF THICK BLOOD SMEARS

1. Place three small drops of blood onto one end of a clean microscope slide.
2. Using the corner of a second clean microscope slide as a stirrer, combine the contents of the three drops of blood by thoroughly mixing and spreading to a circular film approximately the size of a dime or nickel.
3. Let the slide air-dry.
4. Remove the hemoglobin by immersing the slide in a buffer solution before staining or directly during Giemsa staining.

PROCEDURE 2-11 | **PREPARATION OF THIN BLOOD SMEARS**

1. Place a small drop of blood close to the end of a microscope slide.
2. Hold a second slide (spreader slide) on edge at a 30- to 40-degree angle and draw back into the blood drop, allowing it to spread along the edge of the spreader slide.
3. Quickly and steadily push the spreader slide forward so that the blood spreads out into a thin film with a feathered edge.
4. Air-dry and stain.

PROCEDURE 2-12 | **GIEMSA STAIN**

Thick Smears

1. Stain with Giemsa stain (1:50 dilution of Giemsa stock solution with buffered water 7.0 pH) for 30-60 minutes.
2. Wash briefly by immersing the slides in the buffered water for 3-5 minutes and drain.
3. Air-dry in a vertical position and examine under oil.

Thin Smears

1. Immerse the prepared slides for 1 minute in a Coplin jar that contains absolute methyl alcohol.
2. Let air-dry.
3. Stain with Giemsa stain (1:20 dilution) for 20 minutes.
4. Wash by dipping slides in and out of buffered water once or twice.
5. Air-dry in a vertical position and examine under oil.

The Amebas

Hassan Aziz and Elizabeth Zeibig

WHAT'S AHEAD

Focusing In
Morphology and Life Cycle
 Notes
Laboratory Diagnosis
Pathogenesis and Clinical
 Symptoms

Classification of the Amebas
 Entamoeba histolytica
 Entamoeba hartmanni
 Entamoeba coli
 Entamoeba polecki
 Endolimax nana

Iodamoeba bütschlii
Entamoeba gingivalis
Naegleria fowleri
Acanthamoeba species
Looking Back

LEARNING OBJECTIVES

On completion of this chapter and review of its figures and corresponding photomicrographs, the successful learner will be able to:

3-1. Define the following key terms:
   Acanthopodia
   Ameba (*pl.*, amebas)
   Amebiasis
   Amebic
   Amebic colitis
   Amebic dysentery
   Chromatoid bars
   Cyst (*pl.*, cysts)
   Encystation
   Excystation
   Extraintestinal
   Flagellum (*pl.*, flagella)
   Flagellate (*pl.*, flagellates)
   Glycogen mass
   Karyosome (karyosomal chromatin)
   Kernig's sign
   Pathogenicity
   Peripheral chromatin
   Pseudopod (*pl.*, pseudopods)
   Trophozoite (*pl.*, trophozoites; often abbreviated as troph or trophs)
   Vector (*pl.*, vectors)

3-2. State the geographic distribution of the amebas.

3-3. Given a list of parasites, select those organisms belonging to the protozoan group Ameba, subphylum Sarcodina.

3-4. Classify the individual ameba as intestinal or extraintestinal.

3-5. Construct, describe, and compare and contrast the following life cycles:
   A. General intestinal amebas
   B. General extraintestinal amebas
   C. Each specific ameba

3-6. Briefly identify and describe the populations prone to contracting clinically significant disease processes and clinical signs and symptoms associated with each pathogenic ameba.

3-7. Identify and describe each of the following as they relate to the amebas:
   A. Factors responsible for the asymptomatic carrier state of an infected patient
   B. Treatment options
   C. Prevention and control measures

3-8. Determine specimen(s) of choice, alternative specimen type(s) when appropriate, collection protocol(s), and laboratory diagnostic technique(s) required for the recovery of each of the amebas.

3-9. Given the name, description, photomicrograph, and/or diagram of an ameba:

Identify, describe and/or label its characteristic structures, when appropriate

State the purpose of the designated characteristic structure(s).

Name the parasite, including its morphologic form,

3-10. Analyze case studies that include pertinent patient information and laboratory data and:

A. Identify and describe the function of key differential characteristics structures.

B. Identify each responsible amebic organism by category, scientific name, common name, and morphologic form, with justification when indicated.

C. Identify the associated symptoms, diseases, and conditions associated with the responsible parasite.

D. Construct a life cycle associated with each amebic parasite present that includes corresponding epidemiology, route of transmission, infective stage, and diagnostic stage(s).

E. Propose each of the following related to stopping and preventing ameba infections:

1. Treatment options
2. Prevention and control plan

F. Determine the specimen(s) of choice and alternative specimen types, when appropriate, as well as the appropriate

laboratory diagnostic techniques for the recovery of each ameba.

G. Recognize sources of error, including but not limited to those involved in specimen collection, processing, and testing and propose solutions to remedy them.

H. Interpret laboratory data, determine specific follow-up tests that could or should be done, and predict the results of those identified tests.

I. Determine additional morphologic forms, when appropriate, that may also be detected in clinical specimens.

3-11. Compare and contrast the similarities and differences between:

A. The amebas covered in this chapter

B. The amebas covered in this chapter and the other parasites covered in this text.

3-12. Describe the standard, immunologic, and new laboratory diagnostic approaches for the recovery of amebas in clinical specimens.

3-13. Given prepared laboratory specimens, and with the assistance of this manual, the student will be able to:

A. Differentiate amebic parasites from artifacts.

B. Differentiate the amebic organisms from each other and from the other appropriate categories of parasites.

C. Correctly identify each amebic parasite by scientific, common name, and morphologic form based on its key characteristic structure(s).

CASE STUDY 3-1   UNDER THE MICROSCOPE

Eleven-year-old Scooter was admitted to the emergency room with complaints of fever, vomiting, and altered mental status. Patient history revealed that the boy felt fine until 2 days ago, at which time he developed a headache and experienced photophobia. On questioning Scooter, it was discovered that the patient went swimming in a local river 5 days ago. A lumbar puncture was attempted but was unsuccessful because of the child's combativeness. Antibiotics were administered because of suspected meningitis. The patient was then transferred to a tertiary care facility for further evaluation. He suffered a seizure en route, with jerking movements of his right side.

A complete blood count was done, which revealed an increased white blood cell count with a predominance of segmented neutrophils. A second lumbar puncture was attempted at the tertiary care facility. The successful puncture revealed a yellowish, puslike fluid. The spinal fluid's protein, white blood cell, and red blood cell levels were elevated, with a decrease in glucose levels. Examination of the spinal fluid wet mount actively showed motile trophozoites. Within 3 days of being transferred to the tertiary facility, Scooter slipped into a coma and never regained consciousness. He died 5 days after onset of the illness.

Questions for Consideration

1. Which ameba is the most likely cause of Scooter's infection? (Objective 3-10B)
2. Name associated diseases linked with the responsible parasite. (Objective 3-10C)
3. Construct the life cycle of the responsible parasite emphasizing the epidemiology, route of transmission, and infective and diagnostic stages. (Objective 3-10D)
4. What are the treatment options and how can this parasitic infection be prevented or controlled? (Objective 3-10E)
5. What is the specimen of choice for the recovery of this parasite? (Objective 3-10F)
6. Interpret the laboratory data given and propose specific follow-up tests that could aid in the identification of the infection. (Objective 3-10H)

FOCUSING IN

Protozoa are unicellular organisms and the lowest form of animal life. In the subkingdom Protozoa, there are three phyla of medical interest in humans. The phylum Sarcomastigophora, subphylum Sarcodina, includes the pathogenic and nonpathogenic amebas. This chapter describes the morphologic features, laboratory diagnosis, life cycle, epidemiology and clinical symptoms, treatment, and prevention and control of nine ameba species, each of which is known to infect humans.

MORPHOLOGY AND LIFE CYCLE NOTES

The most important feature that separates **amebas** from the other groups of unicellular Protozoa is the means by which they move. Amebas are equipped with the ability to extend their cytoplasm in the form of **pseudopods** (often referred to as false feet), which allows them move within their environment. With one exception, there are two morphologic forms in the amebic life cycle—**trophozoites,** the form that feeds, multiplies, and possesses pseudopods, and **cysts,** the nonfeeding stage characterized by a thick protective cell wall designed to protect the parasite from the harsh outside environment when deemed necessary. It is important to note here that the nuclear characteristics of trophozoites are basically identical to those of their corresponding cysts.

Trophozoites are characteristically delicate and fragile and, because of their ability to produce and use pseudopods, motile. The life cycles of all the intestinal amebas are similar. The most common means whereby amebas are transferred to humans is through ingestion of the infective cyst in contaminated food or water. In most cases, trophozoites are easily destroyed by the gastric juices of the stomach. Trophozoites are also susceptible to the environment outside the host. Therefore, trophozoites are not usually transmitted to humans. **Excystation,** the morphologic conversion from the cyst form into the trophozoite form, occurs in the ileocecal area of the intestine. Replication only occurs in the trophozoite stage; it is accomplished by multiplication of the nucleus via asexual binary fission.

The conversion of trophozoites to cysts, a process known as **encystation,** occurs in the intestine when the environment becomes unacceptable for continued trophozoite multiplication. A number of conditions individually or in combination may trigger encystation, including ameba overpopulation, pH change, food supply (too much or too little), and available oxygen (too much or too little). Contrary to the trophozoites, cysts are equipped with a protective cell wall. The cell wall allows cysts to enter the outside environment with the passage of feces and remain viable for long periods of time. The ingestion of the infective cysts completes the typical intestinal amebic life cycle.

Because the basic life cycle is the same for each of the intestinal amebas, a section dedicated to life cycle notes does not appear under the discussion of each individual parasite. Only notes of interest or importance are noted, when appropriate. The life cycles of the extraintestinal ameba differ from those of the intestinal amebas; these are discussed individually in this chapter.

Quick Quiz! 3-1

Amebas transform from trophozoites to cysts on entry into an unsuspecting human. (Objective 3-5A)
A. True
B. False

LABORATORY DIAGNOSIS

Amebic trophozoites as well as cysts may be seen in stool samples submitted for parasite study. Trophozoites are primarily recovered from stools that are of soft, liquid, or loose consistency. Formed stool specimens are more likely to contain cysts. The morphologic forms present in samples other than stool are noted on an individual basis. It is important to point out that the presence of either or both morphologic forms is diagnostic.

Proper determination of organism size, using the ocular micrometer (see Chapter 2), is essential when identifying the amebas. The appearance of key nuclear characteristics, such as the number of nuclei present and the positioning of the nuclear structures, is crucial to differentiate the amebas correctly. The presence of other amebic structures and characteristics, such as cytoplasmic inclusions and motility, also aids in the identification of the amebas. Standard microscopic procedures include examination of specimens for amebas using saline wet preparations, iodine wet preparations, and permanent stains.

The saline wet preparation and iodine wet preparation each have an advantage that supports their use. Saline wet preparations are of value because they will often show motility of the amebic trophozoites. The internal cytoplasmic, as well as the nuclear structures, may be more readily seen with the use of iodine wet preparations.

It is important to note that permanent smear procedures of samples suspected of having amebas must be performed to confirm parasite identification. In most cases, the key identifying characteristics cannot be accurately distinguished without the permanent stain. The permanent stain allows for many of the otherwise refractive and invisible structures to be more clearly visible and thus easier to identify. The permanent smear procedure may, however, shrink amebic parasites, causing measurements smaller than those typically seen in wet preparations.

Alternative laboratory diagnosis techniques are available for three of the amebas covered in this chapter—*Entamoeba histolytica*, *Naegleria fowleri*, and *Acanthamoeba* spp. Representative laboratory diagnostic methodologies are presented in Chapter 2, as well as in each individual parasite discussion, as appropriate.

Quick Quiz! 3-2

Formed stool specimens are more likely to contain which of the following? (Objective 3-8)
A. Trophozoites
B. Cysts

PATHOGENESIS AND CLINICAL SYMPTOMS

A number of patients infected with intestinal amebas are asymptomatic. Amebas are often discovered, however, in patients suffering from diarrhea without an apparent cause. Diagnosis of nonpathogenic amebas is important because this finding suggests that the ingestion of contaminated food or drink may have occurred. The presence of pathogenic amebas in addition to nonpathogenic amebas is also possible because the transmission route of both amebic groups is identical. Thorough screening of such samples is crucial to ensure proper identification of all parasites that may be present. Infection is most common in people who live in underdeveloped

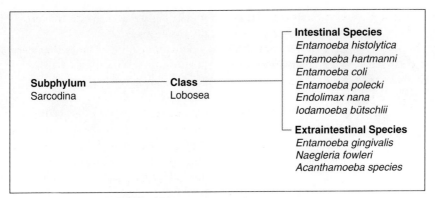

FIGURE 3-1 Parasite classification, the amebas.

countries that have poor sanitary conditions. In the United States, **amebiasis** is often found in immigrants from and people who have traveled to underdeveloped countries. Furthermore, amebas may be present and thus infect individuals in areas and institutions in which crowded conditions prevail.

It is important to note that only one of the intestinal amebas, *E. histolytica*, may produce characteristic symptoms, and is universally considered to be a pathogen. Infections with each of the extraintestinal amebas may cause symptoms that are other than intestinal in nature, often involving such areas as the mouth, eye, and brain.

Quick Quiz! 3-3

Infections with intestinal amebas are prevalent in which of the following? (Objective 3-2)

A. Underdeveloped countries with poor sanitary conditions

B. Beef consumers in the United States

C. People traveling to Europe

D. Japan, because of seafood diet

CLASSIFICATION OF THE AMEBAS

The amebas, members of the subphylum Sarcodina and class Lobosea, may be separated into two categories, intestinal and **extraintestinal** (meaning parasites that migrate and/or take up

residence outside the intestines). The species discussed in this chapter are classified under these categories and are listed in Figure 3-1.

Entamoeba histolytica
(en'tuh-mee'buh/his-toe-lit'i-kuh)

Common associated disease or condition names: Intestinal amebiasis, amebic colitis, amebic dysentery, extraintestinal amebiasis.

Morphology

Trophozoites. The trophozoites (trophs) of *E. histolytica* range in size from 8 to 65 μm, with an average size of 12 to 25 μm (Figs. 3-2 to 3-4; Table 3-1). Note that parasite names are often shortened to just the first letter of the genus followed by the species name; *E. histolytica* is the abbreviated version of *Entamoeba histolytica*. Abbreviations will be used along with the entire parasite names, as appropriate, throughout the rest of this text.

The trophozoite exhibits rapid, unidirectional, progressive movement, achieved with the help of finger-like hyaline pseudopods. The single nucleus typically contains a small central mass of chromatin known as a **karyosome** (also referred to as **karyosomal chromatin**). Variants of the karyosome include eccentric or fragmented karyosomal material. The karyosome of this amebic parasite is surrounded by chromatin material, a

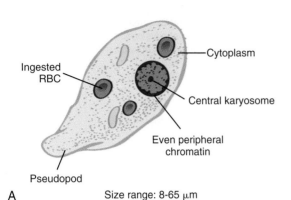

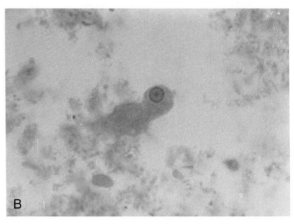

A

Size range: 8-65 μm
Average size: 12-25 μm

B

FIGURE 3-2 A, *Entamoeba histolytica* trophozoite. **B,** *Entamoeba histolytica* trophozoite. **(B** *from Mahon CR, Lehman DC, Manuselis G: Textbook of diagnostic microbiology, ed 4, St Louis, 2011, Saunders.)*

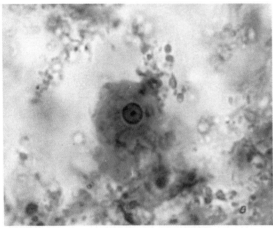

FIGURE 3-3 *Entamoeba histolytica* trophozoite showing typical central karyosome and even peripheral chromatin, resulting in a smooth nuclear perimeter (trichrome stain, ×1000). *(Courtesy of WARD'S Natural Science Establishment, Rochester, NY; http://wardsci.com.)*

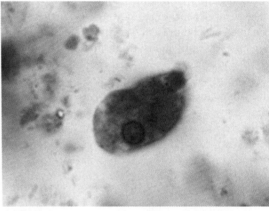

FIGURE 3-4 Atypical *Entamoeba histolytica* trophozoite. Note eccentric karyosome (iron hematoxylin stain, ×1000). *(Courtesy of WARD'S Natural Science Establishment, Rochester, NY; http://wardsci.com.)*

morphologic structure called **peripheral chromatin.** This peripheral chromatin is typically fine and evenly distributed around the nucleus in a perfect circle. Variations, such as uneven peripheral chromatin, may also be seen. Although the karyosome and peripheral chromatin appearance may vary, most trophozoites maintain the more typical features described. The invisible nucleus in unstained preparations becomes apparent when stained. Stained preparations may reveal

TABLE 3-1	*Entamoeba histolytica* Trophozoite: Typical Characteristics at a Glance
Parameters	**Description**
Size range	8-65 μm
Motility	Progressive, finger-like pseudopodia
Number of nuclei	One
Karyosome	Small and central
Peripheral chromatin	Fine and evenly distributed
Cytoplasm	Finely granular
Cytoplasmic inclusions	Ingested red blood cells

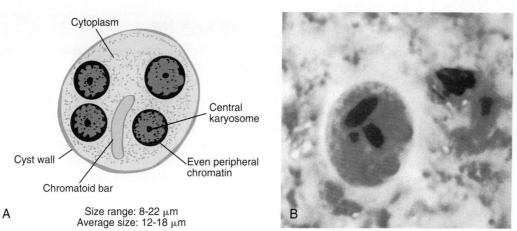

FIGURE 3-5 A, *Entamoeba histolytica* cyst. **B,** *Entamoeba histolytica–Entamoeba dispar* cyst. (**B** *from Forbes BA, Sahm DF, Weissfeld AS: Bailey & Scott's diagnostic microbiology, ed 12, St Louis, 2007, Mosby.)*

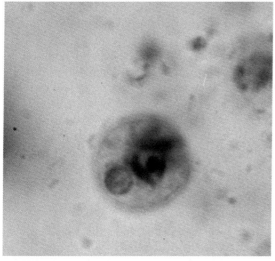

FIGURE 3-6 *Entamoeba histolytica* cyst. Note single nucleus and prominent chromatoid bars (iron hematoxylin stain, ×1000). *(Courtesy of WARD'S Natural Science Establishment, Rochester, NY; http://wardsci.com.)*

TABLE 3-2	*Entamoeba histolytica* Cyst: Typical Characteristics at a Glance
Parameter	**Description**
Size range	8-22 μm
Shape	Spherical to round
Number of nuclei	One to four
Karyosome	Small and central
Peripheral chromatin	Fine and evenly distributed
Cytoplasm	Finely granular
Cytoplasmic inclusions	Chromatoid bars, rounded ends in young cysts
	Diffuse glycogen mass in young cysts

lightly staining fibrils located between the karyosome and peripheral chromatin. The *E. histolytica* trophozoite contains a finely granular cytoplasm, which is often referred to as having a ground glass in appearance. Red blood cells (RBCs) in the cytoplasm are considered diagnostic because *E. histolytica* is the only intestinal ameba to exhibit this characteristic. Bacteria, yeast, and other debris may also reside in the cytoplasm, but their presence, however, is not diagnostic.

◼ **Cysts.** The spherical to round cysts of *E. histolytica* are typically smaller than the trophs, measuring 8 to 22 μm, with an average range of 12 to 18 μm (Figs. 3-5 and 3-6; Table 3-2). The presence of a hyaline cyst wall helps in the recognition of this morphologic form. Young cysts characteristically contain unorganized chromatin material that transforms into squared or round-ended structures call **chromatoid bars,** defined as structures that contain condensed RNA material. A diffuse **glycogen mass,** a cytoplasmic area without defined borders that is believed to represent stored food, is also usually visible in young cysts. As the cyst matures, the glycogen mass usually disappears, a process that likely represents usage of the stored food. One to four nuclei are usually present. These nuclei appear basically the same as those of the trophozoite in all respects but are usually smaller. Nuclear variations do occur, with the most common of these being eccentric (rather than the typical central) karyosomes, thin plaques of peripheral chromatin, or a clump of peripheral chromatin at one side of the nucleus that appears crescent shaped. The nuclei in Figure 3-3 are enlarged to show the nuclear detail. The mature infective cyst is quadrinucleated (containing four nuclei). The cytoplasm remains fine and granular. RBCs, bacteria, yeast, and other debris are not found in the cyst stage.

Laboratory Diagnosis

The diagnosis of *E. histolytica* infection may be accomplished by standard and alternative methods. In addition to performing traditional wet preparation and permanent staining techniques on a suspected stool sample, material collected from a sigmoidoscopy procedure, as well as hepatic abscess material, may be processed and examined in the same manner. A special medium known at TYI-S-33 supports *E. histolytica* in culture. When *E. histolytica* is suspected but not recovered in stool samples, other laboratory tests, including immunologically based procedures, may be used. Methods currently available include antigen tests, enzyme-linked immunosorbent assay (ELISA), indirect hemagglutination (IHA), gel diffusion precipitin (GDP), and indirect immunofluorescence (IIF). Serologic tests designed to detect *E. histolytica* are available and are typically only helpful in cases of extraintestinal infections.

Life Cycle Notes

Once the infective cyst is ingested, excystation occurs in the small intestine. As a result of the nuclear division, a single cyst produces eight motile trophozoites. These motile amebas settle in the lumen of the large intestine, where they replicate by binary fission and feed on living host cells. On occasion, trophozoites migrate to other organs in the body, such as the liver, and may cause abscess formation. Unless these trophozoites return to the lumen of the large intestine, their life cycle ceases and diagnosis in such cases will rely on serologic testing. Encystation occurs in the intestinal lumen, and cyst formation is complete when four nuclei are present. These infective cysts are passed out into the environment in human feces and are resistant to a variety of physical conditions. Survival in a feces-contaminated environment for up to 1 month is common.

It is important to note that in addition to cysts, trophozoites, under the right conditions, may also be present in the stool. Liquid or semiformed samples may show trophozoites if the intestinal motility is rapid. Cysts will form, on the other hand, if the intestinal motility is normal.

Epidemiology

Entamoeba histolytica infection occurs in as many as 10% of the world's population and is considered a leading cause of parasitic deaths after only malaria, the clinical manifestation of infection with *Plasmodium* species parasites, as detailed in Chapter 6, and schistosomiasis, the umbrella term for the disease associated with *Schistosoma* spp. infection, as detailed in Chapter 11. In addition to thriving in subtropical and tropical areas of the world, this parasite exists in colder climates, such as Alaska, Russia, and Canada. Locations at which human waste is used as fertilizer, areas of poor sanitation, hospitals for the mentally ill, prisons, and day care centers tend to harbor *E. histolytica*. This organism has historically been prevalent in homosexual communities because it causes frequent asymptomatic infections in homosexual men, particularly in western countries.

Several means of transmitting *E. histolytica* are known. Ingestion of the infective stage, the cyst, occurs through hand-to-mouth contamination and food or water contamination. In addition, *E. histolytica* may also be transferred via unprotected sex. Flies and cockroaches may also serve as **vectors** (living carriers responsible for transmitting parasites from infected hosts uninfected hosts) of *E. histolytica* by depositing infective cysts on unprotected food. Improperly treated water supplies are additional sources of possible infection.

Clinical Symptoms

Entamoeba histolytica is the only known pathogenic intestinal ameba. The range of symptoms varies and depends on two major factors: (1) the location(s) of the parasite in the host; and (2) the extent of tissue invasion.

◤ **Asymptomatic Carrier State.** Three factors, acting separately or in combination, are responsible for the asymptomatic carrier state of a patient infected with *E. histolytica*: (1) the parasite is a low-virulence strain; (2) the inoculation into the host is low; and (3) the patient's immune system is intact. In these cases, amebas may reproduce but the infected patient shows no clinical symptoms.

◤ **Symptomatic Intestinal Amebiasis.** Patients infected with *E. histolytica* who exhibit symptoms often suffer from **amebic colitis**, defined as an intestinal infection caused by the presence of amebas exhibiting symptoms. In some cases, these patients may transition from amebic colitis into a condition characterized by blood and mucus in the stool known as **amebic dysentery.** Individuals with amebic colitis may exhibit nondescript abdominal symptoms or may complain of more specific symptoms, including diarrhea, abdominal pain and cramping, chronic weight loss, anorexia, chronic fatigue, and flatulence. Secondary bacterial infections may develop after

the formation of flask-shaped amebic ulcers in the colon, cecum, appendix, or rectosigmoid area of the intestine. As noted, stools recovered from patients suffering from amebic dysentery are characterized by the presence of blood and/or pus and mucus.

◤ **Symptomatic Extraintestinal Amebiasis.** *E. histolytica* trophozoites that migrate into the bloodstream are removed by and take up residence in the liver. The formation of an abscess in the right lobe of the liver and trophozoite extension through the diaphragm, causing amebic pneumonitis, may occur. Patients in this state often exhibit symptoms similar to those of a liver infection plus a cough, with the most common of the symptoms being upper right abdominal pain with fever. Weakness, weight loss, sweating, pronounced nausea, and vomiting may occur, as well as marked constipation with or without alternating diarrhea.

In addition to the liver, *E. histolytica* has been known to migrate to and infect other organs, including the lung, pericardium, spleen, skin, and brain. Venereal amebiasis may also occur. Men become infected with penile amebiasis after experiencing unprotected sex with a woman who has vaginal amebiasis. The disease may also be transferred during anal intercourse. It is interesting to note that on examination of these genital areas, the trophozoite form of *E. histolytica* is most commonly encountered.

Treatment

Treatment regimens for patients infected with *E. histolytica* vary by the type of infection present. Because there is concern that an infection with *E. histolytica* may become symptomatic in the intestinal tract only or with subsequent extraintestinal invasion, asymptomatic individuals may be treated with paromomycin, diloxanide furoate (Furamide), or metronidazole (Flagyl). Patients showing symptomatic intestinal amebiasis typically respond well to iodoquinol, paromomycin, or diloxanide furoate. Metronidazole or tinidazole, in combination with a symptomatic intestinal amebiasis treatment, is recommended for patients who have progressed to extraintestinal amebiasis.

Prevention and Control

Several steps may be taken to prevent *E. histolytica* infections. Uncontaminated water is essential; this may be accomplished by boiling or treating with iodine crystals. It is interesting to note that the infective (quadrinucleated) cyst is resistant to routine chlorination. A water treatment regimen that includes filtration and chemical treatment is necessary to ensure a safe water supply. Properly washing food products, avoiding the use of human feces as fertilizer, good personal hygiene and sanitation practices, protection of food from flies and cockroaches, and the avoidance of unprotected sexual practices serve as a means to break the transmission cycle.

Notes of Interest and New Trends

Several discoveries during the late 1880s led to the confirmation that *E. histolytica* was indeed a pathogen. Of particular note was the work of Loesch, who studied the stool of a patient suffering from dysentery. The ameba-infected stool from this patient was transferred to a dog for further study.

The overall prevalence of *Entamoeba* infection in the United States is approximately 4%. *Entamoeba* spp. infect approximately 10% of the world's population. The prevalence of infection is as high as 50% in areas of Central and South America, Africa, and Asia.

Of all of the cases of *E. histolytica* worldwide, only 10% progress to the invasive stage. Invasive and noninvasive strains of *E. histolytica* may be distinguished by performing isoenzyme electrophoresis and examining the zymodemes (isoenzyme patterns). These analyses are conducted primarily for epidemiologic studies of the organism. Applications of isoenzyme electrophoresis are not, however, useful in routine laboratory testing.

The World Health Organization (WHO) recommends that intestinal infection be diagnosed with an *E. histolytica*–specific test, thus rendering the classic stool ova and parasite examination obsolete in this setting. However, finding quadrinucleated cysts or trophozoites containing ingested erythrocytes in stool is considered by many to be diagnostic for amebic colitis.

Several identification methods have been developed, including specific immunologic tests and new techniques (see Chapter 2), all of which have shown promising results. A monoclonal antibody ELISA assay to detect antigen of *E. histolytica* in stool samples has been developed and experimentally tested. Similarly, DNA hybridization probe testing using feces samples has been developed. Molecular analysis by polymerase chain reaction (PCR)–based assays is the method of choice for discriminating between *E. histolytica* and nonpathogenic amebas. In addition, latex agglutination testing for the presence of serum *E. histolytica* antibodies has been studied and appears to be a useful screening method. Epidemiologic studies may benefit from an *E. histolytica* skin test that has been formulated.

A nonpathogenic ameba, known as *Entamoeba dispar,* has been identified that is morphologically identical to *E. histolytica.* Thus, it is often impossible to distinguish these two ameba based on morphology alone. Because of this inability to distinguish these two like parasites, the laboratory often reports both names if trophozoites that lack RBCs and/or cysts are recovered. If however, trophozoites are seen that contain ingested RBCs, it is then appropriate to report them as *E. histolytica.* In cases for which identification is not apparent, speciation requires specialized testing methodologies that include DNA probes and electrophoresis techniques designed to target enzymes.

Quick Quiz! 3-4

Which of the following structures is (are) typical in trophozoites of *E. histolytica*? (Objective 3-9A)
A. Single nucleus with a small karyosome
B. Unevenly distributed peripheral chromatin
C. Chromatoid bars
D. Glycogen mass

Quick Quiz! 3-5

E. histolytica infection is traditionally diagnosed by finding which of the following? (Objective 3-8)

A. Adult and egg forms of the parasite in a suspected stool sample

B. Trophozoites and/or cysts in a suspected stool sample

C. Larvae in a suspected CSF sample

D. Adult form of the parasite in suspected tissue samples

Quick Quiz! 3-6

The infective stage of *E. histolytica* is which of the following? (Objective 3-5)

A. Trophozoite

B. Cyst

Quick Quiz! 3-7

Which of the following factors is not responsible for the asymptomatic carrier state of a patient infected with *E. histolytica*? (Objective 3-7A)

A. Low virulence strain

B. Low inoculation into host

C. Intact patient's immune system

D. Patient's blood type

Quick Quiz! 3-8

Which of the following prevention measures can control the spread of *E. histolytica*? (Objective 3-7C)

A. Drinking tap water

B. Using human feces as fertilizer

C. Boiling water or treat with iodine crystals

D. Practicing unsafe sex

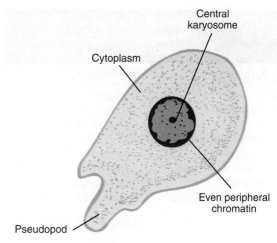

Size range: 5-15 μm
Average size: 8-12 μm

FIGURE 3-7 *Entamoeba hartmanni* trophozoite.

Entamoeba hartmanni
(en'tuh-mee'buh/hart-man'nee)

Common associated disease or condition names: Intestinal amebiasis, amebic colitis, amebic dysentery, extraintestinal amebiasis.

Morphology

Size accounts for the major difference between the trophozoites and cysts of *Entamoeba hartmanni* and *Entamoeba histolytica*.

Trophozoites. The typical *E. hartmanni* trophozoite measures a mere 8 to 12 μm, with a size range of 5 to 15 μm (Fig. 3-7; Table 3-3). Finger-shaped pseudopods exhibiting nonprogressive motility are standard. Trophozoites contain one nucleus that is not typically visible in unstained preparations. The peripheral chromatin is usually present as evenly distributed granules and often has a beaded appearance. The karyosome may be centrally or eccentrically located. Nuclear structure variations identical to those described in the discussion of *E. histolytica* may occur. The finely granular cytoplasm of *E. hartmanni* may contain bacteria. Unlike that of *E. histolytica*, the

TABLE 3-3	*Entamoeba hartmanni* Trophozoite: Typical Characteristics at a Glance
Parameter	**Description**
Size range	5-15 μm
Motility	Nonprogressive, finger-like pseudopods
Number of nuclei	One
Karyosome	Small and central
Peripheral chromatin	Fine and evenly distributed
Cytoplasm	Finely granular
Cytoplasmic inclusions	Ingested bacteria may be present

TABLE 3-4	*Entamoeba hartmanni* Cyst: Typical Characteristics at a Glance
Parameter	**Description**
Size range	5-12 μm
Shape	Spherical
Number of nuclei	One to four
Karyosome	Small and central
Peripheral chromatin	Fine and evenly distributed
Cytoplasm	Finely granular
Cytoplasmic inclusions	Chromatoid bars, rounded ends in young cysts
	Diffuse glycogen mass in young cysts

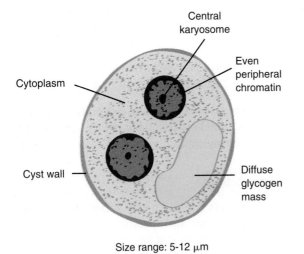

Size range: 5-12 μm
Average size: 7-9 μm

FIGURE 3-8 *Entamoeba hartmanni* cyst.

cytoplasm of *E. hartmanni* does not contain ingested red blood cells.

Cysts. *E. hartmanni* cysts range in size from 5 to 12 μm, with an average size of 7 to 9 μm (Fig. 3-8; Table 3-4). The spherical cysts may have one, two, three, or four nuclei. Nuclei located in the *E. hartmanni* cysts are characteristically smaller in size than the single nucleus of its corresponding trophozoite. The typical nuclear structures of fine and even peripheral chromatin surrounding a small central karyosome, as well as their variations, are consistent with those of *E. histolytica*. The cysts of *E. hartmanni* develop just as those of *E. histolytica*. A diffuse glycogen mass and round-ended chromatoid bars, similar to those seen in *E. histolytica*, are typically seen in a finely granular cytoplasm and are considered characteristic of young cysts.

Laboratory Diagnosis

Laboratory diagnosis is accomplished by examining stool for *E. hartmanni* trophozoites and cysts. It is important to note that the size ranges of *E. histolytica* and *E. hartmanni* overlap. For example, trophozoites that measure 12 μm and cysts that measure 10 μm are within the size range of both parasites. Specific identification based only on size in such cases is impossible. The protocol for reporting such findings varies by laboratory. Proper use of the ocular micrometer (see Chapter 2) is therefore essential to obtain correct measurements of suspected organisms.

Epidemiology

The geographic distribution of *E. hartmanni* is cosmopolitan. The prevalence of *E. hartmanni* appears to be similar to that of *E. histolytica* in areas in which specific and accurate diagnoses have been made. The ingestion of infected cysts present in contaminated food or water accounts for the transmission of *E. hartmanni*. The means whereby food and water become contaminated are similar to those of *E. histolytica*.

Clinical Symptoms

Infections with *E. hartmanni* are typically asymptomatic.

Treatment

Although some questions exist regarding the **pathogenicity** (the ability to produces infectious disease) of *E. hartmanni*, it is generally considered a nonpathogen and treatment is usually not indicated.

Prevention and Control

Good sanitation and personal hygiene practices, as well as protection of food from flies and cockroaches, will help prevent the spread of *E. hartmanni*.

Notes of Interest and New Trends

Entamoeba hartmanni was at one time designated as "small race" *E. histolytica* because of the many similarities between the two organisms.

Serologic differences between *E. hartmanni* and *E. histolytica* have been described.

Quick Quiz! 3-9

A main difference between the trophozoites of *E. hartmanni* and *E. histolytica* is which of the following? (Objective 3-11A)
A. Trophozoites of *E. histolytica* are smaller in size.
B. Presence of pseudopods
C. Trophozoites of *E. hartmanni* do not contain ingested red blood cells.
D. Nuclear structure and peripheral chromatin

Quick Quiz! 3-10

Which of the following is true regarding *E. hartmanni*? (Objectives 3-2, 3-4, 3-5, and 3-7)
A. The organism is found worldwide.
B. It is generally considered a pathogen and treatment is indicated.
C. It is an extraintestinal ameba.
D. The life cycle requires one morphologic form, the trophozoite.

Entamoeba coli
(en'tuh-mee'buh/ko'lye)

Common associated disease or condition names: Intestinal amebiasis, amebic colitis, amebic dysentery, extraintestinal amebiasis.

Morphology

Trophozoites. The trophozoites of *Entamoeba coli* typically measure between 18 and 27 μm (Figs. 3-9 and 3-10; Table 3-5). Some trophozoites may be as small as 12 μm, whereas others may be as large as 55 μm. The trophozoite is equipped with blunt pseudopods and exhibits sluggish, nonprogressive motility. The single

TABLE 3-5	*Entamoeba coli* Trophozoite: Typical Characteristics at a Glance
Parameter	**Description**
Size range	12-55 μm
Motility	Nonprogressive, blunt pseudopods
Number of nuclei	One
Karyosome	Large, irregular shape, eccentric
Peripheral chromatin	Unevenly distributed
Cytoplasm	Coarse and granulated
Cytoplasmic inclusions	Vacuoles containing bacteria often visible

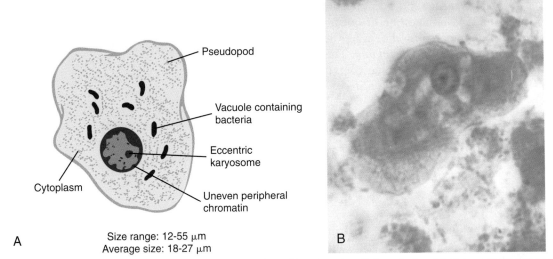

FIGURE 3-9 **A,** *Entamoeba coli* trophozoite. **B,** *Entamoeba coli* trophozoite. (**B** *from Forbes BA, Sahm DF, Weissfeld AS: Bailey & Scott's diagnostic microbiology, ed 12, St Louis, 2007, Mosby.*)

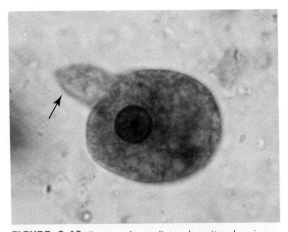

FIGURE 3-10 *Entamoeba coli* trophozoite showing a prominent pseudopod *(arrow).* Note irregular nuclear perimeter and atypical central karyosome (iron hematoxylin stain, ×1000). *(Courtesy of WARD'S Natural Science Establishment, Rochester, NY; http://wardsci.com.)*

nucleus is easily recognizable. In unstained preparations, the karyosome and surrounding peripheral chromatin appear as refractile structures. The nuclear structures are enhanced when the trophozoites are stained. The typical nucleus consists of a large, often irregularly shaped karyosome that is eccentrically located. The karyosome is surrounded by unevenly distributed peripheral chromatin that varies in size and becomes apparent with addition of stain. In some cases, chromatin granules may be visible in the area between the karyosome and peripheral chromatin. Nuclear variations similar to those of *E. histolytica* and *E. hartmanni* may also occur in the trophozoites of *E. coli.* Vacuoles, often containing bacteria, are commonly seen in the coarsely granulated cytoplasm. In contrast to *E. histolytica,* red blood cell inclusions are not present in the trophozoites of *E. coli.*

Cysts. The cysts of *E. coli* vary in size from 8 to 35 μm and average 12 to 25 μm (Fig. 3-11; Table 3-6). A thick cell wall surrounds the round to spherical cyst. As with the trophozoite, the cyst nuclei are readily discernible. One to eight nuclei with the typical nuclear features may be seen in unstained as well as stained preparations. Occasionally, large cysts containing 16 or more nuclei may be present. The granular cytoplasm of young cysts may contain a glycogen mass. On occasion, the glycogen mass may displace the

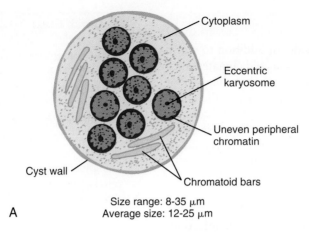

A
Size range: 8-35 μm
Average size: 12-25 μm

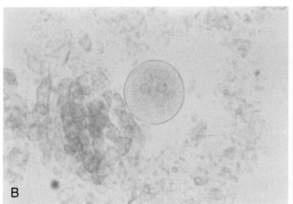

B

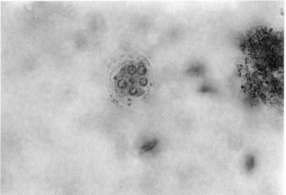

FIGURE 3-11 A, *Entamoeba coli* cyst. **B,** *Entamoeba coli* cyst with five nuclei visible (trichome stain, ×). (**B** from *Mahon CR, Lehman DC, Manuselis G: Textbook of diagnostic microbiology, ed 4, St Louis, 2011, Saunders.*)

TABLE 3-6	*Entamoeba coli* Cyst: Typical Characteristics at a Glance
Parameter	**Description**
Size range	8-35 μm
Shape	Round to spherical
Number of nuclei	One to eight
Karyosome	Large, irregular shape, eccentric
Peripheral chromatin	Unevenly distributed
Cytoplasm	Coarse and granulated
Cytoplasmic inclusions	Diffuse glycogen mass present in young cysts; may displace nuclei (often seen in cysts with two nuclei) to opposite ends of the cyst Thin chromatoid bars with pointed to splintered ends in young cysts

nuclei present to opposite ends of the cyst, a variation often seen in cysts with two nuclei present. Thin chromatoid bars, often with pointed to splintered ends, may also be contained in the cytoplasm of young cysts.

Laboratory Diagnosis

Stool examination is the method of choice for the recovery of *E. coli* trophozoites and cysts. Although not considered as being pathogenic, the presence of *E. coli* suggests ingestion of contaminated food or drink. Laboratory technicians should therefore examine these preparations carefully for the presence of pathogenic parasites in addition to the nonpathogenic *E. coli*.

Epidemiology

E. coli is found worldwide. In addition to warm climates, *E. coli* also occurs in cold climates, such as Alaska. Geographic areas that have poor hygiene and sanitation practices are at the greatest risk of becoming endemic with *E. coli*. As with the other intestinal amebas, *E. coli* is transmitted through the ingestion of the infected cyst through contaminated food or drink.

Clinical Symptoms

As with infections of *E. hartmanni*, infections with *E. coli* are usually asymptomatic.

Treatment

E. coli is considered a nonpathogen. Treatment, therefore, is usually not indicated.

Prevention and Control

The adequate disposal of human feces, as well as proper personal hygiene practices, is crucial for preventing *E. coli* infections. Protection of food and drink from flies and cockroaches is also necessary to break the *E. coli* transmission cycle.

Notes of Interest and New Trends

The morphologic differentiation of *E. coli* from *E. histolytica*, as well as the pathogenicity of each of these parasites, was not established until the early 1900s.

> ### Quick Quiz! 3-11
>
> The trophozoites of *E. coli*: (Objective 3-9A)
> A. Have eight nuclei
> B. Have a typical nucleus consists of a large, often irregularly shaped karyosome that is eccentrically located
> C. Are characterized by a karyosome that is surrounded by evenly distributed peripheral chromatin
> D. Contain red blood cell inclusions

> ### Quick Quiz! 3-12
>
> Which of the following is not true about *E. coli*? (Objectives 3-2, 3-5, and 3-7C)
> A. The parasite is found worldwide.
> B. It is considered to be a pathogen.
> C. The infection is transmitted through the ingestion of the infected cyst through contaminated food or drink.
> D. The infection can be prevented by adequate disposal of human feces and good personal hygiene practices.

Entamoeba polecki
(en'tuh-mee'buh/poh-lek'ee)

Common associated disease or condition names: None (considered as a nonpathogen).

Morphology

 Trophozoites. The average *Entamoeba polecki* trophozoite measures 12 to 20 μm (Fig. 3-12; Table 3-7). The trophozoites may vary in size, however, ranging from 8 to 25 μm. Sluggish, nonprogressive motility is observed in stools of normal consistency containing *E. polecki* trophozoites. In diarrheal stools, *E. polecki* trophozoites exhibit progressive, unidirectional motility,

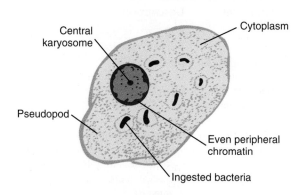

Size range: 8-25 μm
Average size: 12-20 μm

FIGURE 3-12 *Entamoeba polecki* trophozoite.

TABLE 3-7	Entamoeba polecki Trophozoite: Typical Characteristics at a Glance
Parameter	**Description**
Size range	8-25 µm
Motility normal stools	Sluggish, nonprogressive
Motility diarrheal stools	Progressive, unidirectional
Number of nuclei	One
Karyosome	Small and central
Peripheral chromatin	Fine and evenly distributed
Cytoplasm	Granular and vacuolated
Cytoplasmic inclusions	Ingested bacteria Other food particles

TABLE 3-8	Entamoeba polecki Cyst: Typical Characteristics at a Glance
Parameter	**Description**
Size range	10-20 µm
Shape	Spherical or oval
Number of nuclei	One
Karyosome	Small and central
Peripheral chromatin	Fine and evenly distributed
Cytoplasm	Granular
Cytoplasmic inclusions	Chromatoid bars , angular or pointed ends in young cysts Glycogen mass in young cysts Inclusion mass

similar to that of *E. histolytica*. The single nucleus may be slightly visible in unstained preparations. The nuclear structures have features resembling both *E. histolytica* and *E. coli*. The small central karyosome resembles that of *E. histolytica*. The peripheral chromatin may take several forms, some resembling that of *E. coli*. The presence of fine and evenly distributed peripheral chromatin is the most common form seen. Fine granules interspersed with large granules evenly distributed, as well as clumped chromatin at one or both edges of the nuclear membrane, may occur. The granular and vacuolated cytoplasm resembles that of *E. coli*, often containing ingested yeast, bacteria, or other food particles.

◾ **Cysts.** Although the cysts of *E. polecki* range in size from 10 to 20 µm, the average is 12 to 18 µm (Fig. 3-13; Table 3-8). The cysts vary in shape from spherical to oval. Unlike the typical cysts of the other *Entamoeba* discussed, *E. polecki* cysts only contain one nucleus. The typical nucleus consists of a small central karyosome surrounded by fine and evenly distributed peripheral chromatin, just as those of *E. histolytica*. Thin chromatoid bars with pointed or angular ends are often present in the granular cytoplasm of young cysts. Irregularly shaped chromatoid bars may also be seen. A diffuse glycogen mass may be present in the cytoplasm of young cysts. A nondescript oval or round inclusion mass is seen in approximately 50% of

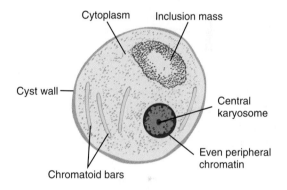

Size range: 10-20 µm
Average size: 12-18 µm

FIGURE 3-13 *Entamoeba polecki* cyst.

the cysts studied. This non–glycogen-containing structure appears elusive and does not have defined borders. The makeup of the inclusion mass is not known.

Laboratory Diagnosis

The trophozoites and cysts of *E. polecki* may be diagnosed by examining stool samples.

Epidemiology

E. polecki has for a number of years been primarily considered a parasite of pigs and monkeys.

Human infections are relatively rare. This ameba is found only in select areas of the world, with the highest prevalence occurring in Papua, New Guinea. Infections with *E. polecki* have also been reported in Southeast Asia, France, and the United States. It is interesting to note that all the reported cases of *E. polecki* documented in the United States in 1985 occurred in Southeast Asian refugees who settled in Rochester, Minnesota. Ingestion of the *E. polecki* cyst is most likely responsible for the onset of infection. Human to human as well as pig to human are the major routes of parasite transmission.

Clinical Symptoms

Most patients with *E. polecki* are asymptomatic. The only documented discomfort associated with symptomatic patients is diarrhea.

Treatment

A combination of metronidazole (Flagyl) and diloxanide furoate (Furamide) has successfully treated patients with *E. polecki*. Metronidazole alone has also been effective.

Prevention and Control

E. polecki may be prevented by improving personal hygiene and sanitation practices. Education programs regarding the routes of transmitting *E. polecki* infection are also essential.

 Quick Quiz! 3-13

Which of the following statements is not true about the cysts of *E. polecki*? (Objective 3-9A)
A. Cysts vary in shape from spherical to oval.
B. Cysts contain at least four nuclei.
C. The typical cyst nucleus resembles that of *E. histolytica*.
D. A diffuse glycogen mass may be present in the cytoplasm of cysts.

 Quick Quiz! 3-14

Infection with *E. polecki* is mainly transmitted to humans via which of the following? (Objective 3-5A)
A. Ingestion of *E. polecki* trophozoite
B. Ingestion of *E. polecki* cysts
C. Humans do not get infected with *E. polecki*.
D. Touching an injected pig or monkey

Endolimax nana
(en'doe-lye'macks/nay'nuh)

Common associated disease or condition names: None (considered as a nonpathogen).

Morphology

Trophozoites. *Endolimax nana* trophozoites vary in size from 5 to 12 μm (Fig. 3-14; Table 3-9). The average trophozoite size range is 7 to 10 μm. *E. nana* trophozoites exhibit sluggish, nonprogressive motility, which is accomplished by blunt, hyaline pseudopods. The single nucleus may or may not be visible in unstained preparations. The karyosome is typically large and irregularly shaped, and is often described as blotlike in appearance. The absence of peripheral chromatin is a key feature that aids in the identification of *E. nana* trophozoites. The cytoplasm of

TABLE 3-9	*Endolimax nana* Trophozoite: Typical Characteristics at a Glance
Parameter	**Description**
Size range	5-12 μm
Motility	Sluggish, nonprogressive, blunt pseudopods
Number of nuclei	One
Karyosome	Large, irregular, blotlike
Peripheral chromatin	Absent
Cytoplasm	Granular and vacuolated
Cytoplasmic inclusion	Bacteria

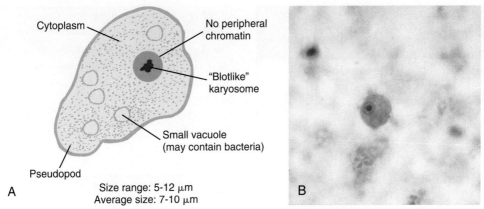

FIGURE 3-14 **A,** *Endolimax nana* trophozoite. **B,** *Endolimax nana* trophozoite. (**B** *from Forbes BA, Sahm DF, Weissfeld AS: Bailey & Scott's diagnostic microbiology, ed 12, St Louis, 2007, Mosby.)*

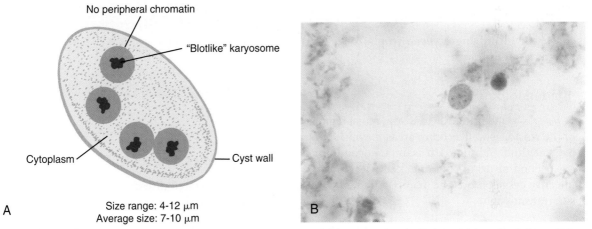

FIGURE 3-15 **A,** *Endolimax nana* cyst. **B,** *Endolimax nana* cyst (trichrome stain, ×). (**B** *from Mahon CR, Lehman DC, Manuselis G: Textbook of diagnostic microbiology, ed 4, St Louis, 2011, Saunders.)*

these trophozoites is granular and vacuolated, and usually contains bacteria.

◗ **Cysts.** The spherical, ovoid, or ellipsoid cysts of *E. nana* typically measure 7 to 10 μm in size (Fig. 3-15; Table 3-10). Some cysts may measure a mere 4 μm, whereas others may be as large as 12 μm. Although there may be one to four nuclei in an *E. nana* cyst, the most commonly seen form is the mature cyst that contains four nuclei. The structures of these cyst nuclei are basically identical to those seen in the trophozoite—a large blotlike karyosome, usually centrally located, and

the absence of peripheral chromatin. The cytoplasm of *E. nana* cysts may contain granules of chromatin material or nondescript small oval masses. Chromatoid bars, such as those often seen in the *Entamoeba* spp. cysts, are not present. A diffuse glycogen mass may be present in young cysts.

Laboratory Diagnosis

As with other intestinal amebas discussed in this chapter, the laboratory diagnostic technique of

TABLE 3-10	*Endolimax nana* Cyst: Typical Characteristics at a Glance
Parameter	**Description**
Size range	4-12 μm
Shape	Spherical, ovoid, ellipsoid
Number of nuclei	One to four; four most common
Karyosome	Large, blotlike, usually central
Peripheral chromatin	Absent
Cytoplasm	Granular and vacuolated
Cytoplasmic inclusions	Chromatin granules Nondescript small mass Diffuse glycogen mass in young cysts

choice for identifying *E. nana* trophozoites and cysts is stool examination.

Epidemiology

E. nana is found primarily in warm, moist regions of the world, as well as other areas in which poor hygiene and substandard sanitary conditions exist. Food or drink contaminated with *E. nana* infective cysts serve as the major sources of parasite transmission.

Clinical Symptoms

E. nana infections are usually asymptomatic.

Treatment

E. nana is considered a nonpathogen. Treatment is generally not indicated.

Prevention and Control

As with other intestinal amebas, protection of food and drink from flies and cockroaches is essential to halt the spread of *E. nana* infections. In addition, good sanitation and personal hygiene practices are also crucial preventive measures.

Quick Quiz! 3-15

The appearance of an *E. nana* karyosome is usually which of the following? (Objective 3-9A)
A. Granular
B. Large and round
C. Small and round
D. Blotlike

Quick Quiz! 3-16

Which of the following statements is true regarding *E. nana*? (Objectives 3-2 and 3-7)
A. *E. nana* is found primarily in cold regions of the world.
B. *E. nana* is prevalent in areas in which poor hygiene and substandard sanitary conditions exist.
C. *E. nana* is considered as a human pathogen, so treatment is mandatory.
D. Humans can obtain protection from *E. nana* via vaccination.

Iodamoeba bütschlii
(eye-o'doh-mee'buh/bootch'lee-eye)

Common associated disease or condition names: None (considered as a nonpathogen).

Morphology

Trophozoites. The trophozoites of *Iodamoeba bütschlii* average 12 to 18 μm but may vary from 8 to 22 μm in size (Fig. 3-16; Table 3-11). These trophozoites characteristically exhibit progressive, sluggish motility. The single nucleus consists of a large, usually central karyosome surrounded by refractive achromatic granules, which are often not distinct, even when the trophozoite is permanently stained. Peripheral chromatin is absent. The coarsely granular and vacuolated cytoplasm may contain bacteria, yeast cells, or other debris.

Cysts. *I. bütschlii* cysts typically measure 8 to 12 μm in size. Some cysts may be as small as

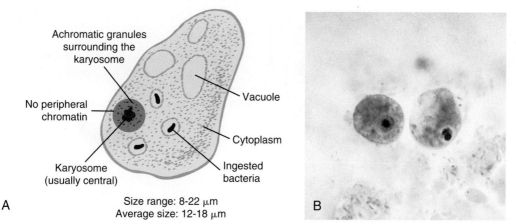

FIGURE 3-16 **A,** *Iodamoeba bütschlii* trophozoite. **B,** *Iodamoeba bütschlii* trophozoites. (**B** *from Forbes BA, Sahm DF, Weissfeld AS: Bailey & Scott's diagnostic microbiology, ed 12, St Louis, 2007, Mosby.*)

TABLE 3-11	*Iodamoeba bütschlii* Trophozoite: Typical Characteristics at a Glance
Parameter	**Description**
Size range	8-22 μm
Motility	Sluggish, usually progressive
Number of nuclei	One
Karyosome	Large, usually central refractive achromatic granules may or may not be present
Peripheral chromatin	Absent
Cytoplasm	Coarsely granular and vacuolated
Cytoplasmic inclusions	Bacteria Yeast cells Other debris

TABLE 3-12	*Iodamoeba bütschlii* Cyst: Typical Characteristics at a Glance
Parameter	**Description**
Size range	5-22 μm
Shape	Ovoid, ellipsoid, triangular, other shapes
Number of nuclei	One
Karyosome	Large, eccentric achromatic granules on one side may be present
Peripheral chromatin	Absent
Cytoplasm	Coarsely granular and vacuolated
Cytoplasmic inclusions	Well-defined glycogen mass Granules may be present

5 μm, whereas others may be as large as 22 μm in size (Fig. 3-17; Table 3-12). *I. bütschlii* cysts vary in shape. Ovoid, ellipsoid, triangular, or other shapes of these cysts may be seen. Just like those of the corresponding trophozoite, *I. bütschlii* cysts contain one nucleus. The large karyosome is typically seen in an eccentric position. Achromatic granules, indistinct in iodine preparations, may be seen on one side of the karyosome. Granules may occasionally be present in the coarsely granulated and vacuolated cytoplasm. Chromatoid bars are absent. A well-defined glycogen mass with definite borders is characteristic and is considered as an important diagnostic feature of the *I. bütschlii* cyst.

Laboratory Diagnosis

The examination of stool samples for the trophozoites and cysts of *I. bütschlii* is the method of

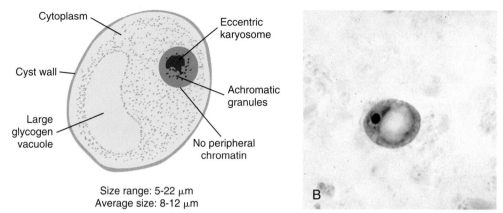

FIGURE 3-17 A, *Iodamoeba bütschlii* cyst. **B,** *Iodamoeba bütschlii* cyst. (**B** *from Forbes BA, Sahm DF, Weissfeld AS: Bailey & Scott's diagnostic microbiology, ed 12, St Louis, 2007, Mosby.)*

choice for laboratory diagnosis. Iodine wet preps often prove to be of benefit, particularly in the identification of *I. bütschlii* cysts. The glycogen mass typically picks up the iodine stain and is thus characteristically recognizable. It is important to point out that the glycogen mass remains unstained following trichrome staining, another feature that aids in the identification of *I. bütschlii* cysts.

Epidemiology

I. bütschlii is found worldwide and has a higher prevalence in tropical regions than in temperate regions. The frequency of *I. bütschlii* infection appears to be much less than that of *E. coli* and *E. nana*. Transmission of *I. bütschlii* occurs when the infective cysts are ingested in contaminated food or drink. Hand-to-mouth transmission may also occur.

Clinical Symptoms

I. bütschlii is a nonpathogenic intestinal ameba that usually does not produce clinical symptoms.

Treatment

Because *I. bütschlii* is considered to be a nonpathogen, treatment is usually not indicated.

Prevention and Control

Upgrading the personal hygiene and sanitation practices in substandard areas, particularly in regions of high prevalence, is critical for the prevention of *I. bütschlii* infections.

Notes of Interest and New Trends

The term *Iodamoeba* was coined to describe an ameba that stains well with iodine. Unlike the other intestinal ameba, the nucleus of *I. bütschlii* does not undergo typical division. The nucleus of the *I. bütschlii* cyst is often described as resembling a basket of flowers in shape. Contaminated hog feces have been implicated as the source of some infections with *I. bütschlii*.

Quick Quiz! 3-17

Iodamoeba bütschlii cysts typically: (Objective 3-9A)
A. Contain four nuclei
B. Have a small karyosome in a central position
C. Lack chromatoid bars
D. Lack a glycogen mass

Entamoeba gingivalis
(en'th-mee'buh/jin-ji-va'lis)

Common associated disease or condition names: None (considered as a nonpathogen).

Morphology

▨ **Trophozoites.** The trophozoite of *Entamoeba gingivalis* ranges in size from 8 to 20 μm and morphologically resembles that of *E. histolytica* (Fig. 3-18; Table 3-13). *E. gingivalis* trophozoites characteristically exhibit active motility. The multiple pseudopods vary in their appearance as the trophozoite moves. The pseudopods may appear long when seen at one point in time and short and blunt the next time that they are seen. The single nucleus contains a central karyosome surrounded by peripheral chromatin that is for the most part fine and evenly distributed. Achromatic granules arranged in strands may be visible, extending from the karyosome to the peripheral chromatin ring. A number of inclusions are typically found in the finely granular cytoplasm, including food vacuoles containing phagocytosed and partially digested white blood cells (leukocytes) and epithelial cells of the host, bacteria, and ingested red blood cells, although not as commonly found as in *E. histolytica* trophozoites. It is important to note that *E. gingivalis* is the only ameba that ingests white blood cells. This distinguishing characteristic is helpful when it is necessary to differentiate *E. gingivalis* from *E. histolytica*.

▨ **Cysts.** There is no known cyst stage of *E. gingivalis*.

Laboratory Diagnosis

An accurate diagnosis of *E. gingivalis* trophozoites may best be made by examining mouth scrapings (see Chapter 2), particularly from the gingival area. Material from the tonsillar crypts

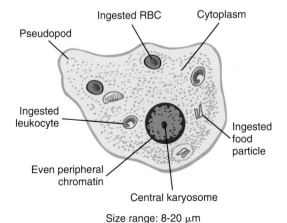

Size range: 8-20 μm

FIGURE 3-18 *Entamoeba gingivalis* trophozoite.

TABLE 3-13	*Entamoeba gingivalis* Trophozoite: Typical Characteristics at a Glance
Parameter	**Description**
Size range	8-20 μm
Motility	Active, varying pseudopod appearance
Number of nuclei	One
Karyosome	Centrally located
Peripheral chromatin	Fine and evenly distributed
Cytoplasm	Finely granular
Cytoplasmic inclusions	Leukocytes Epithelial cells Bacteria

and pulmonary abscess, as well as sputum, may also be examined. Vaginal and cervical material (see Chapter 2) may be examined to diagnose *E. gingivalis* in the vaginal and cervical areas.

Life Cycle Notes

E. gingivalis, as the name implies, typically lives around the gum line of the teeth in the tartar and gingival pockets of unhealthy mouths. In addition, *E. gingivalis* trophozoites have been known to inhabit tonsillar crypts and bronchial mucus. It is particularly important to diagnose *E. gingivalis* and *E. histolytica* correctly because both organisms may be found in the sputum and in pulmonary abscesses. *E. gingivalis* may also be found in the mouths of individuals who practice good oral hygiene. Existing as a scavenger, the *E. gingivalis* trophozoites feed on disintegrated cells and multiply by binary fission. Characteristically delicate, these trophozoites will not survive following contact with stomach juices. *E. gingivalis* trophozoites have also been recovered in vaginal and cervical specimens from women who are using intrauterine devices (IUDs). Spontaneous disappearance of the trophozoites seems to occur following removal of the IUD.

Epidemiology

E. gingivalis is found in all populations that have been studied for its presence. Infections of *E. gingivalis* are contracted via mouth-to-mouth (kissing) and droplet contamination, which may be transmitted through contaminated drinking utensils.

Clinical Symptoms

Infections of *E. gingivalis* occurring in the mouth and in the genital tract typically produce no symptoms. Nonpathogenic *E. gingivalis* trophozoites are frequently recovered in patients suffering from pyorrhea alveolaris. It appears that the trophozoites thrive under disease conditions but do not produce symptoms of their own.

Treatment

Treatment of *E. gingivalis* is typically not indicated because the organism is generally considered a nonpathogen.

Prevention and Control

Improved oral hygiene accomplished by the proper care of the teeth and gums is necessary to prevent the spread of oral *E. gingivalis* infections. Prompt removal of IUDs in infected patients spontaneously removes *E. gingivalis* from the genital tract.

Notes of Interest and New Trends

Discovered in 1849, *E. gingivalis* was the first ameba recovered from a human specimen.

Quick Quiz! 3-19

Which of the following is a unique characteristic of *E. gingivalis*? (Objectives 3-5B, 3-9A, and 3-9C)
A. The trophozoites exhibit active motility via their pseudopods.
B. There is no known cyst form of this parasite.
C. The trophozoite has a single nucleus with characteristics that resemble those of *E. histolytica*.
D. *E. gingivalis* is the only ameba that may ingest white blood cells.

Quick Quiz! 3-20

E. gingivalis: (Objectives 3-4, 3-5, and 3-7)
A. Is an intestinal ameba
B. Is a pathogen and must be treated with metronidazole
C. Can be found in the mouth and in the genital tract
D. Has a typical amebic life cycle (i.e., trophozoites and cysts)

Naegleria fowleri
(nay'gleer-ee'uh/fow-ler'i)

Common associated disease or condition name: Primary amebic meningoencephalitis (PAM).

Morphology

Naegleria fowleri is the only ameba with three known morphologic forms—ameboid trophozoites, **flagellate** (pertains to Protozoa that move by means of flagella) forms, and cysts.

Ameboid trophozoites. The typical ameboid trophozoite of *N. fowleri* appears elongate, measuring from 8 to 22 µm in length (Fig. 3-19; Table 3-14). The anterior end is usually broad, whereas the posterior end is usually tapered. The sluglike motility of the *N. fowleri* ameboid trophozoite is accomplished by blunt pseudopodia. The single nucleus contains a large karyosome that is generally centrally located. Peripheral chromatin is absent. The cytoplasm of the *N. fowleri* ameboid trophozoite is granular and often contains vacuoles.

Flagellate forms. The pear-shaped flagellate form of *N. fowleri* typically measures 7 to 15 µm in size (Fig. 3-20). Two whiplike structures that assist select parasites in locomotion known as **flagella** extend from the broad end of the organism. The typical motility that is seen is accomplished by jerky movements or spinning. The nucleus is basically identical to that of the ameboid trophozoite, a large central karyosome minus peripheral chromatin. The flagellate trophozoites typically have granular cytoplasms that often contain vacuoles.

Cysts. The cysts, measuring from 9 to 12 µm in size, are generally round and have thick cell walls (Fig. 3-21). Similar to both corresponding trophozoite stages, the *N. fowleri* cyst has only one nucleus, consisting of a large, centrally located karyosome lacking peripheral chromatin. The cytoplasm is typically granular and often contains vacuoles.

Laboratory Diagnosis

Microscopic examination of cerebrospinal fluid (CSF) is the method of choice for the recovery

TABLE 3-14	*Naegleria fowleri* Ameboid Trophozoite: Typical Characteristics at a Glance
Parameter	**Description**
Size range	8-22 µm
Motility	Sluglike, blunt pseudopods
Number of nuclei	One
Karyosome	Large and usually centrally located
Peripheral chromatin	Absent
Cytoplasm	Granular, usually vacuolated

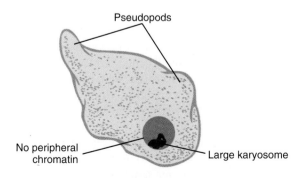

Size range: 8-22 µm

FIGURE 3-19 *Naegleria fowleri* ameboid trophozoite.

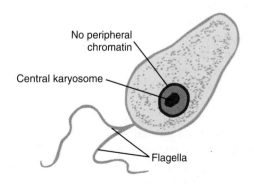

Size range: 7-15 µm

FIGURE 3-20 *Naegleria fowleri* flagellate form.

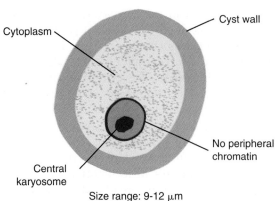

Size range: 9-12 μm

FIGURE 3-21 *Naegleria fowleri* cyst.

of *N. fowleri* ameboid trophozoites (see Chapter 2). Preparing and scanning saline and iodine wet preparations of the CSF are recommended. Samples of tissues and nasal discharge (see Chapter 2) may also be examined. Clinical specimens may be cultured. *N. fowleri* ameboid trophozoites show a characteristic trailing effect when placed on agar plates that have been previously inoculated with gram-negative bacilli.

Life Cycle Notes

The ameboid trophozoites of *N. fowleri* are the only form known to exist in humans. Replication of the ameboid trophozoites occurs by simple binary fission. The ameboid trophozoites transform into flagellate trophozoites in vitro after being transferred to water from a tissue or culture. The flagellate trophozoites do not divide but rather lose their flagella and convert back into the ameboid form, in which reproduction resumes. The cyst form is known to exist only in the external environment.

It appears that the entire life cycle of *N. fowleri*, which consists of the amebic trophozoites converting to cysts and flagellates and then back to amebic trophozoites, occurs in the external environment. Humans primarily contract this ameba by swimming in contaminated water. The ameboid trophozoites enter the human body through the nasal mucosa and often migrate to the brain, causing rapid tissue destruction. Some infections may be caused by inhaling dust infected with *N. fowleri*.

Epidemiology

N. fowleri is primarily found in warm bodies of water, including lakes, streams, ponds, and swimming pools. Prevalence is higher in the summer months of the year. In addition to water sources, there have been cases of contaminated dust. One such case occurred in Nigeria, a country that has a warm climate.

The ameboid trophozoites of *N. fowleri* enter the human body through the nasal mucosa. Inhalation of contaminated dust has accounted for other documented infections. There is also some evidence to suggest that sniffing contaminated water may transmit this ameba.

Clinical Symptoms

▧ **Asymptomatic.** Patients who contract *N. fowleri* resulting in colonization of the nasal passages are usually asymptomatic.

▧ **Primary amebic meningoencephalitis.** Primary amebic meningoencephalitis (PAM) occurs when the ameboid trophozoites of *N. fowleri* invade the brain, causing rapid tissue destruction. Patients may initially complain of fever, headache, sore throat, nausea, and vomiting. Symptoms of meningitis rapidly follow, including stiff neck and seizures. In addition, the patient will often experience smell and taste alterations, blocked nose, and **Kernig's sign** (defined as a diagnostic sign for meningitis, where the patient is unable to fully straighten his or her leg when the hip is flexed at 90 degrees because of hamstring stiffness). In untreated patients, death usually occurs 3 to 6 days after onset. Postmortem brain tissue samples of these patients reveal the typical ameboid trophozoites of *N. fowleri*.

Treatment

Unfortunately, medications used to treat meningitis and amebic infections are ineffective against *N. fowleri*. There is evidence, however, that prompt and aggressive treatment with amphotericin B may be of benefit to patients suffering from infections with *N. fowleri*, despite its known toxicity. In rare cases, amphotericin B in combination with rifampin or miconazole has also proved to be an effective treatment. Amphotericin B and miconazole damage the cell wall of *Naegleria*, inhibiting the biosynthesis of ergosterol and resulting in increased membrane permeability, which causes nutrients to leak out of the cells. Rifampicin inhibits RNA synthesis in the amoeba by binding to beta subunits of DNA-dependent RNA polymerase, which in turn blocks RNA transcription. A person can survive if signs are recognized early but, if not, PAM almost always results in death.

Prevention and Control

Because of the numerous bodies of water that may potentially be infected, total eradication of *N. fowleri* is highly unlikely. Posting off-limits signs around known sources of contamination, as well as educating the medical community and public, may help curb infection rates. It is also important that swimming pools and hot tubs be adequately chlorinated. Cracks found in the walls of pools, hot tubs, and baths should be repaired immediately to prevent the creation of a possible source of contamination.

Notes of Interest and New Trends

The first case of PAM was reported by Carter and Fowleri, for whom the ameba is named, in 1965 in Australia, and by Butt and Patras in 1966 in the United States.

One noteworthy species of *Naegleria* that could possibly infect humans in the future is known as *N. australiensis*. This organism exists in the environment in Asia, Australia, Europe, and United States. *N. australiensis* has been found to be pathogenic in mice that have been exposed to this parasite by intranasal instillation.

A number of methods have been studied in recent years aimed at classifying, identifying and speciating *Naegleria*. These laboratory techniques include PCR assay, monoclonal antibody testing, flow cytometry, and DNA hybridization. In addition, a method designed to aid in taxonomic classification, called DNA restriction fragment length polymorphism (RFLP), has been studied. Results of all of these tests to date have been favorable. Further studies, however, have been recommended.

Quick Quiz! 3-21

The known morphologic forms of *Naegleria fowleri* are: (Objective 3-5B)
A. Ameboid trophozoites, flagellate forms, and cysts
B. Ameboid trophozoites, immature cysts, and mature cysts
C. Eggs, larvae, and adults
D. Flagellate forms, cysts, and larvae

Quick Quiz! 3-22

The specimen of choice for the recovery of *N. fowleri* is which of the following? (Objective 3-8)
A. Sputum
B. Stool
C. Cerebrospinal fluid
D. Urine

Quick Quiz! 3-23

Humans most often contract *N. fowleri* by which of the following? (Objective 3-5B)
A. Swimming in contaminated water
B. Kissing an infected person
C. Practicing unprotected sex
D. Ingestion of contaminated food

Quick Quiz! 3-24

The ameboid trophozoites of *N. fowleri* enter the human body through all of the following routes except: (Objective 3-5B)
A. Entry through the nasal mucosa
B. Inhalation of contaminated dust
C. Sniffing contaminated water
D. Ingesting contaminated food and drink

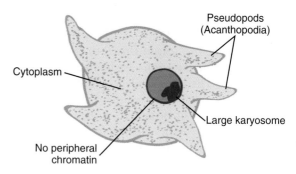

Size range: 12-45 μm
Average size: 25 μm

FIGURE 3-22 *Acanthamoeba* species trophozoite.

Quick Quiz! 3-25

Practical measures for the control and prevention of *N. fowleri* include which of the following? (Objective 3-7C)
A. Banning swimming at all times during the summer months
B. Avoidance of chlorinating swimming pools and hot tubs
C. Providing education and awareness in the medical community
D. Avoidance of consuming contaminated food or water prior to swimming

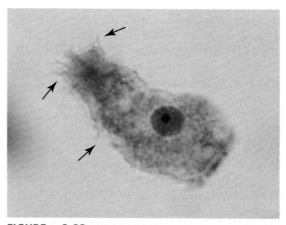

FIGURE 3-23 *Acanthamoeba* species trophozoite showing typical thornlike acanthopodia *(arrows)* (iron hematoxylin stain, ×1000). *(Courtesy of WARD'S Natural Science Establishment, Rochester, NY;* http://wardsci.com.)

Acanthamoeba species
(ay-kanth'uh-mee'buh)

Common associated disease or condition names: Granulomatous amebic encephalitis (GAE), *Acanthamoeba* keratitis

Morphology

▨ **Trophozoites.** The *Acanthamoeba* trophozoite averages 25 μm, with a range of 12 to 45 μm in size (Figs. 3-22 and 3-23; Table 3-15). Motility is sluggish and there is little evidence of progressive motility. Spinelike pseudopods, known as **acanthopodia**, project outward from the base of the organism. *Acanthamoeba* trophozoites contain one nucleus, consisting of a large karyosome similar to that of *N. fowleri*. Obvious

TABLE 3-15	*Acanthamoeba* species Trophozoite: Typical Characteristics at a Glance
Parameter	**Description**
Size range	12-45 μm
Motility	Sluggish, spinelike pseudopods
Number of nuclei	One
Karyosome	Large
Peripheral chromatin	Absent
Cytoplasm	Granular and vacuolated

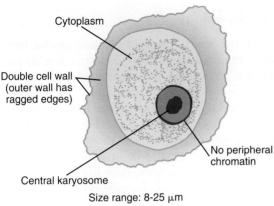

Cytoplasm

Double cell wall
(outer wall has
ragged edges)

No peripheral
chromatin

Central karyosome

Size range: 8-25 μm

FIGURE 3-24 *Acanthamoeba* species cyst.

TABLE 3-16	*Acanthamoeba* species Cyst: Typical Characteristics at a Glance
Parameter	**Description**
Size range	8-25 μm
Shape	Roundish with ragged edges
Number of nuclei	One
Karyosome	Large and central
Peripheral chromatin	Absent
Cytoplasm	Disorganized, granular, sometimes vacuolated
Other features	Double cell wall—smooth inner cell wall and outer jagged cell wall

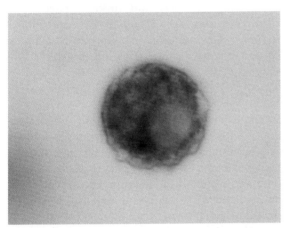

FIGURE 3-25 *Acanthamoeba* species cyst exhibiting a typical disorganized cytoplasm and vacuoles (iron hematoxylin stain, ×1000). *(Courtesy of WARD'S Natural Science Establishment, Rochester, NY; http://wardsci.com.)*

peripheral chromatin is absent. The cytoplasm appears granular and vacuolated.

▶ **Cysts.** The round-shaped *Acanthamoeba* species cyst measures 8 to 25 μm (Figs. 3-24, 3-25; Table 3-16). The cyst is equipped with a double cell wall. The inner smooth cell wall is surrounded by an outer jagged cell wall. This appearance is characteristic and aids in *Acanthamoeba* cyst identification. The single nucleus is similar in appearance to that of the corresponding trophozoite form, a large karyosome and no obvious peripheral chromatin.

A disorganized, granular, and sometimes vacuolated cytoplasm surrounds the nucleus.

Laboratory Diagnosis

As with *N. fowleri*, the specimen of choice for diagnosing *Acanthamoeba* spp. trophozoites and cysts is CSF. Brain tissue may also be examined. Corneal scrapings (see Chapter 2) are the specimen of choice for recovery of *Acanthamoeba* infections of the eye. Suspected corneal scrapings may be cultured on non-nutrient agar plates seeded with gram-negative bacteria (specifically, a viable strain of *E. coli*). The bacteria serve as a source of food for the parasites. As the *Acanthamoeba* organisms feed, they produce a set of marks (known as tracks) on the agar. Histologic examination of corneal scrapings may also recover *Acanthamoeba*. Although primarily used to detect fungi in clinical specimens, calcofluor white may be used to stain *Acanthamoeba* cysts present in corneal scrapings. Indirect immunofluorescent antibody staining (see Chapter 2) is the technique of choice for speciating *Acanthamoeba*.

Life Cycle Notes

The trophozoites and cysts of *Acanthamoeba* convert between these two morphologic forms in the external environment. Humans may acquire

Acanthamoeba in one of two ways. One route consists of aspiration or nasal inhalation of the organisms. Trophozoites and cysts enter via the lower respiratory tract or through ulcers in the mucosa or skin. These organisms often migrate via hematogenous spread—that is, transported through the bloodstream—and invade the central nervous system (CNS), causing serious CNS infections. The second route of infection consists of direct invasion of the parasite in the eye. Two groups of individuals are at risk for direct eye invasion, contact lens wearers and those who have experienced trauma to the cornea. Contact lens wearers who use homemade, nonsterile saline solutions that are contaminated with *Acanthamoeba* typically suffer a serious eye infection, known as *Acanthamoeba* keratitis. It is important to note that unlike *N. fowleri*, which is associated with swimming or bathing in contaminated water, *Acanthamoeba* spp. infection is not associated with water but rather with contaminated saline.

There are currently 10 species of *Acanthamoeba* known to infect humans. *Acanthamoeba castellanii* has been identified as the species responsible for most CNS and eye infections in humans. The names of these species, as well as the type of infection with which each is associated, are listed in Table 3-17.

TABLE 3-17 *Acanthamoeba* species Identified in Humans

Species Name	Associated with	
	CNS Infection	Eye Infection
A. astronyxis	X	
A. castellanii	X	X
A. culbertsoni	X	X
A. divionensis	X	
A. griffini	X	
A. healyi	X	
A. hatchetti		X
A. lugdunensis		X
A. polyphaga		X
A. rhysodes	X	X

Epidemiology

Over the years, cases of *Acanthamoeba* have been reported from many countries worldwide. Both CNS and eye infections of *Acanthamoeba* spp. have been reported in the United States. CNS infections primarily occur in patients who are immunocompromised or debilitated. Contact lens wearers, particularly those wearing soft contacts, may be at risk of contracting *Acanthamoeba* eye infections. Poor hygiene practices, especially the use of homemade saline rinsing solutions, is the major risk factor that may lead to these infections.

Animals, including rabbits, beavers, cattle, water buffalo, dogs, and turkeys, have been known to contract *Acanthamoeba* infections. Just as in humans, immunocompromised animals appear to contract fatal CNS infections.

Clinical Symptoms

Granulomatous amebic encephalitis. CNS infections with *Acanthamoeba* are also known as granulomatous amebic encephalitis (GAE). Symptoms of this condition develop slowly over time and include headaches, seizures, stiff neck, nausea, and vomiting. Granulomatous lesions of the brain are characteristic and may contain both *Acanthamoeba* trophozoites and cysts. On occasion, *Acanthamoeba* spp. invade other areas of the body, including the kidneys, pancreas, prostate, and uterus, and form similar granulomatous lesions.

***Acanthamoeba* keratitis.** *Acanthamoeba* infections of the cornea of the eye are known as amebic keratitis. Common symptoms include severe ocular pain and vision problems. The infected tissue of the cornea may contain *Acanthamoeba* trophozoites and cysts. Perforation of the cornea may result, as well as subsequent loss of vision.

Treatment

Because of the slow progression of GAE, most patients who suffer from it die, not only before an accurate diagnosis may be made, but also before experimental treatments can be administered and studied. There is some evidence to suggest that sulfamethazine might be a suitable treatment. Cases of *Acanthamoeba* keratitis have successfully been treated with several medications that include itraconazole, ketoconazole, miconazole, propamidine isethianate, and rifampin. Of all these agents, propamidine appears to have the best documented success record. The key to successful treatment to eye infections is to begin treatment immediately once the infection has been diagnosed.

Prevention and Control

Strategies designed to keep individuals from contracting *Acanthamoeba* CNS infections are difficult to determine because the life cycle of this ameba is poorly understood. However, eye infections with *Acanthamoeba* may be prevented primarily by following all manufacturer-established protocols associated with the use of contact lenses. One of the most important protocols for contact lens wearers is to avoid using homemade nonsterile saline solutions.

Notes of Interest and New Trends

Acanthamoeba shares many characteristics with the gram-negative bacteria *Pseudomonas aeruginosa*, which frequently occurs in standing water as an eye pathogen, but they are usually not recovered simultaneously from the same patient. It is believed that *P. aeruginosa* inhibits the activity of *Acanthamoeba* spp.

Acanthamoeba has been rarely known to infect areas of the body other than those typically reported. An interesting case involved cutaneous lesions filled with *Acanthamoeba* trophozoites and cysts on the trunk, legs, and arm of a patient suffering from AIDS. The patient also presented with brain lesions that did not show the *Acanthamoeba* organisms. Another case involved *Acanthamoeba* invasion of bone following a

graft procedure. In this case, the patient subsequently developed osteomyelitis.

Several newer testing methods (see Chapter 2) aimed at differentiating the strains of *Acanthamoeba* have been studied, including monoclonal antibodies and flow cytometry. In addition, DNA RFLP tests have been performed to aid in taxonomic classification of *Acanthamoeba* spp. Although additional testing with all these techniques has been suggested, available tests have shown promising results.

Quick Quiz! 3-26

The term *acanthopodia* refers to: (Objective 1)
A. Spinelike pseudopods
B. Hairy projections
C. Double-layer cell wall
D. Large karyosome and no obvious peripheral chromatin

Quick Quiz! 3-27

The specimen of choice for diagnosing *Acanthamoeba* species trophozoites and cysts is which of the following? (Objective 3-8)
A. Urine
B. Sputum
C. Cerebrospinal fluid
D. Stool

Quick Quiz! 3-28

Humans may acquire *Acanthamoeba* species by which of the following? (Objective 3-5B)
A. Aspiration or nasal inhalation of the organisms
B. Direct invasion of the parasites in the eye
C. Swimming or bathing in contaminated water
D. A or B

Quick Quiz! 3-29

Infections with *Acanthamoeba* species are encountered in which of the following anatomical parts? (Objective 3-5)
A. Eye
B. Large intestines
C. Lungs
D. Liver

Quick Quiz! 3-30

To prevent infection with *Acanthamoeba* species, contact lens wearers should avoid which of the following? (Objective 3-7C)
A. Strenuous exercise
B. Foods with high carbohydrate content
C. Wearing clothing made of cotton
D. Using homemade nonsterile saline solutions

LOOKING BACK

The typical characteristics that differentiate the amebas include size, shape, nuclear structure, cytoplasm appearance, and cytoplasmic inclusions. These characteristics may best be compared in the comparison drawings at the end of this chapter: amebic trophozoites found in stool, amebic cysts found in stool, and extraintestinal amebic trophozoites and cysts.

It is important for clinicians to examine all samples sent to the laboratory for parasitology studies carefully. Suspicious amebic forms must be evaluated closely, looking particularly for the typical amebic characteristics. Composite drawings, such as those provided in this chapter, provide a useful resource and to aid in the identification of and distinction between the amebas.

TEST YOUR KNOWLEDGE!

3-1. Match each of the key terms (column A) with its corresponding definition (column B). (Objective 3-1)

Column A

___ **A.** Ameba

___ **B.** Amebic dysentery

___ **C.** Cyst

___ **D.** Encystation

___ **E.** Excystation

___ **F.** Karyosome

___ **G.** Pseudopod

___ **H.** Trophozoite

Column B

1. Transformation of a trophozoite stage into a cyst stage
2. Transformation of a cyst stage into a trophozoite stage
3. Amebic stage with a thick cell wall allowing for survival of the organism in the external environment
4. A motile class of Protozoa equipped with pseudopods
5. Extension of cytoplasm that aids ameba in motility
6. Amebic stage characterized by its ability to move and multiply
7. Small mass of chromatin located within the nucleus of certain protozoan parasites
8. An intestinal amebic infection characterized by blood and mucus in the stool

3-2. Which of the following statements is not true about amebic trophozoites? (Objective 3-1)
A. Trophozoites are delicate and motile.
B. Trophozoites are easily destroyed by gastric juices.
C. Trophozoites are resistant to the environment outside the host.
D. Replication occurs in the trophozoite stage.

3-3. The ingestion of the infective _____ (cysts, trophozoites) completes the typical intestinal amebic life cycle. (Objectives 3-1 and 3-5A)

3-4. Classify the individual ameba as intestinal or extraintestinal. (Objective 3-4)

Entamoeba histolytica   _____

Entamoeba hartmanni   _____

Entamoeba coli   _____

Entamoeba polecki   _____

Endolimax nana   _____

Iodamoeba bütschlii   _____

Entamoeba gingivalis   _____

Naegleria fowleri   _____

Acanthamoeba species   _____

3-5. Describe the typical life cycle of an intestinal ameba. (Objective 3-5 A)

3-6. Compare the life cycles of *Entamoeba gingivalis* and *Naegleria fowleri*. (Objective 3-5C)

3-7. Amebic dysentery is caused by: (Objective 3-6)
A. *Entamoeba histolytica*
B. *Entamoeba coli*
C. *Entamoeba gingivalis*
D. *Endolimax nana*

3-8. Identify and describe the clinical significance associated with each of the following amebas. (Objective 3-6)
A. *Entamoeba histolytica*
B. *Entamoeba coli*
C. *Naegleria fowleri*
D. *Acanthamoeba* species

3-9. True/False. Treatment for patients with asymptomatic intestinal amebiasis is not recommended. (Objective 3-7)
A. True
B. False

3-10. Primary amebic meningoencephalitis is primarily caused by: (Objective 3-6)
A. *Entamoeba histolytica*
B. *Naegleria fowleri*
C. *Entamoeba gingivalis*
D. *Acanthamoeba* spp.

3-11. Match each ameba (column A) with the corresponding specimen of choice for its recovery (column B). (Objective 3-8)

Column A	Column B
1. *Entamoeba histolytica* ___	**A.** Stool
2. *Entamoeba coli* ___	**B.** Spinal fluid
3. *Endolimax nana* ___	**C.** Mouth scrapings
4. *Entamoeba gingivalis* ___	**D.** Corneal scrapings
5. *Acanthamoeba* spp.	
6. *Naegleria fowleri*	

3-12. Describe the standard laboratory approach for the recovery of amebic organisms. (Objective 3-12)

CASE STUDY 3-2   **UNDER THE MICROSCOPE**

Annie, an 11-year-old white girl, was adopted from a downtown Chicago orphanage and brought home to her new family in rural Illinois. Three weeks later, she began to experience severe diarrhea, fever, malaise, and abdominal cramping. Examination by her pediatrician led him to order a stool for culture and parasite examination (commonly known as an ova and parasite examination [O&P]). The stool arrived in the laboratory and the gross appearance was noted as liquid, with mucus and tinges of blood. It was immediately processed by standard techniques (discussed in detail in Chapter 2). The culture was negative for intestinal pathogens.

The direct and concentrated saline wet preps slide showed suspicious, irregularly shaped forms. The laboratory technician on duty, suspicious but not certain that a parasite was present, decided to hold the report pending further studies. The suspicious form seen in the permanent stain is shown in the diagram. This form measured 13 μm.

Continued

CASE STUDY 3-2   UNDER THE MICROSCOPE—cont'd

Questions for Consideration

1. What classification of parasites you suspect? (Objective 3-10B)
2. State the key differential characteristics that will distinguish the parasites in this group. (Objective 3-10A)
3. Given the gross appearance of this specimen, what morphologic form would you suspect to find? Does the diagram demonstrate that form? (Objective 3-10B)
4. What key structure (other than the nucleus) is seen in the cytoplasm of this organism? (Objectives 3-10A)
5. What organism (genus and species) and morphologic form do you suspect? Substantiate your answer by describing the key differential factors used to reach your conclusion. (Objectives 3-10A, 3-10B)

6. Could this organism be the cause of the symptoms described? (Objectives 3-10C)
7. In this sample, are other morphologic forms of this parasite possible? If so, name the form(s) and their typical characteristics. If not, why not? (Objectives 3-10A, 3-10I)

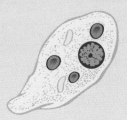

COMPARISON DRAWINGS
Intestinal Amebic Trophozoites Found in Stool

FIGURE 3-2A. *Entamoeba histolytica* trophozoite

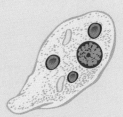

Size range: 8-65 μm
Average size: 12-25 μm

FIGURE 3-7. *Entamoeba hartmanni* trophozoite

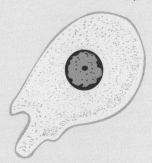

Size range: 5-15 μm
Average size: 8-12 μm

FIGURE 3-9A. *Entamoeba coli* trophozoite

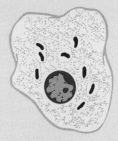

Size range: 12-55 μm
Average size: 18-27 μm

FIGURE 3-12. *Entamoeba polecki* trophozoite

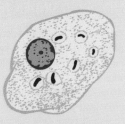

Size range: 8-25 μm
Average size: 12-20 μm

COMPARISON DRAWINGS
Intestinal Amebic Trophozoites Found in Stool—cont'd

FIGURE 3-14A. *Endolimax nana* trophozoite

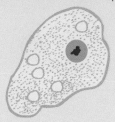

Size range: 5-12 μm
Average size: 7-10 μm

FIGURE 3-16A. *Iodamoeba bütschlii* trophozoite

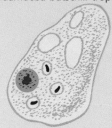

Size range: 8-22 μm
Average size: 12-18 μm

COMPARISON DRAWINGS
Intestinal Amebic Cysts Found in Stool

FIGURE 3-5A. *Entamoeba histolytica* cyst

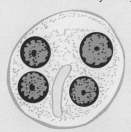

Size range: 8-22 μm
Average size: 12-18 μm

FIGURE 3-8. *Entamoeba hartmanni* cyst

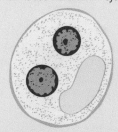

Size range: 5-12 μm
Average size: 7-9 μm

FIGURE 3-11A. *Entamoeba coli* cyst

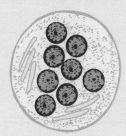

Size range: 8-35 μm
Average size: 12-25 μm

FIGURE 3-13. *Entamoeba polecki* cyst

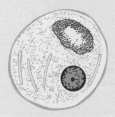

Size range: 10-20 μm
Average size: 12-18 μm

Continued

COMPARISON DRAWINGS
Intestinal Amebic Cysts Found in Stool—cont'd

FIGURE 3-15A. *Endolimax nana* cyst

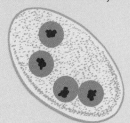

Size range: 4-12 μm
Average size: 7-10 μm

FIGURE 3-17A. *Iodamoeba bütschlii* cyst

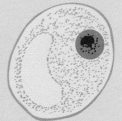

Size range: 5-22 μm
Average size: 8-12 μm

COMPARISON DRAWINGS
Extraintestinal Amebas: Trophozoites and Cysts

FIGURE 3-18. *Entamoeba gingivalis* trophozoite

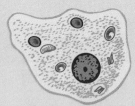

Size range: 8-20 μm

FIGURE 3-19. *Naegleria fowleri* ameboid trophozoite

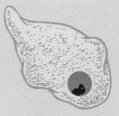

Size range: 8-22 μm

FIGURE 3-22. *Acanthamoeba* spp. trophozoite

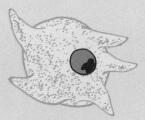

Size range: 12-45 μm
Average size: 25 μm

FIGURE 3-24. *Acanthamoeba* spp. cyst

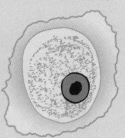

Size range: 8-25 μm

The Flagellates

Linda Graeter and Elizabeth Zeibig

WHAT'S AHEAD

Focusing In
Morphology and Life Cycle
  Notes
Laboratory Diagnosis
Pathogenesis and Clinical
  Symptoms

Flagellate Classification
  Giardia intestinalis
  Chilomastix mesnili
  Dientamoeba fragilis
  Trichomonas hominis
  Enteromonas hominis

Retortamonas intestinalis
Trichomonas tenax
Trichomonas vaginalis
Looking Back

LEARNING OBJECTIVES

On completion of this chapter and review of its figures and corresponding photomicrographs, the successful learner will be able to:

4-1. Define the following key terms:
  Axoneme (*pl.*, axonemes)
  Axostyle
  Costa
  Cytosome
  Flagellum (*pl.*, flagella)
  Flagellate (*pl.*, flagellates)
  Median body (*pl.*, median bodies)
  Undulating membrane

4-2. State the geographic distribution of the flagellates.

4-3. Given a list of parasites, select those organisms belonging to the protozoan group flagellates, subphylum Mastigophora.

4-4. Classify the individual flagellates as intestinal or extraintestinal.

4-5. Construct, describe, and compare and contrast the following life cycles:
  A. General intestinal flagellates
  B. General atrial flagellates
  C. Each specific flagellate

4-6. Briefly identify and describe the populations prone to contracting clinically significant disease processes and clinical signs and symptoms associated with each pathogenic flagellate.

4-7. Identify and describe each of the following as they relate to the flagellates:
  A. Factors responsible for the asymptomatic carrier state of an infected patient
  B. Treatment options
  C. Prevention and control measures

4-8. Determine the specimen of choice, alternative specimen type where appropriate, collection protocol, and laboratory diagnostic technique required for recovery of each of the flagellates.

4-9. Given the name, description, photomicrograph, and/or diagram of a flagellate:
  A. Identify, describe, and/or label its characteristic structures, when appropriate.
  B. State the purpose of the designated characteristic structure(s).
  C. Name the parasite, including its morphologic form.

4-10. Analyze case studies that include pertinent patient information and laboratory data and:

A. Identify and describe the function of key differential characteristic structures.

B. Identify each responsible flagellate organism by category, scientific name, common name, and morphologic form, with justification when indicated.

C. Identify the associated symptoms, diseases, and conditions associated with the responsible parasite.

D. Construct a life cycle associated with each flagellate parasite present that includes corresponding epidemiology, route of transmission, infective stage, and diagnostic stage(s).

E. Propose each of the following related to controlling and preventing flagellate infections:
   1. Treatment options
   2. Prevention and control plan

F. Determine the specimen of choice and alternative specimen types, where appropriate, as well as appropriate laboratory diagnostic technique for the recovery of each flagellate.

G. Recognize sources of error, including but not limited to, those involved in specimen collection, processing, and testing and propose solutions to remedy them.

H. Interpret laboratory data, determine specific follow-up tests to be done, and predict the results of those tests.

I. Determine additional morphologic forms, when appropriate, that may also be detected in clinical specimens.

4-11. Compare and contrast the similarities and differences between:
   A. The flagellates covered in this chapter
   B. The flagellates covered in this chapter and the other parasites covered in this text

4-12. Describe the standard, immunologic, and new laboratory diagnostic approaches for the recovery of flagellates in clinical specimens.

4-13. Given prepared laboratory specimens, and with the assistance of this manual, the learner will be able to:
   A. Differentiate flagellate parasites from artifacts.
   B. Differentiate the flagellate organisms from each other and from the other appropriate categories of parasites.
   C. Correctly identify each flagellate parasite by scientific and common names and morphologic form, based on its key characteristic structure(s).

CASE STUDY 4-1 | **UNDER THE MICROSCOPE**

A 30-year-old man, Bryan, visited his physician complaining of cramping, frequent diarrhea, and weight loss. Patient history revealed that Bryan was a frequent back country hiker and camper who did not always filter his drinking water while on his camping trips. The physician on duty ordered a series of stool samples for ova and parasite (O&P) examination.

Questions for Consideration
1. Indicate how Bryan might have come into contact with parasites and identify the factors that likely contributed to this contact. (Objective 4-10D)
2. Name two other symptoms associated with parasitic infections that people like Bryan may experience. (Objective 4-10C)
3. How should the physician order the O&P analysis in terms of frequency of specimen collection? (Objective 4-10F)

FOCUSING IN

Flagellates belong to the phylum Protozoa and are members of the subphylum Mastigophora. The flagellates can be categorized into two groups, intestinal and atrial. This chapter describes the morphologic features, laboratory diagnosis, life cycle, epidemiology, clinical symptoms, treatment, and prevention and control of eight members of the flagellates, each of which is known to infect humans.

MORPHOLOGY AND LIFE CYCLE NOTES

Movement of the **flagellates** is accomplished by the presence of whiplike structures known as **flagella** in their trophozoite form. It is this characteristic that distinguishes flagellates from the other groups of protozoans. All flagellate life cycles consist of the trophozoite form. Cysts, on the other hand, are not known to exist in several of the flagellate life cycles discussed in this chapter. The morphologic forms of each flagellate life cycle are noted individually for each organism.

The general characteristics of the flagellate trophozoites are similar to those of the amebic trophozoites, with one major exception. In those flagellate life cycles with no known cyst stage, the trophozoite is considered to be more resistant to destructive forces, surviving passage into the stomach following ingestion. In addition, these trophozoites also appear to survive in the outside environment. As with the amebas, nuclear characteristics of trophozoites are basically identical to those of their corresponding cysts.

In flagellate life cycles that consist of both the trophozoite and cyst, the processes of encystation and excystation occur, similar to those of the amebas. Unlike the amebas, however, flagellates reside mainly in the small intestine, cecum, colon and, in the case of *Giardia intestinalis,* the duodenum. The flagellate cysts, like those of the amebas, are equipped with thick, protective cell walls. These cysts may survive in the outside environment, just like those of the amebas.

The typical intestinal flagellate life cycle is similar in process to that of the typical amebas and thus does not appear under the discussion of each individual parasite. Only notes of interest and importance are noted, when appropriate. As with the amebas, the life cycles of the atrial flagellates differ from those of the intestinal flagellates. The atrial flagellate life cycles are, therefore, discussed on an individual basis in this chapter.

LABORATORY DIAGNOSIS

Stools submitted for parasite study that contain flagellates may reveal trophozoites and/or cysts. Like the amebas, flagellate trophozoites are typically seen in loose, liquid, or soft stool specimens, whereas flagellate cysts are more common in formed stools. The morphologic forms seen in specimens other than stool vary and are discussed on an individual basis. As in the case of the amebas, the presence of either or both flagellate morphologic forms is diagnostic.

Nuclear characteristics, such as number of nuclei present and the presence and positioning of the nuclear structures, are helpful in differentiating the flagellates. Proper identification of structures specific to select flagellates, such as a finlike structure connected to the outer edge of some flagellates known as an **undulating membrane** and **axostyle** (a rodlike support structure found in some flagellates), is often even more crucial in determining proper parasite identification. It is important to note that although the flagellate trophozoites technically possess flagella, these structures are not always visible, thus making the other visible flagellate structures important identifying features.

The use of saline and iodine wet preparations, as well as permanent stains, results in the same benefits in flagellate identification as those described for the amebas. Again, it should be noted that the permanent smear procedure may shrink flagellate parasites, resulting in smaller than typical measurements. Representative laboratory diagnostic methodologies are provided in Chapter 2, as well as in individual parasite discussions, as appropriate.

> ### Quick Quiz! 4-1
>
> All flagellate life cycles possess trophozoite and cyst morphologic forms. (Objectives 4-5A and 4-5B)
> A. True
> B. False

> ### Quick Quiz! 4-2
>
> This flagellate morphologic structure is often not visible under microscopic examination. (Objective 4-9A)
> A. Undulating membrane
> B. Pseudopods
> C. Flagella
> D. Axostyle

PATHOGENESIS AND CLINICAL SYMPTOMS

There are many similarities in terms of pathogenesis and clinical symptoms between flagellates and amebas. Although this section is written specifically about flagellates, the information covered pertains to both groups of parasites.

Flagellates are often recovered from patients suffering from diarrhea without an apparent cause. In addition, there are a number of asymptomatic flagellate infections. It is important to identify the nonpathogenic flagellates because this finding suggests the ingestion of contaminated food or drink. Pathogenic flagellates have transmission routes similar to those of the nonpathogenic variety. Careful examination of all samples, especially those containing nonpathogenic flagellates, is essential to proper identification of all possible parasites present.

It is important to note that there is only one intestinal flagellate, *G. intestinalis*, that is considered pathogenic. Infections with *G. intestinalis* may produce characteristic symptoms. Each of the atrial flagellates may cause symptoms in areas such as the mouth and genital tract.

Quick Quiz! 4-3

The presence of nonpathogenic flagellates is important because it suggests that: (Objective 4-5A)
A. The patient will develop clinical signs and symptoms.
B. Only cyst forms will be recovered in corresponding patient samples.
C. The parasites will invade multiple organ systems in the body.
D. Contaminated food or drink was consumed by the patient.

FLAGELLATE CLASSIFICATION

The flagellates belong to the subphylum Mastigophora, class Zoomastigophora. Like the amebas, the flagellates may be separated into two categories, intestinal and extraintestinal. Figure 4-1 identifies the species that fall under each category.

Giardia intestinalis
(gee'are-dee'uh/in-tes-ti-nal-is)

Common associated disease or condition names: Giardiasis, traveler's diarrhea.

Initially known as *Cercomonas intestinalis*, this important flagellate was first discovered in 1859 by French scientist Dr. F. Lambl. In honor of the significant contributions of both Dr. Lambl and Czechoslovakian scientist Dr. Giard to the field of parasitology, Stiles coined the term *Giardia lamblia* (pronounced lamb-bleé uh) in 1915 (see the Notes of Interest and New Trends section for additional historical information). Since the term *Giardia intestinalis* is gaining

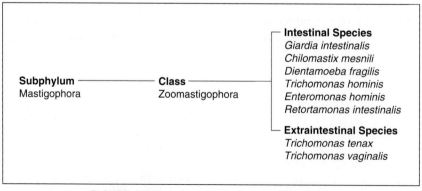

FIGURE 4-1 Parasite classification, the flagellates.

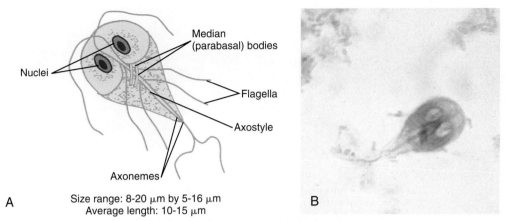

FIGURE 4-2 **A,** *Giardia intestinalis* trophozoite. **B,** *Giardia intestinalis* trophozoite. (**B** *from Forbes BA, Sahm DF, Weissfeld AS: Bailey & Scott's diagnostic microbiology, ed 12, St Louis, 2007, Mosby.)*

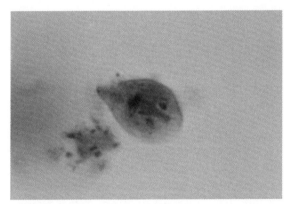

FIGURE 4-3 *Giardia intestinalis* trophozoite. Note red-staining nuclei (trichrome stain, ×1000).

TABLE 4-1	*Giardia intestinalis* Trophozoite: Typical Characteristics at a Glance
Parameter	**Description**
Size range	8-20 μm long 5-16 μm wide
Shape	Pear-shaped, teardrop
Motility	Falling leaf
Appearance	Bilaterally symmetrical
Nuclei	Two ovoid-shaped, each with a large karyosome No peripheral chromatin
Flagella	Four pairs, origination of each: One pair, anterior end One pair, posterior end Two pair, central, extending laterally
Other structures	Two median bodies Two axonemes Sucking disk

popularity (some also consider *Giardia duodenale* as a synonym), its formal name is currently under review by the International Commission on Zoological Nomenclature. For the purposes of this text, this parasite will be referred to as *Giardia intestinalis*.

Morphology

Trophozoites. The typical *G. intestinalis* trophozoite ranges from 8 to 20 μm in length by 5 to 16 μm in width (Figs. 4-2 and 4-3; Table 4-1). The average *G. intestinalis* trophozoite, however, measures 10 to 15 μm long. The *G. intestinalis*

trophozoite is described as pear or teardrop shaped. The broad anterior end of the organism tapers off at the posterior end. The *G. intestinalis* trophozoite characteristically exhibits motility that resembles a falling leaf. The trophozoite is bilaterally symmetrical, containing two ovoid to spherical nuclei, each with a large karyosome,

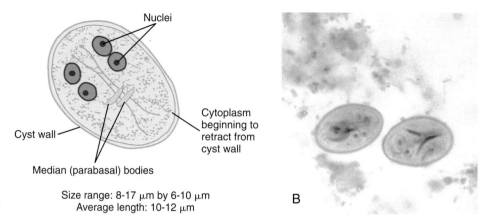

FIGURE 4-4 **A,** *Giardia intestinalis* cyst. **B,** *Giardia intestinalis* cyst. (**B** from Forbes BA, Sahm DF, Weissfeld AS: Bailey & Scott's diagnostic microbiology, ed 12, St Louis, 2007, Mosby.)

usually centrally located. Peripheral chromatin is absent. These nuclei are best detected on permanently stained specimens. The trophozoite is supported by an axostyle made up of two **axonemes,** defined as the interior portions of the flagella. Two slightly curved rodlike structures, known as **median bodies,** sit on the axonemes posterior to the nuclei.

It is important to note that there is some confusion regarding the proper name of the median bodies. Some texts refer to these structures as parabasal bodies rather than median bodies, suggesting that the two structures are different. Other texts consider median bodies and parabasal bodies as two names for the same structure. For the purposes of this text, the term *median body* is used to define structures believed to be associated with energy, metabolism, or support. Their exact function is unclear. Although they are sometimes difficult to detect, the typical *G. intestinalis* trophozoite has four pairs of flagella. One pair of flagella originates from the anterior end and one pair extends from the posterior end. The remaining two pairs of flagella are located laterally, extending from the axonemes in the center of the body. The *G. intestinalis* trophozoite is equipped with a sucking disc. Covering 50% to 75% of the ventral surface, the sucking disk serves as the nourishment point of entry by attaching to the intestinal villi of an infected human.

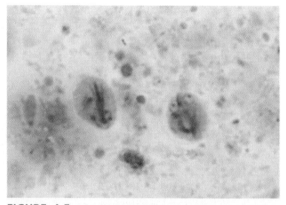

FIGURE 4-5 *Giardia intestinalis* cyst. Note red-staining nuclei (trichrome stain, ×1000).

Cysts. The typical ovoid *G. intestinalis* cyst ranges in size from 8 to 17 μm long by 6 to 10 μm wide, with an average length of 10 to 12 μm (Figs. 4-4 and 4-5; Table 4-2). The colorless and smooth cyst wall is prominent and distinct from the interior of the organism. The cytoplasm is often retracted away from the cyst wall, creating a clearing zone. This phenomenon is especially possible after being preserved in formalin. The immature cyst contains two nuclei and two median bodies. Four nuclei, which may be seen in iodine wet preparations as well as on permanent stains, and four median bodies are present in the fully mature cysts. Mature

TABLE 4-2	*Giardia intestinalis* Cyst: Typical Characteristics at a Glance
Parameter	**Description**
Size range	8-17 µm long 6-10 µm wide
Shape	Ovoid
Nuclei	Immature cyst, two Mature cyst, four Central karyosomes No peripheral chromatin
Cytoplasm	Retracted from cell wall
Other structures	Median bodies: two in immature cyst or four in fully mature cyst Interior flagellar structures*

*Twice as many in mature cyst as compared with immature cyst.

cysts contain twice as many interior flagellar structures.

Laboratory Diagnosis

The specimen of choice for the traditional recovery technique of *G. intestinalis* trophozoites and cysts is stool. It is important to note that *Giardia* is often shed in the stool in showers, meaning that many organisms may be passed and recovered on one day's sample and the following day's sample may reveal no parasites at all. Thus, examination of multiple samples is recommended prior to reporting that a patient is free of *Giardia*. Duodenal contents obtained by aspiration, as well as upper small intestine biopsies, may also be collected for examination. Duodenal contents can identify *G. intestinalis* using the string test, also known as Enterotest.

Several other diagnostic techniques are available for identifying *G. intestinalis,* including fecal antigen detection by enzyme immunoassays (EIA) and enzyme-linked immunosorbent assay (ELISA). Direct Fluorescence detection of both *Giardia* and *Cryptosporidium* (see Chapter 7), as well as a *Giardia* Western immunoblotting (blot) test have shown promising results in recent studies.

The newest form of identifying *Giardia* is using real-time polymerase chain reaction (RT-PCR). This molecular method is sensitive enough for environment monitoring because studies suggest that a single *Giardia* cyst may be detected using molecular methods.

Life Cycle Notes

On ingestion, the infective *G. intestinalis* cysts enter the stomach. The digestive juices, particularly gastric acid, stimulate the cysts to excyst in the duodenum. The resulting trophozoites become established and multiply approximately every 8 hours via longitudinal binary fission. The trophozoites feed by attaching their sucking disks to the mucosa of the duodenum. Trophozoites may also infect the common bile duct and gallbladder. Changes that result in an unacceptable environment for trophozoite multiplication stimulate encystation, which occurs as the trophozoites migrate into the large bowel. The cysts enter the outside environment via the feces and may remain viable for as long as 3 months in water. Trophozoites entering into the outside environment quickly disintegrate.

Epidemiology

G. intestinalis may be found worldwide—in lakes, streams, and other water sources—and are considered to be one of the most common intestinal parasites, especially among children. Ingestion of water contaminated with *G. intestinalis* is considered to be the major cause of parasitic diarrheal outbreaks in the United States. It is interesting to note that *G. intestinalis* cysts are resistant to the routine chlorination procedures carried out at most water plant facilities. Filtration as well as chemical treatment of this water is crucial to obtain adequate drinking water. In addition to contaminated water, *G. intestinalis* may be transmitted by eating contaminated fruits or vegetables. Person-to-person contact through oral-anal sexual practices or via the fecal-oral route may also transfer *G. intestinalis*.

There are a number of groups of individuals at a high risk of contracting *G. intestinalis*, including children in day care centers, people living in poor sanitary conditions, those who travel to and drink contaminated water in known endemic areas, and those who practice unprotected sex, particularly homosexual males. There are several known animal reservoir hosts, including beavers, muskrats, and water voles. In addition, there is evidence to suggest that domestic sheep, cattle, and dogs may also harbor the parasite, and perhaps may even transmit the parasite directly to humans.

Clinical Symptoms

G. intestinalis was for many years considered to be a nonpathogen. This organism is now considered to be the only known pathogenic intestinal flagellate.

> **Asymptomatic Carrier State.** Infections with *G. intestinalis* are often completely asymptomatic.

> **Giardiasis (Traveler's Diarrhea).** Symptomatic infections with *Giardia* may be characterized by a wide variety of clinical symptoms, ranging from mild diarrhea, abdominal cramps, anorexia, and flatulence to tenderness of the epigastric region, steatorrhea, and malabsorption syndrome. Patients suffering from a severe case of giardiasis produce light-colored stools with a high fat content that may be caused by secretions produced by the irritated mucosal lining. Fat-soluble vitamin deficiencies, folic acid deficiencies, hypoproteinemia with hypogammaglobulinemia, and structural changes of the intestinal villi may also be observed in these cases. It is interesting to note that blood rarely, if ever, accompanies the stool in these patients.

The typical incubation period for *G. intestinalis* is 10 to 36 days, after which symptomatic patients suddenly develop watery, foul-smelling diarrhea, steatorrhea, flatulence, and abdominal cramping. In general, *Giardia* is a self-limiting condition that typically is over in 10 to 14 days after onset. In chronic cases, however, multiple relapses may occur. Patients with intestinal diverticuli or an immunoglobulin A (IgA) deficiency appear to be particularly susceptible to reoccurring infections. It has been suggested that hypogammaglobulinemia may predispose to *Giardia* as well as achlorhydria. An in-depth study of the immunologic and chemical mechanics behind these suggestions, as well as other possible immunologic roles in giardiasis, is beyond the scope of this chapter.

Treatment

The primary choice of treatments for *G. intestinalis* infections, according to the Centers for Disease Control and Prevention (CDC), are metronidazole (Flagyl), tinidazole (Tindamax) and nitazoxanide (Alinia). According to the Food and Drug Administration (FDA) metronidazole, however, is not approved for *G. intestinalis* infections due to a proven increased incidence of carcinogenicity in mice and rats. Tinidazole is approved by the FDA for *G. intestinalis* infections, but is potentially carcinogenic in rats and mice due to the similar structure and biologic effects to that of metronidazole. Tinidazole is as effective as metronidazole and shows to be well tolerated in patients. Nitazoxanide is very efficient in treating adults and children and is similar in use to metronidazole, but is approved by the FDA for the treatment of diarrhea related to *Giardia* infections.

Prevention and Control

The steps necessary to prevent and control *G. intestinalis* are similar to those for *Entamoeba histolytica*. Proper water treatment that includes a combination of chemical therapy and filtration, guarding water supplies against contamination by potential reservoir hosts, exercising good personal hygiene, proper cleaning and cooking of food, and avoidance of unprotected oral-anal sex are among the most important steps to prevent and control *G. intestinalis*. Campers and hikers are encouraged to be equipped with bottled water. Double-strength saturated iodine solution may be added to potentially contaminated water prior to consuming. Portable water purification systems are also available and appear to be effective. It is imperative that individuals follow the manufacturer's directions when treating water with iodine or when using the purification system to ensure the safest drinking water possible.

Notes of Interest and New Trends

Giardia intestinalis was discovered in 1681 by Anton van Leeuwenhoek when he examined a sample of his own stool. The first known rough description of *Giardia* was, however, written later by the Secretary of the Royal Society of London, Robert Hooke.

The first recorded water outbreak of *G. intestinalis* occurred in St. Petersburg, Russia, and involved a group of visiting travelers. *Giardia* was also recognized during World War I as being responsible for diarrheal epidemics that occurred among the fighting soldiers. Increased travel in the 1970s allowed for Americans traveling to the former Soviet Union to become infected with *Giardia*. Between 1965 and 1984, over 90 water outbreaks (occurring in town and city public water supplies) were recorded in the United States.

There are several documented reports suggesting that a marked increase in the prevalence of *G. intestinalis* has occurred in the male homosexual population in recent years.

A series of two studies on the prevalence of parasites in the St. Louis area from 1988 through 1993 concluded that *G. intestinalis* was the most common parasite reported. It is interesting to note that in both studies accurate epidemiologic information regarding parasite prevalence was difficult to obtain, partly because many parasitic infections are never reported to the proper authorities.

Giardia trophozoites have often been referred to as resembling an old man with whiskers, a cartoon character, and/or a monkey's face.

A number of studies have suggested that several zymodemes of *G. intestinalis* exist. This may prove to be valuable information in the future as more so-called secrets about *Giardia* are revealed.

G. intestinalis and *E. histolytica* cysts, as well as a host of other parasites, were isolated in samples acquired from the Hudson River and East River in New York City in the early 1980s. Almost 25% of scuba divers in the New York City police and fire departments, who have been known to dive in these waters, tested positive for both parasites.

G. intestinalis and *Trichomonas vaginalis* (see later) are both known to be carriers of double-stranded RNA viruses.

Quick Quiz! 4-4

The proposed function(s) of the median bodies seen in *G. intestinalis* is (are) which of the following? (Objective 4-9 B)

A. Support
B. Energy
C. Metabolism
D. All of the above

Quick Quiz! 4-5

Which specimen type and collection regimen would be most appropriate for the diagnosis of *G. intestinalis*? (Objective 4-8)

A. One stool sample
B. Two stool samples
C. Multiple stool samples collected on subsequent days
D. One stool sample and one blood sample

Quick Quiz! 4-6

G. intestinalis trophozoites attach to the mucosa of the duodenum and feed with the assistance of this morphologic structure. (Objective 4-9B)

A. Sucking disk
B. Axostyle
C. Axoneme
D. Nucleus

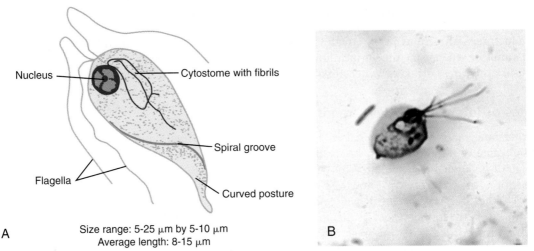

FIGURE 4-6 **A,** *Chilomastix mesnili* trophozoite. **B,** *Chilomastix mesnili* trophozoite. (*B from Forbes BA, Sahm DF, Weissfeld AS: Bailey & Scott's diagnostic microbiology, ed 12, St Louis, 2007, Mosby.*)

Quick Quiz! 4-7

Individuals become infected with *G. intestinalis* by which of the following? (Objective 4-5C)
A. Swimming in contaminated water
B. Ingesting contaminated food or drink
C. Inhalation of infective cysts
D. Walking barefoot on contaminated soil

Quick Quiz! 4-8

Individuals at risk for contracting *G. intestinalis* when camping and hiking are encouraged to take which of these steps to prevent infection? (Objective 4-7C)
A. Treat potentially infected water with a double-strength saturated saline solution prior to consuming.
B. Use only bottled water for drinking, cooking & appropriate personal hygiene.
C. Avoid swimming in contaminated water.
D. Wear shoes at all times.

Chilomastix mesnili
(ki″lo-mas′tiks/mes′nil′i)

Common associated disease and condition names: None (considered a nonpathogen).

TABLE 4-3	*Chilomastix mesnili* Trophozoite: Typical Characteristics at a Glance
Parameter	**Description**
Size range	5-25 µm long 5-10 µm wide
Shape	Pear-shaped
Motility	Stiff, rotary, directional
Nuclei	One with small central or eccentric karyosome No peripheral chromatin
Flagella	Four: Three extending from anterior end One extending posteriorly from cytostome region
Other structures	Prominent cytostome extending 1/3 to 1/2 body length Spiral groove

Morphology

Trophozoites. The pear-shaped *Chilomastix mesnili* trophozoite ranges from 5 to 25 µm long by 5 to 10 µm wide, with an average length of 8 to 15 µm (Fig. 4-6; Table 4-3). The broad anterior end tapers toward the posterior end of the organism. Stiff rotary motility in a directional

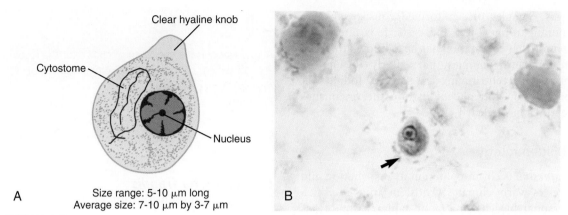

Clear hyaline knob

Cytostome

Nucleus

A   Size range: 5-10 μm long
Average size: 7-10 μm by 3-7 μm

B

FIGURE 4-7 A, *Chilomastix mesnili cyst.* **B,** *Chilomastix mesnili cyst.* (***B*** *from Mahon CR, Lehman DC, Manuselis G: Textbook of diagnostic microbiology, ed 4, St Louis, 2011, Saunders.*)

pattern is typical of the *C. mesnili* trophozoite. The single nucleus, which is usually not visible in unstained preparations, is located in the anterior end of the trophozoite. The typical small karyosome may be found located centrally or eccentrically in the form of chromatin granules that form plaques against the nuclear membrane. Peripheral chromatin is absent. *C. mesnili* trophozoites characteristically have four flagella. Three of the flagella, which seldom stain, extend out of the anterior end of the organism. The fourth flagellum is shorter than the others and extends posteriorly from a rudimentary mouth referred to as a **cytostome.** Extending one third to one half of the body length, the cytostome is prominently located to one side of the nucleus. The structure bordering the cytostome resembles a shepherd's crook and is the most prominent of several supporting cytostomal fibrils found in this area. The ventral surface indentation located toward the center of the body that extends down toward the posterior end of the trophozoite is known as a typical spiral groove. The presence of this spiral groove results in a curved posture at the posterior end.

◼ **Cysts.** The cysts of *C. mesnili* are usually lemon-shaped and possess a clear anterior hyaline knob. The average cyst measures 7 to 10 μm long and 3 to 7 μm in width, but may range in

TABLE 4-4	*Chilomastix mesnili* **Cyst: Typical Characteristics at a Glance**
Parameter	**Description**
Size range	5-10 μm long
Shape	Lemon-shaped, with a clear hyaline knob extending from the anterior end
Nuclei	One, with large central karyosome No peripheral chromatin
Other structures	Well-defined cytostome located on one side of the nucleus

length from 5 to 10 μm (Fig. 4-7; Table 4-4). A large single nucleus, consisting of a large central karyosome and no peripheral chromatin, is usually located toward the anterior end of the cyst. The well-defined cytostome, with its accompanying fibrils, may be found to one side of the nucleus.

Laboratory Diagnosis

Traditional examination of freshly passed liquid stools from patients infected with *C. mesnili* typically reveals only trophozoites. Formed stool samples from these patients usually reveal only cysts. Samples of semiformed consistency may contain trophozoites and cysts. It is interesting to note that encystation has been known to occur in unformed samples, particularly during the process of centrifuging the sample. Iodine wet preparations often demonstrate the organism's features most clearly.

Epidemiology

C. mesnili is cosmopolitan in its distribution and prefers warm climates. Those in areas in which personal hygiene and poor sanitary conditions prevail are at the greatest risk of *C. mesnili* introduction. The transmission of *C. mesnili* occurs when infective cysts are ingested. This may occur primarily through hand-to-mouth contamination or via contaminated food or drink.

Clinical Symptoms

Infections with *C. mesnili* are typically asymptomatic.

Treatment

Treatment for persons infected with *C. mesnili* is usually not indicated because this organism is considered to be a nonpathogen.

Prevention and Control

Proper personal hygiene and public sanitation practices are the two primary prevention and control measures necessary to eradicate future infections with *C. mesnili*.

Quick Quiz! 4-9

Which of the following are key morphologic characteristics of *C. mesnili*? (Objective 4-9A)
A. Round and four to eight nuclei
B. Oval and presence of a cytosome
C. Round and presence of an axoneme
D. Lemon-shaped and presence of a cytosome

Quick Quiz! 4-10

A liquid stool is the specimen of choice for the recovery of which of these morphologic forms of *C. mesnili*? (Objective 4-8)
A. Trophozoites only
B. Cysts only
C. Trophozoites and cysts

Dientamoeba fragilis
(dye-en'tuh-mee'buh/fradj"i-lis)

Common associated disease and condition names: *Dientamoeba fragilis* infection (symptomatic).

Morphology

D. fragilis was initially classified as an ameba because this organism moves by means of pseudopodia and does not have external flagella. Further investigation using electron microscopy studies has suggested that *D. fragilis* does have flagellate characteristics. It is interesting to note that the specific findings of these studies are not included in a number of texts under the discussion of this organism. Some authorities classify this organism as strictly a flagellate, whereas others list it in the flagellate section but consider it in a group of its own as an ameba-flagellate. Needless to say, there appears to still be some controversy over the correct classification of *D. fragilis*. For our purposes, *D. fragilis* will be considered as a member of the flagellates.

Trophozoites. The typical *D. fragilis* trophozoite is irregular and roundish in shape and ranges in size from 5 to 18 μm, with an average size of 8 to 12 μm (Fig. 4-8; Table 4-5). The trophozoite's progressive motility, seen primarily in freshly passed stool samples, is accomplished by broad hyaline pseudopodia that possess characteristic serrated margins. The typical *D. fragilis* trophozoite has two nuclei, each consisting of four to eight centrally located massed chromatin granules that are usually arranged in a symmetrical fashion. Peripheral chromatin is absent. The nuclei are generally only observable with

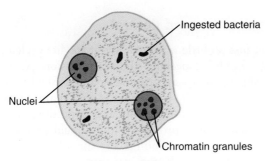

Size range: 5-18 μm
Average size: 8-12 μm

FIGURE 4-8 *Dientamoeba fragilis* trophozoite.

TABLE 4-5	*Dientamoeba fragilis* Trophozoite: Typical Characteristics at a Glance
Parameter	**Description**
Size range	5-18 μm
Shape	Irregularly round
Motility	Progressive, broad hyaline pseudopodia
Number of nuclei	Two, each consisting of massed clumps of four to eight chromatin granules No peripheral chromatin
Cytoplasm	Bacteria-filled vacuoles common

permanent stain. The stain of choice for distinguishing the individual chromatin granules is iron hematoxylin. Although most trophozoites are binucleated—hence, the name *Dientamoeba*—mononucleated forms may also exist. In addition, trophozoites containing three or even four nuclei may occasionally be seen. Vacuoles containing bacteria may be present in the cytoplasm of these trophozoites.

◗ **Cysts.** There is no known cyst stage of *D. fragilis*.

Laboratory Diagnosis

Examination of stool samples for the presence of trophozoites is the method of choice for the laboratory diagnosis of *D. fragilis*. Multiple samples

may be necessary to rule out the presence of this organism because the amount of parasite shedding may vary from day to day. In addition, it is important to note that *D. fragilis* may be difficult to find, much less identify, in typical stool samples. This organism has the ability to blend in well with the background material in the sample. In some cases, the organisms stain faintly and may not be recognized. As noted, care should be exercised when screening all unknown samples. *D. fragilis* may be missed if the sample is not properly examined.

More recently, both conventional and real-time polymerase chain reaction (RT-PCR) methods have been used to diagnose *D. fragilis* in patients. A recent study evaluated methods of detection for *D. fragilis* and RT-PCR was shown to be the most sensitive of all diagnostic methods.

Life Cycle Notes

The complete life cycle of *D. fragilis* is not well understood. Once inside the human body, however, it is known that *D. fragilis* resides in the mucosal crypts of the large intestine. There is no evidence to suggest that *D. fragilis* trophozoites invade their surrounding tissues. *D. fragilis* has only rarely been known to ingest red blood cells. Other specific information regarding the organism's life cycle remains unclear.

Epidemiology

The exact mode of *D. fragilis* transmission remains unknown. One unproven theory suggests that *D. fragilis* is transmitted via the eggs of helminth parasites such as *Enterobius vermicularis* and *Ascaris lumbricoides* (both of these organisms are discussed in detail in Chapter 8). Several studies aimed at answering this question have concluded that a notable frequency of organisms resembling *D. fragilis* were identified in patients who were also infected with *E. vermicularis* (pinworm). Data collected and studied to date indicated that this organism is most likely distributed in cosmopolitan areas. Partly because the mode of transmission remains a mystery, the specific geographic distribution of *D. fragilis* is unknown.

Demographic information collected during studies and surveys in the last 10 to 15 years has indicated that the following individuals appear to be at risk of contracting *D. fragilis:* children, homosexual men, those living in semicommunal groups, and persons who are institutionalized. These data may support the theory that *D. fragilis* transmission may occur by the fecal-oral and oral-anal routes, as well as by the person-to-person route, as the unproven theory described earlier indicates.

Other factors that may potentially inhibit accurate *D. fragilis* epidemiologic information include the fact that infection, when it occurs, is often not reported; in some cases, samples are rarely collected for study and clinicians may experience difficulty in correctly identifying the organism because of its ability to blend in with the background material of the sample.

Clinical Symptoms

 Asymptomatic Carrier State. It is estimated that most people with *D. fragilis* infection remain asymptomatic.

 Symptomatic. Patients who suffer symptoms associated with *D. fragilis* infections often present with diarrhea and abdominal pain. Other documented symptoms that may occur include bloody or mucoid stools, flatulence, nausea or vomiting, weight loss, and fatigue or weakness. Some patients experience diarrhea alternating with constipation, low-grade eosinophilia, and pruritus.

Treatment

Although there is some controversy over the pathogenicity of *D. fragilis,* symptomatic cases of infection may indicate treatment. The treatment of choice for such infections is iodoquinol. Tetracycline is an acceptable alternative treatment. Paromomycin (Humatin) may be used in cases when the treatments listed earlier, for whatever reason, are not appropriate.

Prevention and Control

Because so little is known about the life cycle of *D. fragilis*, especially the transmission phase, designing adequate prevention and control measures is difficult. It is believed that maintaining personal and public sanitary conditions and avoidance of unprotected homosexual practices will at least help minimize the spread of *D. fragilis* infections. If the unproven transmission theory is valid, the primary prevention and control measure would be the eradication of the helminth eggs, especially those of the pinworm.

Notes of Interest and New Trends

D. fragilis differs from the amebic trophozoites when mounted in water preparations. Although both types of organisms swell and rupture under these conditions, only *D. fragilis* returns to its normal size. Numerous granules are present in this stage and exhibit Brownian motion. This is known as the Hakansson phenomenon; it is a feature diagnostic for the identification of *D. fragilis*.

 Quick Quiz! 4-11

A flagellate trophozoite that could be described as 9 to 12 μm with one or two nuclei, each with four symmetrically positioned chromatin granules and vacuoles containing bacteria in the cytoplasm, would most likely be which of the following? (Objective 4-9C)
A. *Giardia intestinalis*
B. *Dientamoeba fragilis*
C. *Chilomastix mesnilli*
D. *Blastocystis hominis*

 Quick Quiz! 4-12

The permanent stain of choice for observing the nuclear features of *D. fragilis* is which of the following? (Objective 4-12)
A. Trichrome
B. Iodine
C. Saline
D. Iron hematoxylin

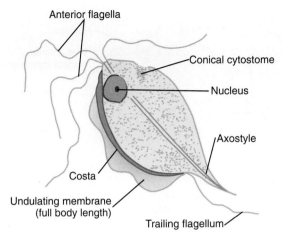

Size range: 7-20 μm by 5-18 μm
Average length: 10-12 μm

FIGURE 4-9 *Trichomonas hominis* trophozoite.

TABLE 4-6	*Trichomonas hominis* Trophozoite: Typical Characteristics at a Glance	
Parameter	**Description**
Size range	7-20 μm long 5-18 μm wide
Shape	Pear-shaped
Motility	Nervous, jerky
Nuclei	One, with a small central karyosome No peripheral chromatin
Flagella	Three to five anterior One posterior extending from the posterior end of the undulating membrane
Other features	Axostyle that extends beyond the posterior end of the body Full body length undulating membrane Conical cytostome cleft in anterior region ventrally located opposite the undulating membrane

Trichomonas hominis

(trick″o-mo′nas/hŏm′ĭ-nĭs)

Common associated disease and condition names: None (considered as a nonpathogen).

Morphology

▨ **Trophozoites.** Ranging in size from 7 to 20 μm long by 5 to 18 μm wide, with an average length of 10 to 12 μm, the typical *Trichomonas hominis* trophozoite is pear-shaped (Fig. 4-9; Table 4-6). The characteristic nervous, jerky motility is accomplished with the assistance of a full body-length undulating membrane. The rodlike structure located at the base of the undulating membrane, known as the **costa**, connects the undulating membrane to the trophozoite body. The single nucleus, not visible in unstained preparations, is located in the anterior region of the organism. The small central karyosome is surrounded by a delicate nuclear membrane. Peripheral chromatin is absent. The trophozoite is supported by an axostyle that extends beyond the posterior end of the body. A cone-shaped cytostome cleft may be seen in the anterior region of the organism lying ventrally opposite the undulating membrane. The typical *T. hominis*

trophozoite has three to five flagella that originate from the anterior end. The single posterior flagellum is an extension of the posterior end of the undulating membrane.

▨ **Cysts.** There is no known cyst form of *T. hominis.*

Laboratory Diagnosis

Stool examination is the method of choice for the recovery of *T. hominis* trophozoites.

Epidemiology

T. hominis is found worldwide, particularly in cosmopolitan areas of warm and temperate climates. It is interesting to note that the frequency of infections is higher in warm climates and that children appear to contract this parasite more often than adults. Transmission most likely occurs by ingesting trophozoites. Contaminated milk is suspected of being one of the sources of infection. It is suspected that in patients suffering from achlorhydria, the milk acts as a shield for the *T. hominis* trophozoites upon entry into the stomach. This may account for the organism's ability to survive passage through the stomach area and to settle in the small intestine. Fecal-oral transmission may also occur.

Clinical Symptoms

Infections with *T. hominis* are generally asymptomatic.

Treatment

T. hominis is considered to be a nonpathogen. Treatment, therefore, is usually not indicated.

Prevention and Control

Improved personal and public sanitary practices are crucial to the prevention and control of *T. hominis*.

Quick Quiz! 4-13

The specimen of choice for the recovery of *T. hominis* is which of the following? (Objective 4-8)
A. Stool
B. Urine
C. Intestinal contents
D. Gastric contents

Quick Quiz! 4-14

Trichomonas hominis can be transmitted by which of the following? (Objective 4-5C)
A. Contaminated milk
B. Bite of an infected mosquito
C. Ingestion of an embryonated ovum
D. Ingestion of undercooked meat

Enteromonas hominis
(ĕn′tĕr-mō′năs/hōm′ĭ-nĭs)

Common associated disease and condition names: None (considered as a nonpathogen).

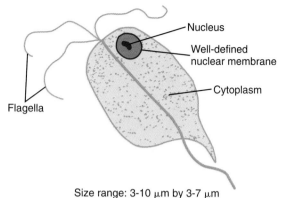

Size range: 3-10 μm by 3-7 μm
Average length: 7-9 μm

FIGURE 4-10 *Enteromonas hominis* trophozoite.

TABLE 4-7	*Enteromonas hominis* Trophozoite: Typical Characteristics at a Glance
Parameter	**Description**
Size range	3-10 μm long
	3-7 μm wide
Shape	Oval; sometimes half-circle
Motility	Jerky
Nuclei	One with central karyosome
	No peripheral chromatin
Flagella	Four total:
	Three directed anteriorly
	One directed posteriorly
Other structures	None

Morphology

Trophozoites. *Enteromonas hominis* trophozoites typically range from 3 to 10 μm long by 3 to 7 μm wide, with an average length of 7 to 9 μm (Fig. 4-10; Table 4-7). The typical *E. hominis* trophozoite is oval in shape. This organism may also be seen in the form of a half-circle. In this case, the body is flattened on one side. *Enteromonas hominis* trophozoites usually exhibit jerky motility. The single nucleus, visible only in stained preparations, consists of a large central karyosome surrounded by a well-defined nuclear membrane. Peripheral chromatin is absent. The nucleus is located in the anterior end

TABLE 4-8	*Enteromonas hominis* Cyst: Typical Characteristics at a Glance
Parameter	**Description**
Size range	3-10 μm long
	4-7 μm wide
Shape	Oval, elongated
Nuclei	One to four
	Binucleated and quadrinucleated nuclei located at opposite ends
	Central karyosome
	No peripheral chromatin
Other structures	None

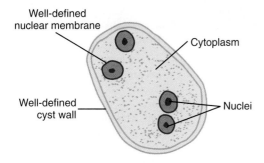

Well-defined nuclear membrane

Cytoplasm

Well-defined cyst wall

Nuclei

Size range: 3-10 μm by 4-7 μm
Average length: 5-8 μm

FIGURE 4-11 *Enteromonas hominis* cyst.

of the trophozoite. Four flagella originate from the organism's anterior end. Three of these flagella are directed anteriorly; the fourth is directed posteriorly. The posterior end of the organism comes together to form a structure resembling a small tail. These trophozoites are simple, relatively speaking, in that structures such as an undulating membrane, costa, cytostome, and axostyle are absent.

Cysts. The typical oval to elongated *E. hominis* cyst measures 3 to 10 μm long by 4 to 7 μm wide, with an average length of 5 to 8 μm (Fig. 4-11; Table 4-8). On first inspection of these organisms, yeast cells may often be suspected.

Further investigation, however, reveals one to four nuclei. When more than one nucleus is present, these structures are typically located at opposite ends of the cell. Although binucleated cysts appear to be the most commonly encountered, quadrinucleated forms may also occur. The nuclei resemble those of the trophozoites in that each consists of a well-defined nuclear membrane surrounding a central karyosome. Peripheral chromatin is again absent. The cysts of *E. hominis* are protected by a well-defined cell wall. Fibrils and internal flagellate structures are also not seen in the cyst form. It is important to note that the size range of *E. hominis* cysts overlaps that of *Endolimax nana* cysts. A high frequency of binucleated cysts seen on a stained preparation indicates probable *E. hominis* because the probability of finding binucleated *E. nana* cysts is extremely rare.

Laboratory Diagnosis

Examination of stool samples is the laboratory diagnostic technique of choice for identifying *E. hominis* trophozoites and cysts. Unfortunately, this organism is difficult to identify accurately because of its small size. Careful screening of samples is recommended to prevent missing an *E. hominis* organism.

Epidemiology

E. hominis is distributed worldwide in warm and temperate climates. Ingestion of infected cysts appears to be the primary cause of *E. hominis* transmission.

Clinical Symptoms

Infections with *E. hominis* are characteristically asymptomatic.

Treatment

E. hominis is considered to be a nonpathogen. Treatment for *E. hominis* infections is, therefore, not indicated.

Prevention and Control

The observance of proper personal hygiene and public sanitation practices will undoubtedly result in the prevention and control of future infections with *E. hominis*.

Quick Quiz! 4-15

When *E. hominis* cysts contain more than one nuclei, where do they tend to be positioned within the cytoplasm? (Objective 4-9A)
A. Center
B. Around the periphery of the organism
C. At opposite ends of the cell
D. Throughout the organism

Quick Quiz! 4-16

Treatment is always indicated for patients when *E. hominis* is present on parasite examination. (Objective 4-7B)
A. True
B. False

Retortamonas intestinalis

(rē-tort′ă-mō′năs/ĭn″-tĕs-ti′nă-lĭs)

Common associated disease and condition names: None (considered as a nonpathogen).

Morphology

Trophozoites. The body length of a typical *Retortamonas intestinalis* trophozoite measures 3 to 7 μm, with an average of 3 to 5 μm (Fig. 4-12; Table 4-9). Ranging from 5 to 6 μm in width, the ovoid trophozoite exhibits characteristic jerky motility. A single large nucleus is present in the anterior portion of the organism. The nucleus has a somewhat small and compact central karyosome. A fine and delicate ring of chromatin granules may be visible on the nuclear membrane. Opposite the nucleus in the anterior portion of the trophozoite lies a cytostome that extends approximately half of the body length.

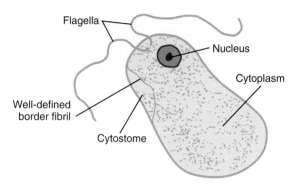

Size range: 3-7 μm by 5-6 μm
Average length: 3-5 μm

FIGURE 4-12 *Retortamonas intestinalis* trophozoite.

TABLE 4-9	*Retortamonas intestinalis* Trophozoite: Typical Characteristics at a Glance
Parameter	**Description**
Size range	3-7 μm long 5-6 μm wide
Shape	Ovoid
Motility	Jerky
Nuclei	One, with small central karyosome Ring of chromatin granules may be on nuclear membrane
Flagella	Two; anterior
Other structures	Cytostome extending halfway down body length with well-defined fibril border opposite the nucleus in the anterior end

A well-defined fibril borders this structure. The *R. intestinalis* trophozoite is equipped with only two anterior flagella.

Cysts. The lemon- to pear-shaped *R. intestinalis* cysts measure from 3 to 9 μm in length and up to 5 μm wide, with an average length of 5 to 7 μm (Fig. 4-13; Table 4-10). The single nucleus, consisting of a central karyosome, may be surrounded by a delicate ring of chromatin granules and is located in the anterior region or closer toward the center of the organism. Two fused fibrils originate anterior to the nuclear region,

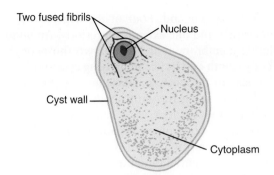

Size range: 3-9 μm by up to 5 μm
Average length: 5-7 μm

FIGURE 4-13 *Retortamonas intestinalis* cyst.

TABLE 4-10	*Retortamonas intestinalis* Cyst: Typical Characteristics at a Glance
Parameter	**Description**
Size range	3-9 μm long Up to 5 μm wide
Shape	Lemon-shaped, pear-shaped
Nuclei	One, located in anterior-central region with central karyosome May be surrounded by a delicate ring of chromatin granules
Other structures	Two fused fibrils resembling a bird's beak in the anterior nuclear region, only visible in stained preparations

splitting up around the nucleus, and extend separately posterior to the nucleus, forming a characteristic bird's beak. This structure, along with the nucleus itself, is often difficult to see, especially in unstained preparations.

Laboratory Diagnosis

A stained stool preparation is the best sample to examine for the presence of *R. intestinalis* trophozoites and cysts. Unfortunately, accurate identification is difficult, in part because of the small size of this organism. In addition, the small number of diagnostic features may sometimes not stain well enough to recognize. Stools suspected of containing *R. intestinalis*, as well as the other smaller flagellates, should be carefully screened before reporting a negative test result.

Epidemiology

Although *R. intestinalis* is rarely reported in clinical stool samples, its existence has been documented in warm and temperate climates throughout the world. Transmission is accomplished by ingestion of the infected cysts. A select group of individuals, including patients in psychiatric hospitals and others living in crowded conditions, have been known to contract *R. intestinalis* infections because of poor sanitation and hygiene conditions.

Clinical Symptoms

Infections with *R. intestinalis* typically do not produce symptoms.

Treatment

Because *R. intestinalis* is considered a nonpathogen, treatment is usually not indicated.

Prevention and Control

The most important *R. intestinalis* prevention and control measures are improved personal and public hygiene conditions. ·

Quick Quiz! 4-17

The traditional technique and specimen of choice for identifying *Retortamonas intestinalis* is which of the following? (Objectives 4-8 and 4-12)
A. Permanently stained blood
B. Iodine prep of urine
C. Saline prep of bronchial wash
D. Permanently stained stool

Quick Quiz! 4-18

Individuals contract *R. intestinalis* by which of the following? (Objective 4-5C)
A. Ingesting infective cysts in contaminated food or drink
B. Consuming trophozoites in contaminated beverages
C. Stepping barefoot on infective soil
D. Inhaling infective dust particles

Trichomonas tenax

(trick"o-mo'nas/těn'ăx)

Common associated disease and condition names: None (considered as a nonpathogen).

Morphology

■ **Trophozoites.** The typical *Trichomonas tenax* trophozoite is described as being oval to pear-shaped, measuring 5 to 14 μm long, with an average length of 6 to 9 μm (Fig. 4-14; Table 4-11). The single, ovoid, vesicular nucleus is filled with several chromatin granules and is usually located in the central anterior portion of the organism. The *T. tenax* trophozoite is equipped with five flagella, all of which originate at the anterior end. Four of the flagella extend anteriorly and one extends posteriorly. An undulating membrane that extends two thirds of the body length and its accompanying costa typically lie next to the posterior flagellum. A thick axostyle runs along the entire body length, curving around the nucleus, and extends posteriorly beyond the body of the organism. A small anterior cytostome is located next to the axostyle, opposite the undulating membrane.

■ **Cyst.** There is no known cyst stage of *T. tenax*.

Laboratory Diagnosis

The specimen of choice for diagnosing *T. tenax* trophozoite is mouth scrapings. Microscopic examination of tonsillar crypts and pyorrheal pockets (see Chapter 2) of patients suffering from *T. tenax* infections often yields typical trophozoites. Tartar between the teeth and gingival margin of the gums are the primary areas of the mouth that may also potentially harbor this organism. Samples suspected of containing *T. tenax* may also be cultured onto appropriate media.

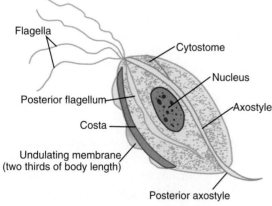

Size range: 5-14 μm long
Average length: 6-9 μm

FIGURE 4-14 *Trichomonas tenax* trophozoite.

TABLE 4-11	*Trichomonas tenax* Trophozoite: Typical Characteristics at a Glance
Parameter	**Description**
Size range	5-14 μm long
Shape	Oval, pear-shaped
Nuclei	One, ovoid nucleus; consists of vesicular region filled with chromatin granules
Flagella	Five total, all originating anteriorly: Four extend anteriorly One extends posteriorly
Other structures	Undulating membrane extending two thirds of body length with accompanying costa Thick axostyle curves around nucleus; extends beyond body length Small anterior cytostome opposite undulating membrane

However, this method is rarely used in most clinical laboratories.

Life Cycle Notes

T. tenax trophozoites survive in the body as mouth scavengers that feed primarily on local microorganisms. Located in the tartar between the teeth, tonsillar crypts, pyorrheal pockets, and gingival margin around the gums, *T. tenax* trophozoites multiply by longitudinal binary fission. These trophozoites are unable to survive the digestive process.

Epidemiology

Although the exact mode of transmitting *T. tenax* trophozoites is unknown, there is evidence suggesting that the use of contaminated dishes and utensils, as well as introducing droplet contamination through kissing, may be the routes of transmission. The trophozoites appear to be durable, surviving several hours in drinking water. Infections with *T. tenax* occur throughout the world almost exclusively in patients with poor oral hygiene.

Clinical Symptoms

The typical *T. tenax* infection does not produce any notable symptoms. On a rare occasion, *T. tenax* has been known to invade the respiratory tract, but this appears to have mainly occurred in patients with underlying thoracic or lung abscesses of pleural exudates.

Treatment

T. tenax is considered to be a nonpathogen and no chemical treatment is normally indicated. The *T. tenax* trophozoites seem to disappear in infected persons following the institution of proper oral hygiene practices.

Prevention and Control

Practicing good oral hygiene is the most effective method of preventing and controlling the future spread of *T. tenax* infections.

Quick Quiz! 4-19

How far down the body length does the *Trichomonas tenax* undulating membrane extend? (Objective 4-9A)
A. One fourth
B. One half
C. Three fourths
D. Full body

Quick Quiz! 4-20

The specimen of choice for the recovery of *Trichomonas tenax* is which of the following? (Objective 4-8)
A. Stool
B. Urine
C. Mouth scrapings
D. Cerebrospinal fluid

Trichomonas vaginalis
(trick″o-mo′nas/vadj-i-nay′lis)

Common associated disease and condition names: Persistent urethritis, persistent vaginitis, infant *Trichomonas vaginalis* infection.

Morphology

Trophozoites. Although typical *T. vaginalis* trophozoites may reach up to 30 μm in length, the average length is 8 to 15 μm (Fig. 4-15; Table 4-12). The trophozoites may appear ovoid, round, or pearlike in shape. Rapid jerky motility is accomplished with the aid of the organism's four to six flagella, all of which originate from the anterior end. Only one of the flagella extends posteriorly. The flagella may be difficult to find on specimen preparations. The characteristic undulating membrane is short, relatively speaking, extending only half of the body length. The single nucleus is ovoid, nondescript, and not visible in unstained preparations. *T. vaginalis* trophozoites are equipped with an easily recognizable axostyle that often curves around the nucleus and extends posteriorly beyond the body. Granules may be seen along the axostyle.

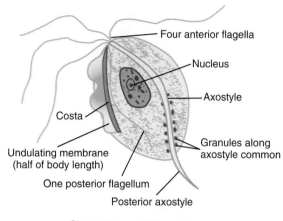

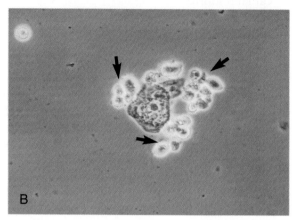

FIGURE 4-15 A, *Trichomonas vaginalis* trophozoite. **B,** Phase contrast wet mount micrograph of a vaginal discharge revealing the presence of *Trichomonas vaginalis* protozoa surrounding a squamous epithelial cell. (**B** *from Mahon CR, Lehman DC, Manuselis G: Textbook of diagnostic microbiology, ed 4, St Louis, 2011, Saunders; courtesy Centers for Disease Control and Prevention, Atlanta.*)

TABLE 4-12	*Trichomonas vaginalis* Trophozoite: Typical Characteristics at a Glance
Parameter	**Description**
Size range	Up to 30 μm long
Shape	Ovoid, round or pear-shaped
Motility	Rapid, jerky
Nuclei	One, ovoid, nondescript
Flagella	All originating anteriorly: Three to five extending anteriorly One extending posteriorly
Other features	Undulating membrane extending half of body length Prominent axostyle that often curves around nucleus; granules may be seen along axostyle

◣ **Cyst.** There is no known *T. vaginalis* cyst stage.

Laboratory Diagnosis

T. vaginalis trophozoites may be recovered using standard processing methods (see Chapter 2) in spun urine, vaginal discharges, urethral discharges, and prostatic secretions. Although permanent stains may be performed, examination of saline wet preparations is preferred in many cases. Not only does the prompt examination of saline wet preparations allow the practitioner to observe the organism's active motility readily, as well as the other typical characteristics, the testing may be performed in a relatively short amount of time. Additional diagnostic tests available include phase contrast microscopy, Papanicolaou (Pap) smears, fluorescent stains, monoclonal antibody assays, enzyme immunoassays, and cultures.

A DNA-based assay has been developed for *T. vaginalis* detection using Affirm VPIII (BD Diagnostics, Sparks, MD). The sensitivity and specificity of this method of testing is much greater than with standard processing methods.

Another diagnostic tool used by laboratories today is InPouch TV (BioMed Diagnostics, White City, OR) culture system. This method can be used with vaginal swabs from women, urethral swabs from men, urine sediment and semen sediment. This method requires incubation time and takes up to 3 days before a result is determined.

Life Cycle Notes

T. vaginalis trophozoites reside on the mucosal surface of the vagina in infected women. The growing trophozoites multiply by longitudinal binary fission and feed on local bacteria and leukocytes. *T. vaginalis* trophozoites thrive in a slightly alkaline or slightly acidic pH environment, such as that commonly seen in an unhealthy vagina. The most common infection site of *T. vaginalis* in males is the prostate gland region and the epithelium of the urethra. The detailed life cycle in the male host is unknown.

Epidemiology

Infections with *T. vaginalis* occur worldwide. The primary mode of transmission of the *T. vaginalis* trophozoites is sexual intercourse. These trophozoites may also migrate through a mother's birth canal and infect the unborn child. Under optimal conditions, *T. vaginalis* is known to be transferred via contaminated toilet articles or underclothing. However, this mode of transmission is rare. The sharing of douche supplies, as well as communal bathing, are also potential routes of infection. *T. vaginalis* trophozoites, which are by nature hardy and resistant to changes in their environment, have been known to survive in urine, on wet sponges, and on damp towels for several hours, as well as in water for up to 40 minutes.

Clinical Symptoms

◗ **Asymptomatic Carrier State.** Asymptomatic cases of *T. vaginalis* most frequently occur in men.

◗ **Persistent Urethritis.** Persistent or recurring urethritis is the condition that symptomatic men experience as a result of a *T. vaginalis* infection. Involvement of the seminal vesicles, higher parts of the urogenital tract, and prostate may occur in severe cases of infection. Symptoms of severe infection include an enlarged tender prostate, dysuria, nocturia, and epididymitis. These patients often release a thin, white urethral discharge that contains the *T. vaginalis* trophozoites.

◗ **Persistent Vaginitis.** Persistent vaginitis, found in infected women, is characterized by a foul-smelling, greenish-yellow liquid vaginal discharge after an incubation period of 4 to 28 days. Vaginal acidity present during and immediately following menstruation most likely accounts for the exacerbation of symptoms. Burning, itching, and chafing may also be present. Red punctate lesions may be present upon examining the vaginal mucosa of infected women. Urethral involvement, dysuria, and increased frequency of urination are among the most commonly experienced symptoms. Cystitis is less commonly observed but may occur.

◗ **Infant Infections.** *T. vaginalis* has been recovered from infants suffering from both respiratory infection and conjunctivitis. These conditions were most likely contracted as a result of *T. vaginalis* trophozoites migrating from an infected mother to the infant through the birth canal and/or during vaginal delivery.

Treatment

With few exceptions, the treatment of choice for *T. vaginalis* infections is metronidazole (Flagyl). Because this parasite is sexually transmitted, treatment of all sexual partners is recommended.

Prevention and Control

The primary step necessary to prevent and control *T. vaginalis* infections is the avoidance of unprotected sex. In addition, the prompt diagnosis and treatment of asymptomatic men is also essential. Although the risk of contracting *T. vaginalis* by these means is relatively low, the avoidance of sharing douche equipment and communal bathing, as well as close contact with potentially infective underclothing, toilet articles, damp towels, and wet sponges, is recommended.

Notes of Interest and New Trends

Infections with *T. vaginalis* are generally considered to be a nuisance and not a major pathogenic process.

There is evidence to suggest a connection between *T. vaginalis* infections and cervical carcinoma.

Quick Quiz! 4-21

This prominent structure found in *T. vaginalis* trophozoites that often extends beyond the body provides the parasite with support. (Objective 4-9A)
A. Nucleus
B. Axostyle
C. Axoneme
D. Granule

Quick Quiz! 4-22

The cyst morphologic form is not known to exist in the life cycle of *T. vaginalis*. (Objective 4-5C)
A. True
B. False

Quick Quiz! 4-23

T. vaginalis may be recovered in which of the following specimen types? (Objective 4-8)
A. Spun urine
B. Vaginal discharge
C. Stool
D. Urethral discharge
E. More than one of the above: _____ (specify)

Quick Quiz! 4-24

All cases of *T. vaginalis* infection result in symptomatic vaginitis in women and urethritis in men. (Objectives 4-6 and 4-7)
A. True
B. False

Quick Quiz! 4-25

Infant infections with *T. vaginalis* tend to affect which of the following of these body areas? (Objective 4-6)
A. Respiratory and genital
B. Genital and intestinal
C. Intestinal and eye
D. Respiratory and eye

LOOKING BACK

The typical characteristics common to all flagellates include size, shape, and nuclear structures. In addition, most have structures specific to one or just a few of the flagellates, such as varying lengths of the undulating membrane, axonemes, or a spiral groove. In summary, three comparison drawings are included at the end of this chapter for easy reference—the flagellate trophozoites found in stool, the flagellate cysts found in stool, and atrial flagellate trophozoites.

The importance of careful and thorough screening of all samples for the presence of parasites cannot be emphasized enough. Just as amebas may be diagnosed by characteristics typical to their class, so also may flagellates. The composite drawings are provided to serve as a resource tool to help practitioners in the identification of the intestinal and atrial flagellates.

TEST YOUR KNOWLEDGE!

4-1. Match each of these flagellate parasites (column A) with its corresponding description (column B). (Objective 4-9)

Column A	Column B
___ **A.** *Dientamoeba fragilis*	**1.** Lemon-shaped cyst
___ **B.** *Trichomonas tenax*	**2.** Trophozoite has a ventrally located sucking disc
___ **C.** *Giardia intestinalis*	**3.** Transmitted by helminth ova

Column A	Column B
___ **D.** *Retortamonas intestinalis*	**4.** Specimen of choice is a mouth scraping
___ **E.** *Chilomastix mesnili*	**5.** Specimen of choice can be a urethral swab
___ **F.** *Trichomonas vaginalis*	**6.** Fibrils form a characteristic bird's beak

4-2. List the intestinal and then the atrial flagellates. (Objective 4-4)

4-3. Which of the flagellates are commonly found in the United States? (Objective 4-2)

4-4. Which of the flagellates is(are) considered to be sexually transmitted infections? (Objective 4-6)

4-5. Describe the life cycles of *Giardia intestinalis*, *Dientamoeba fragilis*, and *Trichomonas vaginalis*. (Objective 4-5C)

4-6. Other than size, list three major morphologic characteristics that are visible with routine staining preparations of each of the flagellates. (Objective 4-9A)

4-7. List the flagellates that have both trophozoite and cyst stages, and list those that have one or the other. (Objectives 4-5A, 4-5B, and 4-11)

4-8. Which of the flagellates can cause gastrointestinal distress? (Objectives 4-6, 4-11A)

4-9. Define the following terms: (Objective 4-1)
  A. Axoneme
  B. Axostyle
  C. Costa
  D. Cytosome
  E. Median bodies
  F. Undulating membrane

4-10. Why can *Giardia intestinalis* and *Dientamoeba fragilis* be difficult to diagnose? Which specimen collection regimen should be used? (Objectives 4-8, 4-11A, and 4-12)

4-11. Which of the flagellates can be contracted by ingesting the cyst form of the organism? (Objective 4-5C, 4-11A)

4-12. Which of the flagellates are considered to be nonpathogens? (Objective 4-11A)

4-13. An infection caused by which of the flagellates can be a result of poor oral hygiene? (Objective 4-5C)

CASE STUDY 4-2   UNDER THE MICROSCOPE

Marcy took her two young children, Justin, age 4 years, and Shannon, age 6 years, to their pediatrician for evaluation. Both children had been ill for several days. Their symptoms included diarrhea with mucoid stools, weakness, flatulence, nausea, and abdominal cramping. Stool samples from both children were sent to the laboratory for parasite examination (O&P), culture, and sensitivity. The culture showed no intestinal pathogens.

Standard O&P processing techniques were carried out, and the organisms shown in the diagram were observed on the permanent stain. The roundish organisms each measured approximately 12 µm in diameter and had two somewhat discrete nuclei.

Questions for Consideration
1. Based on the morphology of the organism depicted here, which parasite do you suspect is present? State the full name of the parasite (i.e., genus and species). (Objective 4-10B)

2. Which permanent stain was likely used in this case? (Objective 4-10F)
3. Name the structures that are shown in the diagram. (Objective 4-10A)
4. What structures allow this parasite to move? (Objective 4-10A)
5. What other morphologic forms, if any, may be seen in clinical samples of patients infected with this parasite? (Objective 4-10I)
6. By what means is it suspected that this parasite may be transmitted to unsuspecting humans? (Objective 4-10D)

COMPARISON DRAWINGS
Flagellate Trophozoites Found in Stool

FIGURE 4-2A. *Giardia intestinalis* trophozoite

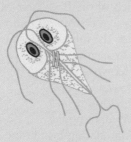

Size range: 8-20 μm by 5-16 μm
Average length: 10-15 μm

FIGURE 4-6A. *Chilomastix mesnili* trophozoite

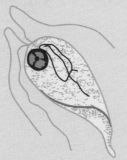

Size range: 5-25 μm by 5-10 μm
Average length: 8-15 μm

FIGURE 4-8. *Dientamoeba fragilis* trophozoite

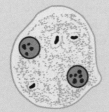

Size range: 5-18 μm
Average size: 8-12 μm

FIGURE 4-9. *Trichomonas hominis* trophozoite

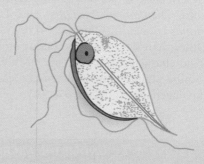

Size range: 7-20 μm by 5-18 μm
Average length: 10-12 μm

FIGURE 4-10. *Enteromonas hominis* trophozoite

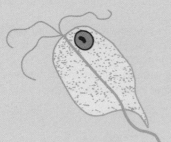

Size range: 3-10 μm by 3-7 μm
Average length: 7-9 μm

FIGURE 4-12. *Retortamonas intestinalis* trophozoite

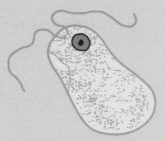

Size range: 3-7 μm by 5-6 μm
Average length: 3-5 μm

COMPARISON DRAWINGS
Flagellate Cysts Found in Stool

FIGURE 4-4A. *Giardia intestinalis* cyst

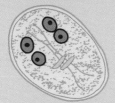

Size range: 8-17 μm by 6-10 μm
Average length: 10-12 μm

FIGURE 4-7A. *Chilomastix mesnili* cyst

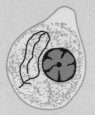

Size range: 5-10 μm long
Average size: 7-10 μm by 3-7 μm

FIGURE 4-9. *Enteromonas hominis* cyst

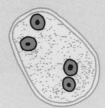

Size range: 3-10 μm by 4-7 μm
Average length: 5-8 μm

FIGURE 4-11. *Retortamonas intestinalis* cyst

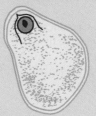

Size range: 3-9 μm by up to 5 μm
Average length: 5-7 μm

COMPARISON DRAWINGS
Atrial Flagellate Trophozoites

FIGURE 4-14. *Trichomonas tenax* trophozoite

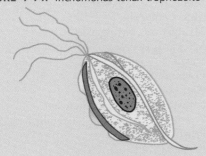

Size range: 5-14 μm long
Average length: 6-9 μm

FIGURE 4-15A. *Trichomonas vaginalis* trophozoite

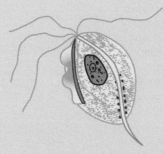

Size range: up to 30 μm long
Average length: 8-15 μm

The Hemoflagellates

Michelle Mantooth and Elizabeth Zeibig

WHAT'S AHEAD

Focusing In
Morphology and Life Cycle
  Notes
Hemoflagellate Classification
Historical Perspective of
  Leishmaniasis
    Leishmania braziliensis
    complex

Leishmania donovani
  complex
Leishmania mexicana
  complex
Leishmania tropica complex
**Historical Perspective of
  Trypanosomiasis**

Trypanosoma brucei
  gambiense
Trypanosoma brucei
  rhodesiense
Trypanosoma cruzi
Trypanosoma rangeli
Looking Back

LEARNING OBJECTIVES

On completion of this chapter and review of its figures and corresponding photomicrographs, the successful learner will be able to:

5-1. Define the following key terms:
Amastigote (*pl.*, amastigotes)
Anergic
Arthralgia (*pl.*, arthralgias)
Baghdad boil (*pl.*, Baghdad boils)
Bay sore
Blepharoplast
Cardiomegaly
Chagas' disease
Chagoma
Chancre
Chiclero ulcer
Congenital transmission
Cutaneous
Dum dum fever
Edema
Epimastigote (*pl.*, epimastigotes)
Erythematous
Espundia
Forest yaws
Glomerulonephritis
Hemoflagellate (*pl.*, hemoflagellates)

Hepatosplenomegaly
Kala-azar
Kerandel's sign
Kinetoplast
Leishmaniasis
Lymphadenopathy
Megacolon
Megaesophagus
Montenegro skin test
Mucocutaneous
Myalgia (*pl.*, myalgias)
Myocarditis
Nagana
Oriental sore
Pian bois
Parasitemia (*pl.*, parasitemias)
Promastigote (*pl.*, promastigotes)
Pruritis
Romaña's sign
Schizodeme analysis
Somnolence
Trypanosomiasis
Trypomastigote (*pl.*, trypomastigotes)
Uta
Visceral

Winterbottom's sign
Xenodiagnosis
Zymodeme analysis

5-2. State the geographic distribution of the hemoflagellates.

5-3. State the common name of the conditions and diseases associated with each of the hemoflagellates.

5-4. Given a list of parasites, select those belonging to the class Zoomastigophora.

5-5. Construct, describe, and compare and contrast the life cycle of each hemoflagellate.

5-6. Identify and describe the populations prone to contracting clinically significant symptoms and disease processes associated with each of the pathogenic hemoflagellates.

5-7. Identify and describe each of the following as they relate to the hemoflagellates:
   A. Treatment options
   B. Prevention and control measures

5-8. Determine the specimen of choice, alternative specimen type where appropriate, collection protocol, and laboratory diagnostic technique required for the recovery of each of the hemoflagellates.

5-9. Given the name, description, photomicrograph, and/or diagram of a hemoflagellate:
   A. Identify, describe, and/or label characteristic structures, when appropriate.
   B. State the purpose of the designated characteristic structure(s).
   C. Name the parasite, including its morphologic form.

5-10. Analyze case studies that include pertinent patient information and laboratory data and:
   A. Identify and describe the function of key differential characteristic structures.
   B. Identify each responsible hemoflagellate organism by scientific name, common name, and morphologic form, with justification, when indicated.
   C. Identify the associated symptoms, diseases, and conditions associated with the responsible parasite.

D. Construct a life cycle associated with each hemoflagellate parasite present that includes corresponding epidemiology, route of transmission, infective stage, and diagnostic stage.

E. Propose each of the following related to stopping and preventing hemoflagellate infections:
   1. Treatment options
   2. Prevention and control plan

F. Determine the specimen of choice and alternative specimen types, where appropriate, as well as the appropriate laboratory diagnostic technique for the recovery of each hemoflagellate.

G. Recognize sources of error, including but not limited to, those involved in specimen collection and processing and specimen testing, and propose solutions to remedy them.

H. Interpret laboratory data, determine specific follow-up tests that could or should be done, and predict the results of those tests.

I. Determine additional morphologic forms, when appropriate, that may also be detected in clinical specimens.

5-11. Compare and contrast the similarities and differences between:
   A. The hemoflagellates covered in this chapter
   B. The hemoflagellates covered in this chapter and the other parasites covered in this text

5-12. Identify and describe the standard, immunologic, and new laboratory diagnostic approaches for the recovery of hemoflagellates in clinical specimens.

5-13. Given prepared laboratory specimens and, with the assistance of this manual, the learner will be able to:
   A. Differentiate hemoflagellate organisms from artifacts.
   B. Differentiate the hemoflagellate organisms from each other and from the other appropriate categories of parasites.
   C. Correctly identify each hemoflagellate parasite by scientific, common name, and morphologic form based on its key characteristic structure(s).

CASE STUDY 5-1   UNDER THE MICROSCOPE

Nine-year-old Charles, an African boy, recently emigrated to the United States from Kenya with his family. He began complaining of chills and diarrhea 2 weeks prior to the office visit. After taking his temperature, which revealed a fever, his mother took him into his pediatrician's office. During the examination, the doctor found a skin lesion on his right arm and marked hepatosplenomegaly. A complete blood count (CBC) was ordered, which revealed that Charles was anemic. The doctor, afraid that the child was experiencing dum dum fever (kala-azar), ordered a biopsy of the infected skin lesion and blood for parasite study.

When the specimens were received in the laboratory, the laboratory technician on duty made slides of the skin lesion material and blood, stained them with Giemsa stain, and carefully examined the slides. No parasites were found in the blood slide. The biopsy slide revealed an oval organism (see diagram); it contained one nucleus, a parabasal body, and an axoneme-like structure.

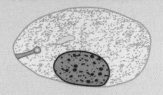

Questions for Consideration
1. What parasite do you suspect? (Objective 5-10B)
2. Which morphologic form of the parasite was described in the biopsy slide? (Objective 5-10B)
3. Indicate where Charles might have come into contact with parasites and identify the factors that most likely contributed to this contact. (Objectives 5-10D)
4. Name two other geographic populations at risk of contracting parasitic infections. (Objectives 5-10D)
5. Name two other symptoms associated with parasitic infections that individuals such as the patient in this case study may experience. (Objective 5-10C)
6. Why did the physician additionally order blood to be examined for parasites? (Objectives 5-10F)

FOCUSING IN

Members of the clinically significant group of parasites located in blood and tissue that move by means of flagella, known as the hemoflagellates, belong to the genera *Leishmania* and *Trypanosoma*. There are four morphologic forms of clinical significance associated with these **hemoflagellates:** amastigote, promastigote, epimastigote, and trypomastigote, all of which are defined and described in detail in this chapter. Although the specific life cycle may vary, all the organisms in these two genera involve some combination of the four morphologic forms. The transmission of all hemoflagellates is via the bite of an arthropod vector. The major difference between the two genera is the primary diagnostic form found in each; for *Leishmania* it is the amastigote and for *Trypanosoma* it is the trypomastigote, with the exception of *Trypanosoma cruzi,* in which amastigotes may also be found. Speciation within the genera usually depends heavily on the patient history and clinical symptoms. Because of the

importance of this information, this text provides a discussion of the geographic distribution and symptomatology of each hemoflagellate.

Suspicions of hemoflagellate disease processes are typically confirmed by more advanced diagnostic techniques, such as serologic tests. Because the initial diagnosis of hemoflagellate infections relies primarily on the detection of the morphologic forms, this text will begin with a detailed discussion of the morphologic forms.

MORPHOLOGY AND LIFE CYCLE NOTES

Morphology

Amastigotes. The average roundish to oval **amastigote** measures 5 by 3 μm in size (Figs. 5-1 and 5-2; Table 5-1). The amastigote contains a nucleus, a basal body structure (called a **blepharoplast**), and a small parabasal body. The large single nucleus is typically located off-center, sometimes present more toward the edge of the organism. The dotlike blepharoplast gives rise to and is attached to an axoneme. The axoneme extends to the edge of the organism. The single parabasal body is located adjacent to the blepharoplast. **Kinetoplast** is an umbrella term often used to refer to the blepharoplast and small parabasal body.

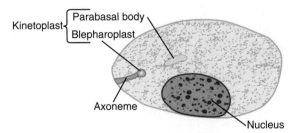

Average size: 5 μm by 3 μm

FIGURE 5-1 Amastigote.

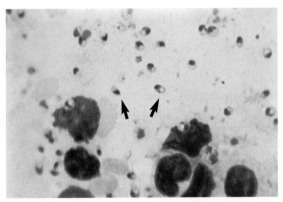

FIGURE 5-2 Amastigotes of *Leishmania* spp. *(From Mahon CR, Lehman DC, Manuselis G: Textbook of diagnostic microbiology, ed 4, St Louis, 2011, Saunders.)*

Promastigotes. The typical **promastigote** measures 9 to 15 μm in length (Figs. 5-3; Table 5-2). The large single nucleus is located in or near the center of the long slender body. The kinetoplast is located in the anterior end of the organism. A single free flagellum extends anteriorly from the axoneme.

Epimastigotes. The average **epimastigote** measures approximately 9 to 15 μm in length (Fig. 5-4; Table 5-3). The body is slightly wider than

TABLE 5-1	Amastigote: Typical Characteristics at a Glance
Parameter	**Description**
Size	5 by 3 μm
Shape	Round to oval
Nucleus	One, usually off center
Other features	Kinetoplast present, consisting of dotlike blepharoplast from which emerges a small axoneme
	Parabasal body located adjacent to the blepharoplast

TABLE 5-2	Promastigote: Typical Characteristics at a Glance
Parameter	**Description**
Size	9-15 μm long
Appearance	Long and slender
Nucleus	One, located in or near center
Other features	Kinetoplast, located in anterior end
	Single free flagellum, extending from anterior end

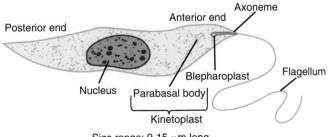

Size range: 9-15 μm long

FIGURE 5-3 Promastigote.

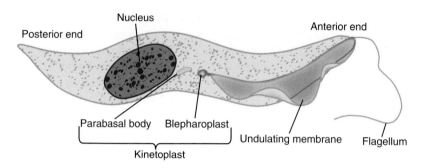

Size range: 9-15 μm long

FIGURE 5-4 Epimastigote.

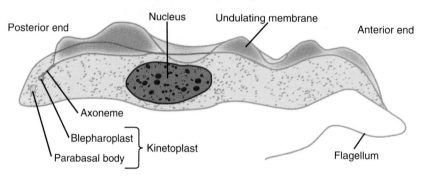

Size range: 12-35 μm by 2-4 μm

FIGURE 5-5 Trypomastigote.

TABLE 5-3	Epimastigote: Typical Characteristics at a Glance
Parameter	**Description**
Size	9-15 μm long
Appearance	Long and slightly wider than promastigote form
Nucleus	One, located in posterior end
Other features	Kinetoplast located anterior to the nucleus
	Undulating membrane, extending half of body length
	Free flagellum, extending from anterior end

Trypomastigotes. The typical **trypomastigote** measures 12 to 35 μm long by 2 to 4 μm wide, and may often assume the shape of the letters C, S or U in stained blood films (Figs. 5-5 to 5-7; Table 5-4). The trypomastigote in Figure 5-5 is represented in its straight form for comparison purposes because it clearly denotes the individual structures. The long slender organism is characterized by a posteriorly located kinetoplast from which emerges a full body length undulating membrane. The single large nucleus is located anterior to the kinetoplast. An anterior free flagellum may or may not be present.

that of the promastigote. The large single nucleus is located in the posterior end of the organism. The kinetoplast is located anterior to the nucleus. An undulating membrane, measuring half the body length, forms into a free flagellum at the anterior end of the epimastigote.

General Morphology and Life Cycle Notes

The amastigote and trypomastigote are the two forms routinely found in human specimens. Amastigotes are found primarily in tissue and

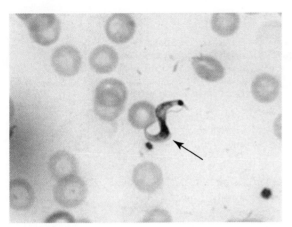

FIGURE 5-6 *Trypanosoma cruzi* trypomastigote exhibiting a characteristic full body length undulating membrane *(arrow)*. Note the S shape of the organism (Giemsa stain, ×1000). *(Courtesy of WARD'S Natural Science Establishment, Rochester, NY;* http://wardsci.com.*)*

TABLE 5-4	Trypomastigote: Typical Characteristics at a Glance
Parameter	**Description**
Size	12-35 μm long by 2-4 μm wide
Shape	C, S or U shape often seen in stained blood films
Appearance	Long and slender
Nucleus	One, located anterior to the kinetoplast
Other features	Kinetoplast located in the posterior end
	Undulating membrane, extending entire body length
	Free flagellum, extending from anterior end when present

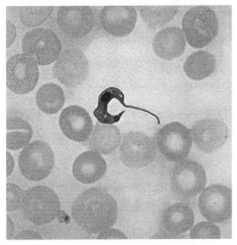

FIGURE 5-7 *Trypanosoma cruzi* C-shaped trypomastigote in a blood smear. *(From Mahon CR, Lehman DC, Manuselis G: Textbook of diagnostic microbiology, ed 4, St Louis, 2011, Saunders.)*

muscle, as well as the central nervous system (CNS) within macrophages, where they multiply. Trypomastigotes reproduce and are visible in the peripheral blood. The promastigote stage may be seen only if a blood sample is collected immediately after transmission into a healthy individual or when the appropriate sample is cultured. Although they may be seen in human blood

samples, epimastigotes are found primarily in the arthropod vector. Specific life cycle information is found under the discussion of each individual hemoflagellate.

> *Quick Quiz! 5-1*
>
> This is the only hemoflagellate morphologic form that does not have an external flagellum. (Objective 5-11A)
> A. Trypomastigote
> B. Amastigote
> C. Promastigote
> D. Epimastigote

Laboratory Diagnosis

Blood, lymph node and ulcer aspirations, tissue biopsies, bone marrow, and cerebrospinal fluid (CSF) are the specimens of choice for diagnosing the hemoflagellate morphologic forms. In addition, serologic and molecular tests are also available for confirming the presence of these organisms. Representative laboratory diagnosis methodologies are presented in Chapter 2, as well as in each individual parasite discussion, as appropriate.

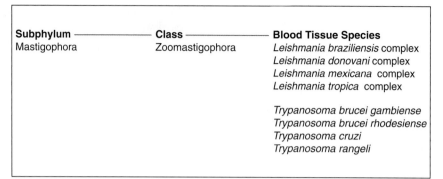

Subphylum —————————	Class —————————	Blood Tissue Species
Mastigophora	Zoomastigophora	*Leishmania braziliensis* complex
		Leishmania donovani complex
		Leishmania mexicana complex
		Leishmania tropica complex
		Trypanosoma brucei gambiense
		Trypanosoma brucei rhodesiense
		Trypanosoma cruzi
		Trypanosoma rangeli

FIGURE 5-8 Parasite classification—the hemoflagellates.

Quick Quiz! 5-2

Hemoflagellates are typically found in stool samples. (Objective 5-8)
A. True
B. False

Pathogenesis and Clinical Symptoms

The symptoms associated with hemoflagellate infections range from a small red papule at the infection site, with intense itching, secondary bacterial infections, fever, and diarrhea, to kidney involvement, mental retardation, a comatose state, and death. In some cases, the initial skin lesions spontaneously heal, whereas in others they may remain dormant for months or even years.

Quick Quiz! 5-3

The symptoms of hemoflagellate infections range from minor, such as irritation at the infection site, to serious (comatose state and death). (Objective 5-6)
A. True
B. False

HEMOFLAGELLATE CLASSIFICATION

There are a number of hemoflagellate species known to cause human infections, some of which have only been known to occur on rare occasions. A discussion of each of these organisms is beyond the scope of this chapter. For the purpose of discussing the *Leishmania* species, this chapter will address them within the classification complexes of more popular texts and literature, as opposed to the individual species. Only those hemoflagellates known to cause more frequent human disease are covered. The individual species are identified and classified in Figure 5-8.

HISTORICAL PERSPECTIVE OF LEISHMANIASIS

Leishmaniasis is a general term used to describe diseases caused by the hemoflagellate genus *Leishmania*. Although its origins remain unclear, what is obvious is that the organisms in this genus and their respective vectors have made successful migrations and adaptations to many environments worldwide. Leishmaniasis has a long history, as evidenced by the depictions on pottery from Ecuador and Peru around the first century AD. The different groups of people exposed to the organism have provided us with a number of common names for the diseases caused by *Leishmania* spp. (e.g., **Baghdad boils, bay sore, chiclero ulcer, dum dum fever, espundia, forest yaws, kala-azar, oriental sore, pian bois,** and **uta**). Table 5-5 describes each of these conditions. Increased travel and exposure to different environments has resulted in the transmission of the various **parasitemias,** a general term

TABLE 5-5	Diseases and Conditions Associated with Leishmaniasis
Disease or Condition	**Description**
Baghdad boils	A common name for an infection with *Leishmania tropica*; it is a cutaneous form of leishmaniasis presenting with pus-containing ulcers
Bay sore	A common name for a cutaneous form of infection caused by *Leishmania mexicana*
Chiclero ulcer	A form of cutaneous leishmaniasis cased by *L. mexicana*; it is commonly found in Belize, Guatemala, and the Yucatan peninsula in areas where chicle sap is harvested for making chewing gum
Dum dum fever	A common name for the visceral leishmaniasis caused by *Leishmania donovani*
Espundia	Another name for an infection resulting from *Leishmania braziliensis*, the principle cause of mucocutaneous disease in Central and South America, particularly in Brazil
Forest yaws	Another name for an infection with *Leishmania guyanensis*, the principle cause of mucocutaneous leishmaniasis in the Guianas, parts of Brazil and Venezuela; also known as pian bois
Kala-azar	Another name for the most severe form of visceral leishmaniasis caused by members of the *Leishmania donovani* complex
Oriental sore	A common reference for the cutaneous leishmaniasis caused by the infecting agents comprising the *Leishmania tropic* complex
Pian bois	Another name for infection with *L. guyanensis*; also known as forest yaws
Uta	A reference to mucocutaneous leishmaniasis in the Peruvian Andes

describing parasitic infection of the blood, into new environments, finding new host organisms and new vectors.

Leishmania spp. are generally grouped for discussion in one of several ways—in complexes of organisms or taxonomic groupings, their vectors, or the clinical nature of the disease caused. The four main complexes considered and described herein are the *Leishmania braziliensis*, *Leishmania donovani*, *Leishmania mexicana*, and *Leishmania tropica* complexes.

Leishmania braziliensis complex
(leesh-may' nee-uh/bra-zil" i-en'sis)

Common associated disease and condition names: Mucocutaneous leishmaniasis, chiclero ulcer, espundia, forest yaws, pian bois, uta.

The *Leishmania braziliensis* complex of organisms is found in Mexico, Argentina, Panama, Colombia, the Peruvian Andes, Guiana, Brazil, Bolivia, Paraguay, Ecuador, and Venezuela. This group of parasites is comprised of *Leishmania braziliensis*, *Leishmania panamensis*, *Leishmania peruviana*, and *Leishmania guyanensis*. This

leishmanial complex and the diseases for which its organisms are the causative agent may also be referred to as New World because of their geographic location in what is commonly considered the New World.

Laboratory Diagnosis

The specimen of choice for identifying the amastigotes of *L. braziliensis* complex is a biopsy of the infected ulcer. Microscopic examination of the Giemsa-stained preparations should reveal the typical amastigotes. Promastigotes may be present when the sample is collected immediately after introduction into the patient. Other more commonly used diagnostic methods include culturing the infected material, which often demonstrates the promastigote stage, and serologic testing. As enzyme analysis and molecular techniques have become more widely available, diagnostic criteria have begun to change as well. However, restriction analysis of kinetoplast DNA, a technique referred to as **schizodeme analysis**, nuclear DNA hybridization, and isoenzyme patterns, known as **zymodeme analysis**, still tend to remain research procedures and are

TABLE 5-6	*Leishmania braziliensis* Complex: Epidemiology		
Subspecies	**Geographic Distribution**	**Vector**	**Reservoir Hosts**
L. braziliensis	Mexico to Argentina	*Lutzomyia* and *Psychodopygus* sandflies for all species comprising this complex	Dogs and forest rodents for all species comprising this complex
L. panamensis	Panama and Colombia		
L. peruviana	Peruvian Andes		
L. guyanensis	Guiana, Brazil, Venezuela		

not currently performed in mainstream clinical diagnostic testing environments.

Life Cycle Notes

Sandflies of the genera *Lutzomyia* and *Psychodopygus* are responsible for transmitting the promastigotes of the species of the *L. braziliensis* complex into unsuspecting humans via a blood meal, resulting in a skin bite. The promastigotes quickly invade the reticuloendothelial cells and transform into amastigotes, which actively reproduce, causing tissue destruction. Reproduction and invasion of additional cells then occur. The skin and mucous membrane areas of the body are primarily affected. The diagnostic stage for the species of the *L. braziliensis* complex is the amastigote. In addition, the amastigote serves as the infective stage for the sandfly. On ingestion, during a blood meal of an infected human, the amastigotes transform back into promastigotes in the fly midgut. These promastigotes multiply and the resulting developed forms eventually migrate into the salivary gland of the fly, where they are ready to be transferred to a new human during a blood meal. Thus, the cycle repeats itself.

Epidemiology

The *L. braziliensis* complex is composed of *L. braziliensis* (found from Mexico to Argentina), *L. panamensis* (found in Panama and Colombia), *L. peruviana* (found in the Peruvian Andes), and *L. guyanensis* (found in Guiana, parts of

Brazil, and Venezuela). The organisms in this complex may also be found in Ecuador, Bolivia, Paraguay, and other Central and South American countries, particularly in the rain forest regions, where chicle sap for chewing gum is harvested (known under these circumstances as chiclero ulcer). Transmission is generally through the bite of the *Lutzomyia* or *Psychodopygus* sandfly and there are numerous reservoir hosts, including a variety of forest rodents and domestic dogs. Table 5-6 illustrates the relationships among the members of this complex, the geographic region in which they tend to thrive, vectors, and host reservoirs.

Clinical Symptoms

▓ **Mucocutaneous Leishmaniasis.** Symptoms of an infection with a member of the *L. braziliensis* complex typically occur within a few weeks to months after transmission into a previously uninfected human. Large ulcers in the oral or nasal mucosa areas (**mucocutaneous**) develop in a number of these patients after the initial invasion of the reticuloendothelial cells. There may be large cutaneous lesions, mucosal lesions, or a combination of both. A **cutaneous (meaning affecting or relating to the skin)** lesion may heal on its own. However, untreated cases of mucosal lesions result in the eventual destruction of the nasal septum. The lips, nose, and other surrounding soft parts may also be affected in these infections. Edema and secondary bacterial infections, combined with numerous mucosal lesions, may cause disfigurement of the patient's face. Death is usually attributed to a secondary bacterial infection.

Treatment

The most widely used antileishmanial agent for the treatment of mucocutaneous leismaniasis is with antimony compounds. However, *L. braziliensis* has shown an increased resistance to pentavalent antimonials such as sodium stibogluconate (Pentosam). Even with drug resistance and the adverse side effects, these classes of drugs are still considered the most effective treatment for *L. braziliensis* complex infections. Alternative treatments for *L. braziliensis* complex infections include liposomal amphotericin B (Ambisome) and oral antifungal drugs such as fluconazole (Diflucan), ketoconazole (Nizoral) and itraconazole (Sporonox).

Prevention and Control

Public awareness through education programs in endemic areas and exercising personal protection against contact with sandflies (e.g., protective clothing, repellents, screening) are preventive measures against infections with *L. braziliensis* complex members. In addition, prompt treatment and eradication of infected ulcers, and control of the sandfly population and reservoir hosts, help prevent the spread of future disease. Work to produce a vaccine against members of the *L. braziliensis* complex and other *Leishmania* spp. is ongoing, with some vaccines for animals (dogs) presently in experimental trials.

 Quick Quiz! 5-4

Of the following laboratory diagnostic methods, which is the most commonly used for the recovery of members of the *L. braziliensis* complex? (Objective 5-8)
A. Schizodeme analysis
B. Culture of infected material
C. Identifying amastigotes in infected material
D. Zymodeme analysis

 Quick Quiz! 5-5

The organism causing chiclero ulcer is most likely found in: (Objectives 5-1 and 5-2)
A. Texas
B. South American rainforest region
C. Nova Scotia
D. Egypt

 Quick Quiz! 5-6

Which of the following is not an acceptable treatment for mucocutaneous leishmaniasis caused by *L. braziliensis*? (Objective 5-7A)
A. Amoxicillin
B. Pentosam
C. Ambisome
D. Fungizone

Leishmania donovani complex
(leesh-may′ nee-uh/don″ o-vay′ nigh)

Common associated disease and condition names: Visceral leishmaniasis, kala-azar, dum dum fever.

The *Leishmania donovani* complex of organisms is found in India, Pakistan, Thailand, Africa, the Peoples Republic of China, the Mediterranean, Europe, Africa, the Near East, parts of the former Soviet Union, the Middle East, Yemen, Oman, Iraq, Kuwait, Saudi Arabia, United Arab Emirates, Bahrain, and Central and South America. This group is comprised of *L. donovani*, *Leishmania infantum*, and *Leishmania chagasi*. This leishmanial complex and the diseases for which its organisms are the causative agent may also be referred to as Old or New World, depending on the geographic location of the species of *Leishmania* involved.

Laboratory Diagnosis

The **Montenegro skin test** is a screening test similar to that of the tuberculin skin test; it is

TABLE 5-7	*Leishmania donovani* Complex: Epidemiology		
Subspecies	**Geographic Distribution**	**Vector**	**Reservoir Hosts**
L. donovani chagasi	Central America, especially Mexico, West Indies, South America	*Lutzomyia* sandfly	Dogs, cats, foxes
L. donovani donovani	Parts of Africa, India, Thailand, Peoples Republic of China, Burma, East Pakistan	*Phlebotomus* sandfly	India, none; China, dogs
L. donovani infantum	Mediterranean Europe, Near East, Africa; also in Hungary; Romania, southern region of former Soviet Union, northern China, southern Siberia	*Phlebotomus* sandfly	Dogs, foxes, jackals, porcupines

used for screening large populations at risk for infections caused by *Leishmania* spp. Its reliability in detecting exposure to the organisms causing leishmaniasis is related to the patient's disease status. It is not a good method for diagnosing active disease. Giemsa-stained slides of blood, bone marrow, lymph node aspirates, and biopsies of the infected areas are better choices for demonstrating the diagnostic amastigote forms. Some consider the sternal marrow aspirate to be the specimen of choice, but the organism can be seen in Giemsa-stained buffy coat films prepared from venous blood, a safer, less invasive procedure. Blood, bone marrow, and other tissues may also be cultured; these samples often show the promastigote forms. Serologic testing is available using IFA (indirect fluorescent antibody), ELISA (enzyme-linked immunosorbent assay), and DAT (direct agglutination test). In addition, schizodeme analysis, zymodeme analysis, and nuclear DNA hybridization are primarily available on a research basis; these may become a more popular diagnostic method in the future.

Life Cycle Notes

The life cycle of the members of the *L. donovani* complex is identical to that of *L. braziliensis*, with only two exceptions. First, the specific sandfly species responsible for *L. donovani* transmission vary with each of the three subspecies

(Table 5-7). Second, *L. donovani* primarily affects the visceral tissue of the infected human.

Epidemiology

The *L. donovani* complex is composed of *L. donovani* (found in India, Pakistan, Thailand, parts of Africa, and the Peoples Republic of China), *L. infantum* (found in the Mediterranean area, Europe, Africa, the Near East, and parts of the former Soviet Union), and *L. chagasi* (found in Central and South America). *L. donovani* and *L. infantum* are known to be endemic in areas of the Middle East, including Yemen, Oman, Kuwait, Iraq, Saudi Arabia, the United Arab Emirates, and Bahrain. The vector species and reservoir hosts vary among the three subspecies of the *L. donovani* complex and are listed in Table 5-7.

Clinical Symptoms

▧ Visceral Leishmaniasis. Patients suffering from **visceral** (pertaining to the internal organs of the body) leishmaniasis, also known as kala-azar or dum dum fever, often present with a nondescript abdominal illness and **hepatosplenomegaly** (enlargement of the spleen and liver). Early stages of disease may resemble malaria (see Chapter 6) or typhoid fever with the development of fever and chills. The onset of these symptoms is gradual and follows an incubation period ranging from

2 weeks to 18 months. Diarrhea, as well as anemia, may often be present. Additional symptoms, including weight loss and emaciation, tend to occur following parasitic invasion of the liver and spleen. Other than a rare papule, which most likely occurs at the bite site, skin lesions are absent. Advanced stages of disease result in kidney damage (e.g., **glomerulonephritis**, inflammation of the glomeruli of the kidney) and granulomatous areas of skin. A characteristic darkening of the skin may be noted. This symptom is referred to by the common disease name, kala-azar, which means black fever. Chronic cases usually lead to death in 1 or 2 years, whereas acute disease debilitates the patient and becomes lethal in a matter of weeks.

Treatment

Liposomal amphotericin B (Ambisome) is the drug of choice for treating visceral leishmaniasis. Sodium stibogluconate (Pentosam) is also an effective treatment for infections with *L. donovani* complex, but resistance has been demonstrated by organisms in India and the Mediterranean. Successful treatment has been accomplished with the use of gamma interferon combined with pentavalent antimony. Infected patients suffering from AIDS appear to respond well to allopurinol. It is further recommended that HIV-infected persons receive secondary prophylaxis as part of their treatment plan.

In the past decade two new drugs have been added to the treatment regimen for visceral leishmaniasis which include a combination of paramomycin and miltefosine. Neither of these drugs is available in the United States at this time.

Prevention and Control

Protection against sandflies by repellents, protective clothing, and screening are essential measures to reduce future *L. donovani* complex infections. Prompt treatment of human infections, as well as control of the sandfly population and reservoir hosts, will also help halt the spread of disease.

Notes of Interest and New Trends

It is important to note that *L. donovani* is capable of being transmitted person to person via blood transfusions. Particular concern over this mode of leishmaniasis transmission arose during and following the Gulf War. It is still of concern today because of the number of armed forces personnel stationed in the Persian Gulf region. Persons who are in and around this region may have been or are presently at risk of contracting the disease. The potential for those presently in the area to contract and bring home these organisms has resulted in the deferment of persons having spent time there for a minimal period of 12 months following their departure.

Research has been done to investigate the persistent levels of galactosyl-alpha(1-3)galactose antibodies in patients successfully treated for visceral leishmaniasis. There is some suspicion that these high levels may indicate parasite remnants, which remain even after the disease is cured. Further studies into this mystery may provide scientists with additional valuable information in the understanding and treatment of *L. donovani*.

Quick Quiz! 5-7

A common name for disease caused by *L. donovani* is: (Objective 5-3)
A. Visceral leishmaniasis
B. Kala-azar
C. Dum dum fever
D. All of the above

Quick Quiz! 5-8

The vector responsible for the transmission of *L. donovani* is: (Objective 5-5)
A. *Lutzomyia* sandfly
B. *Phlebotomus* sandfly
C. *Psychodopygus* sandfly
D. None of the above

TABLE 5-8	*Leishmania mexicana* Complex: Epidemiology		
Subspecies	**Geographic Distribution**	**Vector**	**Reservoir Hosts**
L. mexicana	Belize, Guatemala, Yucatan Peninsula	*Lutzomyia* sandfly for all species comprising this complex	Forest rodents for all species comprising this complex
L. pifanoi	Amazon River Basin, Brazil, Venezuela		
L. amazonensis	Amazon River Basin, Brazil		
L. garnhami	Venezuelan Andes		
L. venezuelensis	Venezuela		

Quick Quiz! 5-9

Which of the following items does not describe kala-azar? (Objectives 5-2, 5-5, and 5-12)
A. Commonly found in Iraq
B. Transmitted by the *Phlebotomus* and *Lutzomyia* sandfly species
C. Is not transmitted by blood transfusion
D. Can be serologically determined by ELISA, IFA, and DAT methods

Leishmania mexicana complex
(leesh-may′ nee-uh/mek-si-kah-nuh)

Common associated disease and condition names: New World cutaneous leishmaniasis, chiclero ulcer, bay sore.

The *Leishmania mexicana* complex of organisms is found in Belize, Guatemala, the Yucatan Peninsula, the Amazon River Basin, Venezuela, Brazil, and the Venezuelan Andes. *L. mexicana, Leishmania pifanoi, Leishmania amazonensis, Leishmania venezuelensis,* and *Leishmania garnhami* are the members of this group. This leishmania complex and the diseases for which its organisms are the causative agent may also be referred to as New World because of the geographic location of its members.

Laboratory Diagnosis

Definitive diagnosis of disease caused by members of the *L. mexicana* complex is made by demonstrating the amastigote form in Giemsa-stained preparations of lesion biopsy material. Culture on NNN medium demonstrates the promastigote stage of these organisms. Serologic testing using monoclonal antibodies and other techniques are available. Schizodeme analysis, zymodeme analysis, and nuclear DNA hybridization are available on a research basis.

Life Cycle Notes

The life cycle of the members of the *L. mexicana* complex is identical to that of *L. braziliensis.* The primary vectors are sandfly species of the genus *Lutzomyia.* Table 5-8 lists the organisms of this complex, geographic location of each species, vector for each organism, and reservoir host.

Epidemiology

The *L. mexicana* complex is composed of *L. mexicana* (found in Belize, Guatemala, and the Yucatan peninsula), *L. pifanoi* (found in the Amazon River basin and parts of Brazil and Venezuela), *L. amazonensis* (found in the Amazon basin of Brazil), *L. venezuelensis* (found in the forested areas of Venezuela), and *L. garnhami* (found in the Venezuelan Andes). Members of this complex are often transmitted by the bite of a *Lutzomyia* sandfly, with forest rodents serving as the reservoir host.

Clinical Symptoms

◼ **New World Cutaneous Leishmaniasis.** Also known as bay sore and chiclero ulcer, **cutaneous** leishmaniasis is usually characterized by a single pus-containing ulcer, which is generally self-healing. Approximately 40% of infections affect the ear and can cause serious damage to the surrounding cartilage. Infected patients initially develop a small red papule, located at the bite site, which is typically 2 cm or larger in diameter and may cause **pruritis** (intense itching). The incubation time and appearance of the papule vary with each subspecies. On occasion, because of **anergic** (the inability of an individual to mount an adequate immune response) and hypersensitivity immunologic responses, spontaneous healing of the ulcers does not occur. Diffuse cutaneous leishmaniasis (DCL) is rare in the New World, but incidents have been reported with all species comprising this complex. In diffuse cutaneous infections with *L. pifanoi*, the initial lesion appears, ulcerates or disappears and, after a period of months to years, appears in local and distant areas from the bite site with lepromatous-appearing lesions. *L. amazonensis* infections have been known to progress to an incurable diffuse cutaneous form of the disease. This latter form of cutaneous leishmaniasis usually occurs when the patient is anergic. A detailed discussion of the associated immunologic details relating to this disease process is beyond the scope of this chapter.

Treatment

Pentavalent antimonials, such as sodium stibogluconate (Pentosam), are considered the drug of choice for treating infections related to the species comprising the *L. mexicana* complex. Antimony combined with pentoxifylline taken orally three times a day for 30 days has been shown to be superior to antimony alone. Amphotericin B and liposomal amphotericin B (Ambisome) have also proven to be effective.

Prevention and Control

Protection against sandflies by repellents, protective clothing, and screening are essential measures to reduce future *L. mexicana* complex infections. Prompt treatment of human infections, as well as control of the sandfly and reservoir host populations, will also help halt the spread of disease.

> *Quick Quiz! 5-10*
>
> The specimen of choice for the recovery of *L. mexicana* complex members is: (Objective 5-8)
> A. CSF
> B. Stool
> C. Lesion biopsy material
> D. Duodenal contents

> *Quick Quiz! 5-11*
>
> Which of the following is not a reservoir host for *L. mexicana* complex? (Objective 5-5)
> A. Squirrels
> B. Chipmunks
> C. Rats
> D. Snakes

> *Quick Quiz! 5-12*
>
> Which of the following best describe disease caused by the *L. mexicana* complex? (Objective 5-6)
> A. Can disseminate into a diffuse cutaneous form
> B. Appears around the ears in approximately 40% of patients
> C. Both A and B are correct.
> D. None of the above

Leishmania tropica complex
(leesh-may′ née-uh/trop′i-kuh)

Common associated disease and condition names: Old World cutaneous leishmaniasis, oriental sores, Delhi boils, Baghdad boils, dry or urban cutaneous leishmaniasis.

The *Leishmania tropica* complex of organisms is found in the Mediterranean, Middle East, Armenia, Caspian region, Afghanistan, India, Kenya, Ethiopian highlands, southern Yemen, Turkmenistan deserts, Uzbekistan, Kazakhstan,

TABLE 5-9	*Leishmania tropica* Complex: Epidemiology		
Subspecies	**Geographic Distribution**	**Vector**	**Reservoir Hosts**
L. aethiopica	Highlands of Ethiopia, Kenya, perhaps Southern Yemen	*Phlebotomus* sandfly for all species comprising this complex	Rock hyrax
L. major	Former Soviet Union, Iran, Israel, Jordan, parts of Africa, Syria (esp. in rural areas)		Gerbils, other rodents
L. tropica	Mediterranean, parts of the former Soviet Union, Afghanistan, India, Kenya, Middle East (especially in urban areas)		Possibly dogs

northern Africa, the Sahara, Iran, Syria, Israel, and Jordan. It is comprised of *L. tropica, Leishmania aethiopica,* and *Leishmania major.* This leishmania complex and the diseases for which its organisms are the causative agent may also be referred to as Old World.

Laboratory Diagnosis

The laboratory diagnosis of *L. tropica* consists of microscopic examination of Giemsa-stained slides of aspiration of fluid underneath the ulcer bed for the typical amastigotes. Culture of the ulcer tissue may also reveal the promastigote forms. Serologic tests, such as IFA testing, are available. Schizodeme analysis, zymodeme analysis, and nuclear DNA hybridization are also available on a research basis.

Life Cycle Notes

With the exception of the specific sandfly species and the area of the body most affected, the life cycle of *L. tropica* complex is basically identical to that of *L. braziliensis.* All three of the *L. tropica* subspecies are transmitted by the *Phlebotomus* sandfly. *L. tropica* complex primarily attacks the human lymphoid tissue of the skin.

Epidemiology

The Leishmania tropica complex is composed of *L. tropica* (found in the Mediterranean region,

Middle East, Armenia, Caspian region, Afghanistan, India, and Kenya), *L. aethiopica* (found in the highlands of Ethiopia, Kenya, and Southern Yemen), and *L. major* (found in the desert regions of Turkmenistan, Uzbekistan, and Kazakhstan, Northern Africa, the Sahara, Iran, Syria, Israel, and Jordan). Members of this complex are often transmitted by the bite of the *Phlebotomus* sandfly, but the reservoir hosts for each of the three members of this complex differ (Table 5-9).

Clinical Symptoms

■ **Old World Cutaneous Leishmaniasis.** Also known as Old World leishmaniasis, oriental sore, and Baghdad or Delhi boil, cutaneous leishmaniasis is characterized by one or more ulcers containing pus that generally self-heal. Infected patients initially develop a small red papule, located at the bite site, which is typically 2 cm or larger in diameter and may cause intense itching. The incubation time and appearance of the papule vary with each subspecies (Table 5-10). On occasion, because of anergic and hypersensitivity immunologic responses, spontaneous healing of the ulcers does not occur. DCL occurs especially on the limbs and face when an immune response fails to take place. Thick plaques of skin, along with multiple lesions or nodules, usually result. A detailed discussion of the associated immunologic details relating to this disease process is beyond the scope of this chapter.

TABLE 5-10	*Leishmania tropica* Complex: Clinical Symptoms
Subspecies	**Clinical Symptoms**
L. aethiopica	Incubation: 2 mo-3 yr; small dry, red papule with possible intense itching; ulceration of papule occurs after several months
L. major	Incubation: as little as 2 wk; small red papule covered with serous exudate; possible intense itching; ulceration of papule occurs early
L. tropica	Incubation: 2 mo-3 yr; small dry, red papule with possible intense itching; papule ulcerates after several months

Treatment

As with the other leishmaniases, an effective treatment of *L. tropica* complex is sodium stibogluconate (Pentosam). The use of steroids, application of heat to the infected lesions, meglumine antimonate (Glucantime), pentamidine, and oral ketoconazole may be indicated for treating *L. tropica* complex infections. Paromomycin ointment may also be given to aid in healing.

Prevention and Control

In addition to controlling the sandfly and reservoir host populations, protection by the use of protective clothing, repellents, and screening are essential to prevent future *L. tropica* complex infections. In addition, the prompt treatment and eradication of infected ulcers are crucial to halt disease transmission. A vaccine has been developed and the preliminary results are promising; however, the clinical trials for this vaccine are still ongoing.

Notes of Interest and New Trends

A number of troops who participated in the Gulf War were stationed in Saudi Arabia and neighboring areas known to be endemic for *L. tropica*.

It is estimated that there are approximately 16,000 cases of leishmaniasis reported in Saudi Arabia every year. Following the war, a number of veterans, as well as members of their families, began to experience vague symptoms, including joint and muscle pains (**arthralgias** and **myalgias**, respectively), headaches, bleeding gums, hair loss, and intestinal disorders. Although a skin test (the Montenegro skin test) for leishmaniasis has been developed, patients in active disease will test negative. There is still a great deal of concern that undiagnosed patients may actually have leishmaniasis and are unknowingly spreading the disease.

Quick Quiz! 5-13

All the following are geographic regions in which the members of the *L. tropica* complex can be found except: (Objective 5-2)
A. Brazil
B. Uzbekistan
C. Iran
D. Syria

Quick Quiz! 5-14

The specimen of choice for the recovery of *L. tropica* complex members is: (Objective 5-8)
A. CSF
B. Fluid underneath the ulcer bed
C. Blood
D. Tissue biopsy

Quick Quiz! 5-15

The most common morphologic form seen in samples positive for *L. tropica* complex members is: (Objective 5-5)
A. Trypomastigote
B. Promastigote
C. Epimastigote
D. Amastigote

HISTORICAL PERSPECTIVE OF TRYPANOSOMIASIS

Trypanosomiasis is a general term used to refer to human diseases caused by hemoflagellates of the genus *Trypanosoma*. These diseases have been well documented through the ages. Ancient papyri discussed the disease from veterinary and human perspectives. In 1895, David Bruce, a Scottish pathologist, identified *Trypanosoma brucei* as the causative agent of the trypanosomal diseases known as **nagana** (a form of the disease often found in cattle) and sleeping sickness. The *T. brucei* first described has become known as *Trypanosoma brucei gambiense* (often abbreviated as *T.b. gambiense*). *Trypanosoma brucei rhodesiense* (*T.b. rhodesiense*) was not described until 1910 by Stephens and Fantham. *Trypanosoma cruzi*, the causative agent of **Chagas' disease**, was later described in 1909 by a young medical student in Brazil named Carlos Chagas.

Trypanosoma brucei gambiense
(trip-an″ o-so′ muh/broo′sye/ gam-bee-en′see)

Common associated disease and condition names: West African sleeping sickness, Gambian trypanosomiasis.
  T. brucei gambiense is found in the tropical areas of western and central Africa. Commonly called West African sleeping sickness or Gambian trypanosomiasis, the disease course for the illness caused by this organism is less aggressive than that of its East African counterpart.

Laboratory Diagnosis

Blood, lymph node aspirations, and CSF are the specimens of choice for diagnosing *T.b. gambiense*. Giemsa-stained slides of blood and lymph node aspirations from infected patients reveal the typical trypomastigote morphologic forms. Several tests may be performed on CSF—microscopic examination of the sediment for trypomastigotes, detection of the presence of

immunoglobulin M (IgM), and detection of the presence of proteins. Infected patients typically have high levels of both IgM and proteins in their CSF. In addition, serum IgM testing may be indicated. The presence of IgM in serum and/or CSF is generally considered diagnostic. A number of serologic tests are also available.

Life Cycle Notes

Humans become infected with *T.b. gambiense* following the injection of trypomastigotes by the tsetse fly during its blood meal. The entering trypomastigotes migrate through the bloodstream and into the lymphatic system, multiplying by binary fission. Although the healthy host's immune system is activated and some of the circulating trypomastigotes are destroyed, mutations of the parasite manage to escape and continue to reproduce. Eventually, invasion of the CNS may occur. The trypomastigotes are transmitted back to the tsetse fly vector when it feeds on an infected human. Once ingested by the tsetse fly, the trypomastigotes continue to multiply and eventually migrate back to the salivary gland, converting into epimastigotes along the way. Once in the salivary gland, the epimastigotes transform back into trypomastigotes, thus completing the cycle.

Epidemiology

T.b. gambiense is found in tropical West Africa and Central Africa, especially in shaded areas along stream banks where the tsetse fly vector breeds. The two species of tsetse flies responsible for the transmission of *T.b. gambiense* are *Glossina palpalis* and *Glossina tachinoides*. There are no known animal reservoir hosts.

Clinical Symptoms

◤ **West African (Gambian) Sleeping Sickness.** Symptoms associated with West African sleeping sickness begin to occur after an asymptomatic incubation period of a few days to several weeks. The first notable symptom that may appear is the development of a painful **chancre** (ulcer), surrounded by a white halo at the bite site. Fever, malaise, headache, generalized weakness, and anorexia are often experienced when the trypomastigotes settle into the lymphatic system. In addition, lymph node enlargement (**lymphadenopathy**) may be apparent during this time. A condition known as **Winterbottom's sign** refers to the enlargement of the cervical lymph nodes in reference to this trypanosomal disease. Other symptoms that may be seen during the glandular phase of the disease include **erythematous** (red) rash, pruritis, localized **edema** (swelling), and **Kerandel's sign** (a delayed sensation to pain). In patients in whom the central nervous system (CNS) becomes involved, mental retardation, tremors, meningoencephalitis, **somnolence** (excessive sleepiness), and character changes may develop. In the final stage of disease, the patient slips into a coma and death occurs, resulting from damage to the CNS, which is often coupled with other conditions, such as pneumonia or malaria. The course of the disease can last as long as several years.

Treatment

There are several medications available for the treatment of *T.b. gambiense* infections. These include melarsoprol, suramin, pentamidine, and eflornithine. The treatment of choice is situation-dependent and is dictated by a number of factors, including patient age (adult, child), stage of disease, and whether the patient is pregnant at the time. In addition, the toxicity levels of these medications are high; caution must be used when selecting the specific treatment and appropriate dosage.

Prevention and Control

The control of tsetse flies may be accomplished by destroying their breeding areas via chemical treatment and clearing of brush. Proper protective clothing, repellents, and screening, as well as prompt treatment of infected persons, will reduce the risk of future *T.b. gambiense* infections.

Notes of Interest and New Trends

T.b. gambiense has also been shown to be acquired through blood transfusion, organ transplantation, and **congenital transmission** (from pregnant mother to fetus).

Quick Quiz! 5-16

Of the following, which tests are considered diagnostic for trypanosomiasis? (Objectives 5-8 and 5-12)
A. Giemsa-stained blood slides revealing the trypomastigote
B. Giemsa-stained blood slides revealing the amastigote
C. Increased serum and CSF IgM levels
D. Both A and C are correct.
E. All of the above

Quick Quiz! 5-17

There are no known animal reservoir hosts for *T.b. gambiense*. (Objective 5-5)
A. True
B. False

Quick Quiz! 5-18

The enlargement of cervical lymph nodes in reference to trypanosomal disease caused by *T.b. gambiense* is referred to as: (Objective 5-1)
A. Chancre
B. Kerandel's sign
C. Winterbottom's sign
D. Somnolence

Trypanosoma brucei rhodesiense
(trip-an″ o-so′muh/broo′sye/ ro-dee″zee-en′see)

Common associated disease and condition names: East African sleeping sickness, Rhodesian trypanosomiasis.

Trypanosoma brucei rhodesiense is found in eastern and central Africa. Commonly called

East African sleeping sickness or Rhodesian trypanosomiasis, the disease course for the illness caused by this organism is much more aggressive than that of its West African counterpart.

Laboratory Diagnosis

The specimens of choice for the detection of the typical *T.b. rhodesiense* trypomastigotes are blood slides stained with Giemsa and microscopic examination of CSF sediment. Protein and IgM studies on CSF may also be performed. As with *T.b. gambiense*, the presence of IgM in the CSF is diagnostic for *T.b. rhodesiense*. In addition, serologic tests are available.

Life Cycle Notes

The only difference in the life cycles of *T.b. rhodesiense* and *T.b. gambiense* are the species of tsetse fly vector. The two primary species of tsetse fly vectors responsible for transmitting *T.b. rhodesiense* are *Glossina morsitans* and *Glossina pallidipes*. Additional species noted for attacking game animals may also transmit this organism.

Epidemiology

T.b. rhodesiense is found in East and Central Africa, especially in brush areas. Cattle and sheep, as well as wild game animals, are known reservoir hosts of this organism.

Clinical Symptoms

East African (Rhodesian) Sleeping Sickness. *T.b. rhodesiense* is a much more virulent organism than *T.b. gambiense*. Following a short incubation period, patients suffering from acute East African sleeping sickness experience fever, myalgia, and rigors. Winterbottom's sign may or may not be present. Lymphadenopathy is absent. Rapid weight loss is common and the CNS becomes involved early in the disease course. In addition, mental disturbance, lethargy, and anorexia may also be present. A rapid and fulminating disease results, with large numbers of trypanosomes circulating in the blood. Death, in part caused by subsequent kidney damage (glomerulonephritis) and **myocarditis** (inflammation of the heart), usually occurs within 9 to 12 months in untreated patients.

Treatment

The treatment of *T.b. rhodesiense* is identical to that for *T.b. gambiense*.

Prevention and Control

Because infections with *T.b. rhodesiense* tend to be more rapid in their course and often involve the neurologic system, extremely early treatment is crucial to halt further transmission of the disease. Additional measures include prompt medical treatment of infected domestic animals, as well as protective clothing, screening, and repellents. The vast species of potential reservoir hosts, coupled with the fact that breeding may occur wherever brush is abundant, primarily away from water sources, complicates prevention and control efforts. The clearing of brush areas and control of the tsetse fly population may reduce the risk of future disease transmission.

Quick Quiz! 5-19

The diagnostic stage of *T.b. rhodesiense* is the: (Objective 5-5)

A. Trypomastigote
B. Epimastigote
C. Promastigote
D. Amastigote

Quick Quiz! 5-20

Which of the following trypanosomal parasites that causes sleeping sicknesses is the more aggressive form? (Objective 5-11)

A. *Trypanosoma brucei gambiense*
B. *Trypanosoma brucei rhodesiense*
C. *Trypanosoma cruzi*
D. *Trypanosoma rangeli*

Trypanosoma cruzi
(trip-an"o-so'muh/kroo'zye)

Common associated disease and condition names: Chagas' disease, American trypanosomiasis.

Trypanosoma cruzi is found in southern portions of the United States, Mexico, and Central and South America. Commonly referred to as Chagas' disease or American trypanosomiasis, the disease course for this illness often presents itself with cardiac and gastrointestinal distress.

Laboratory Diagnosis

Giemsa-stained blood slides are the specimen of choice for detection of the typical *T. cruzi* trypomastigotes. Epimastigotes may rarely be seen in the circulating blood; however, this form is primarily found only in the arthropod vector. Lymph node biopsy Giemsa-stained slides, as well as blood culture, may reveal the typical amastigotes. A number of serologic tests, including complement fixation (CF), DAT, and indirect immunofluorescence (IIF), are also available for diagnostic purposes. The polymerase chain reaction (PCR) and ELISA testing methods are also available for diagnosing infections with *T. cruzi*; ELISA is presently used in blood donor screening to help ensure the safety of transfusable blood and transplantable organs.

Life Cycle Notes

T. cruzi is most frequently transferred to a human host when a reduviid bug vector defecates infective trypomastigotes near the site of its blood meal. The presence of the bite produces an itching sensation in the host. As the host scratches the bite area, the trypomastigotes conveniently gain entry into the host by literally being rubbed into the bite wound. Additional routes of transferring *T. cruzi* include blood transfusions, sexual intercourse, transplacental transmission, and entry through the mucous membranes when the bug bite is near the eye or mouth.

Following entry into the host, the trypomastigotes invade surrounding cells, where they transform into amastigotes. The amastigotes proceed to multiply, destroy the host cells, and then convert back into trypomastigotes. The resulting trypomastigotes migrate through the blood, penetrate additional cells in the body, and transform back into amastigotes, and the replication and destruction cycle repeats. A number of areas in the body may become infected, including the heart muscle, liver, and brain.

The *T. cruzi* trypomastigotes are transmitted back to the reduviid bug when it feeds, via a blood meal, on an infected human. On ingestion, the trypomastigotes transform into epimastigotes in the midgut. Multiplication of the epimastigotes produces thousands of additional parasites that convert back into trypomastigotes when they reach the hindgut. These trypomastigotes are then passed with the feces when the bug defecates near the site of its next blood meal, and thus the cycle begins again.

Epidemiology

T. cruzi is found primarily in South and Central America and only rarely in North America. The highest known prevalence of disease is in Brazil. Although first isolated in a *Panstrongylus megistus*, there are additional reduviid bug species that may serve as vectors. Also known as the kissing bug, conenose bug, and triatomid bug, the reduviid bug nests in human homes that are open in design. Although there are a number of known mammalian hosts, dogs and cats are of particular importance as reservoir hosts in Brazil.

Clinical Symptoms

🔹 **Chagas' Disease.** Named after its discoverer, Carlos Chagas, a Brazilian researcher who was a medical student at the time, Chagas' disease may be asymptomatic, chronic, or acute in nature. The most common initial symptom is the development of an erythematous nodule, known as a **chagoma,** at the site of infection produced by the proliferation of the *T. cruzi* organisms. This lesion may be present anywhere on the body, but it is most frequently located on the face. Edema as well as a rash around the eyes and face may subsequently occur. The painful chagoma may last 2 to 3 months before subsiding. Patients who contract *T. cruzi* through the ocular mucosa develop a characteristic conjunctivitis and unilateral edema of the eyelids, a condition known as **Romaña's sign.**

Chronic Chagas' disease may occur after the initial diagnosis of an acute disease or years to decades after being initially asymptomatic. The destruction of multiple tissues in this phase of infection results in patients who present with myocarditis, enlargement of the colon (sometimes referred to as **megacolon**) and esophagus (sometimes referred to as **megaesophagus**), and hepatosplenomegaly. In addition, CNS involvement, **cardiomegaly** (enlargement of the heart), and electrocardiographic changes may be seen. Complete blockage of the heart, as well as brain damage, may result, causing sudden death. The invasion and destruction of various other organs, including those already mentioned, may also contribute to death in chronic patients.

Patients suffering from acute Chagas' disease typically experience fever, chills, fatigue, myalgia, and malaise. An attack of acute infection may result in one of the following scenarios: (1) recovery; (2) transition to the chronic stage of disease; or (3) death, which usually occurs a few weeks after the attack.

The frequency and form of Chagas' disease seen in small children versus older children and adults vary. In general, Chagas' disease is most commonly seen in children younger than 5 years. These patients characteristically present with symptoms of CNS involvement and experience the most severe form of the disease. After experiencing an initial acute attack, adults and children older than 5 years usually develop a milder chronic or subacute form of the disease.

Treatment

The treatment of choice for infections with *T. cruzi* is nifurtimox (Lampit). Other medications include benznidazole, allopurinol, and the antifungal agent ketoconazole.

Prevention and Control

The eradication of reduviid bug nests and the construction of homes without open design are crucial measures necessary to help alleviate the future spread of the disease. DDT has proved to be useful, not only to control the reduviid population but also to decrease the incidence of malaria (see Chapter 6) when used in bug-infested homes. Educational programs designed to inform people, especially in endemic areas, of the disease, its transmission, and possible reservoir hosts may also prove to be helpful in the fight against *T. cruzi* transmission. In addition, the prospects for developing a vaccine appear to be promising.

Notes of Interest and New Trends

Because of the recent increase of *T. cruzi* infections among persons from the known endemic continent of South America, concern over the safety of donated blood from these individuals has emerged. In 1992, efforts were implemented to minimize the risk of transfusion transmission. All natives of and persons traveling to South America were prohibited from donating blood for transfusion purposes. Travel deferrals are generally 12 months after the departure date.

The traditional method of diagnosing *T. cruzi* trypomastigotes in endemic areas of South America is known as **xenodiagnosis.** In this procedure, a noninfected reduviid bug is allowed to feed on a person suspected of having Chagas' disease. Several weeks later, the feces of the bug is examined for the presence of trypomastigotes.

The PCR method has successfully detected *T. cruzi* in a number of studies conducted in recent years. One study has suggested that this assay may replace xenodiagnosis in patients with chronic disease and that it can be used in the screening of blood bank donors.

Quick Quiz! **5-22**

The specimen of choice for the detection of *T. cruzi* is: (Objective 5-8)
A. Stool
B. Blood
C. Tissue
D. Ulcer

Quick Quiz! **5-23**

Which of the following is the vector first identified as responsible for transmitting *T. cruzi*? (Objective 5-5)
A. *Phlebotomus* spp.
B. *Lutzomyia* spp.
C. *Panstrongylus megistus*
D. *Glossina* spp.

Quick Quiz! **5-24**

Which of the following is not a characteristic finding in Chagas' disease? (Objective 5-6)
A. Romaña's sign
B. Megacolon
C. Cardiomegaly
D. Somnolence

Trypanosoma rangeli
(trip-an″o-so′muh/ran-jel-ee)

Common associated disease and condition names: None known.

Trypanosoma rangeli is found in many of the same geographic regions as *T. cruzi*. There are presently no common names known for disease caused by this organism. Infections are generally asymptomatic and tend to show no pathologic changes or signs of disease.

Laboratory Diagnosis

Giemsa-stained blood slides are the specimen of choice for the detection of the typical *T. rangeli* trypomastigotes. *T. rangeli* trypomastigotes can be seen in the peripheral blood throughout the course of the illness. It can also be diagnosed by xenodiagnosis and serologic testing methods. PCR-based methods are also available.

Life Cycle Notes

The life cycle for *T. rangeli* is similar to that of *T. cruzi*. The vector responsible for transmitting *T. rangeli* is the reduviid bug, *Rhodius prolixus*. This vector actually transmits the parasitic infection via its saliva. *T. rangeli* can be viewed in the blood throughout the course of the infection.

Epidemiology

T. rangeli is commonly found in the same geographic areas as *T. cruzi*—regions of South and Central America, particularly in the areas surrounding Brazil, Venezuela, Colombia, Panama, El Salvador, Costa Rica, Honduras, and Guatemala. Its vector, *Rhodius prolixus,* is attracted to the same open house design as other reduviid bug species. It has numerous reservoir hosts such as monkeys, raccoons, dogs, cats, armadillos, and rodents.

Clinical Symptoms

Patients infected by *T. rangeli* are generally asymptomatic and demonstrate no evidence of illness. It is generally thought to be a benign infection.

Treatment

The treatment of *T. rangeli* infection is similar to that of *T. cruzi*. Nifurtimox and benzimidazole are the drugs of choice for treating *T. rangeli* infections.

Prevention and Control

Prevention and control measures for *T. rangeli* are the same as those for *T. cruzi*.

Quick Quiz! 5-25

The diagnostic testing methods for *T. rangeli* are the same as those for identifying and confirming and infection with *T. cruzi*. (Objectives 5-8, 5-11)
A. True
B. False

Quick Quiz! 5-26

The phrase that best describes the infection associated with *T. rangeli* is that it: (Objective 5-6)
A. Mimics that of individuals infected with *T. cruzi*
B. Causes South American sleeping sickness
C. Is considered a benign infection
D. Produces Winterbottom's sign

Quick Quiz! 5-27

Which of the following is not a prevention and control measure for *T. rangeli*? (Objective 5-7)
A. Use of DDT to control reduviid bug populations
B. Better housing construction
C. Removing overgrown vegetation
D. Educational programs in endemic areas

LOOKING BACK

The hemoflagellates have long been known to cause disease in humans and animals, with both *Leishmania* and *Trypanosoma* spp. dating back to prehistoric times. Increased travel and immigration are resulting in these organisms adjusting to and finding new environments in which to thrive, which they have been doing for many years. Diagnostic methods are rapidly changing how laboratory technicians identify these disease-causing parasites. While the new testing methods are evolving and becoming more clinically mainstream, good microscopy and staining techniques are still necessary diagnostic skills. It is also important to remember that these parasites are starting to show resistance to some common treatment modalities, many of which have adverse side effects. Education, prevention and control measures, and rapid treatment of infected persons are key to the health and well-being of those living in areas endemic for these parasites. The development of vaccines and better treatment methods is paramount.

TEST YOUR KNOWLEDGE!

5-1. Match each of the key terms (column A) with its corresponding definition (column B): (Objective 5-1)

Column A	Column B
A. Somnolence	**1.** The inability to mount an adequate immune response
B. Uta	**2.** Delayed sensation to pain
C. Kerandel's sign	**3.** Inflammation and painful ulceration at the insect bite site
D. Anergic	**4.** Excessive sleepiness
E. Chancre	**5.** Mucocutaneous leishmaniasis in the Peruvian Andes

5-2. The diagnostic stage for *Trypanosoma* spp. is the: (Objective 5-5)
A. Amastigote
B. Epimastigote
C. Trypomastigote
D. Promastigote

5-3. American trypanosomiasis is commonly referred to as: (Objective 5-3)
A. Cruzon's syndrome
B. Chiclero ulcer
C. Bay sore
D. Chagas' disease

5-4. Which of the following organisms is the causative agent of Baghdad boils? (Objective 5-3)
  A. *Leishmania donovani*
  B. *Trypanosoma brucei gambiense*
  C. *Trypanosoma brucei rhodesiense*
  D. *Trypanosoma cruzi*
  E. *Leishmania tropica*

5-5. Which of the following organisms is the causative agent of West African sleeping sickness? (Objective 5-3)
  A. *Leishmania donovani*
  B. *Trypanosoma brucei gambiense*
  C. *Trypanosoma brucei rhodesiense*
  D. *Trypanosoma cruzi*
  E. *Leishmania tropica*

5-6. Which of the following best describes the geographic region in which *Trypanosoma rangeli* is found? (Objective 5-2)
  A. Near East
  B. South and Central America
  C. Middle East
  D. Southeastern United States

5-7. The vector responsible for the transmission of chiclero ulcer is: (Objective 5-5)
  A. *Lutzomyia* and *Psychodopygus* sandflies
  B. *Phlebotomus* and *Psychodopygus* sandflies
  C. *Glossina* spp.
  D. *Lutzomyia* and *Phlebotomus* sandflies

5-8. Choose the best description of zymodeme analysis: (Objective 5-1)
  A. Nuclear DNA hybridization
  B. Restriction analysis of the kinetoplast DNA

  C. Analysis of the isoenzyme patterns of an organism
  D. None of the above

5-9. Winterbottom's sign is associated with which of the following hemoflagellates? (Objective 5-6)
  A. *Leishmania donovani*
  B. *Trypanosoma brucei gambiense*
  C. *Trypanosoma brucei rhodesiense*
  D. *Trypanosoma cruzi*
  E. *Leishmania tropica*

5-10. The reduviid bug is the vector for transmitting which of the following parasites? (Objective 5-5)
  A. *Leishmania donovani*
  B. *Trypanosoma brucei gambiense*
  C. *Trypanosoma brucei rhodesiense*
  D. *Trypanosoma cruzi*
  E. *Leishmania tropica*

5-11. Which of the following organisms causes the less aggressive form of sleeping sickness? (Objective 5-6)
  A. *Trypanosoma brucei gambiense*
  B. *Trypanosoma cruzi*
  C. *Trypanosoma brucei rhodesiense*
  D. *Trypanosoma rangeli*

5-12. Name three geographic regions in which *Leishmania mexicana* complex can be found. (Objective 5-2)

5-13. Describe Winterbottom's sign. (Objective 5-1)

5-14. Name three reservoir hosts for *T.b. rhodesiense*. (Objective 5-5)

5-15. Name three serologic testing methods used for diagnosing *T. cruzi* infections. (Objective 5-12)

CASE STUDY 5-2   **UNDER THE MICROSCOPE**

Martin, a 19-year-old college student, recently returned from a mission trip to Côte d'Ivoire in West Africa. He presented in the emergency room with severe myalgia, abdominal discomfort, diarrhea, vomiting, fever, chills, sweats, enlarged cervical lymph nodes, and diminished reactions to pain. A tender erythematous lesion was found on the calf of his right leg.

Questions for Consideration
1. What are the two specimens that typically reveal the morphologic forms of the responsible parasite? (Objective 5- 10F)
2. Which morphologic form do you suspect will be seen in this case? (Objective 5-10B)

Continued

CASE STUDY 5-2   UNDER THE MICROSCOPE—cont'd

3. Which two conditions are described by enlarged cervical lymph nodes and diminished reaction to pain ? (Objective 5-10C)
4. Name the responsible parasite in this case. (Objective 5-10B)
5. What are the two disease or condition names associated with the presence of this parasite? (Objective 5-10C)

6. Describe the life cycle for this organism. (Objective 5-10D)
7. Discuss the treatment for this infection. (Objective 5-10E)

COMPARISON DRAWINGS
Hemoflagellate Morphologic Forms

FIGURE 5-1. Amastigote

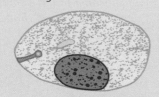

Average size: 5 μm by 3 μm

FIGURE 5-3. Promastigote

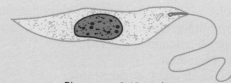

Size range: 9-15 μm long

FIGURE 5-4. Epimastigote

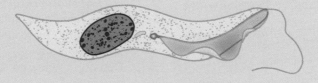

Size range: 9-15 μm long

FIGURE 5-5. Trypomastigote

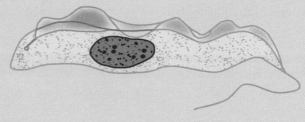

Size range: 12-35 μm by 2-4 μm

Select Sporozoa:
Plasmodium and *Babesia*

Michelle Mantooth and Elizabeth Zeibig

WHAT'S AHEAD

Focusing In
Plasmodium Species
  Historical Perspective
  Morphology and Life
    Cycle Notes
  Laboratory Diagnosis
  Pathogenesis and Clinical
    Symptoms
  Classification

  Plasmodium vivax
  Plasmodium ovale
  Plasmodium malariae
  Plasmodium falciparum
  Plasmodium knowlesi
Babesia Species
  Historical Perspective
  Morphology and Life Cycle
    Notes

  Laboratory Diagnosis
  Pathogenesis and Clinical
    Symptoms
  Classification
    Babesia microti
    Babesia divergens
Looking Back

LEARNING OBJECTIVES

On completion of this chapter and review of its figures and corresponding photomicrographs, the successful learner will be able to:

6-1. Define the following key terms:
Accolé
Aestivoautumnal malaria
Appliqué
Benign tertian malaria
Black water fever
Developing trophozoite (*pl.*, trophozoites)
Erythrocytic cycle
Exoerythrocytic cycle
Gametocyte (*pl.*, gametocytes)
Hemoglobinuria
Hemozoin
Hypnozoite (*pl.*, hypnozoites)
Immature schizont (*pl.*, schizonts)
Ischemia
Macrogametocyte (*pl.*, macrogametocytes)
Malarial Malaria
Malignant tertian malaria
Mature schizont (*pl.*, schizonts)

Maurer's dot (*pl.*, dots)
Merozoite (*pl.*, merozoites)
Microgametocyte (*pl.*, microgametocytes)
Oocyst (*pl.*, oocysts)
Ookinete
Paroxysm (*pl.*, paroxysms)
Quartan malaria
Recrudescence
Red water fever
Rigor
Ring form (*pl.*, forms)
Schizogony
Schizont (*pl.*, schizonts)
Schüffner's dot (*pl.*, dots)
Sporogony
Sporozoa
Sporozoite (*pl.*, sporozoites)
Texas cattle fever
Ziemann's dot (*pl.*, dots)
Zygote

6-2. State the geographic distribution of each *Plasmodium* and *Babesia* species.

6-3. State the common name of the conditions and diseases associated with each of the *Plasmodium* and *Babesia* species.

6-4. Given a list of parasites, select those belonging to the protozoan genus *Plasmodium*.

6-5. Given a list of parasites, select those belonging to the protozoan genus *Babesia*.

6-6. Briefly summarize the life cycle of each of the *Plasmodium* and *Babesia* species.

6-7. For each of the *Plasmodium* species:
   A. State the age of red blood cells most likely to become infected.
   B. State which morphologic forms are typically seen in the peripheral blood of patients with a mild infection, as well as those growth stages seen in a severe infection, where appropriate.

6-8. Identify and describe the populations prone to contracting, clinically significant symptoms, and disease processes associated with each of the pathogenic *Plasmodium* and *Babesia* species.

6-9. Identify and describe each of the following as they relate to the *Plasmodium* and *Babesia* species:
   A. Treatment options
   B. Prevention and control measures

6-10. Select the specimen of choice, collection protocol, and laboratory diagnostic techniques for the recovery of each of the *Plasmodium* and *Babesia* species.

6-11. Compare and contrast the *Plasmodium* and *Babesia* species from each other and from other groups of parasites in terms of the key features that the parasites have in common, as well as the features that distinguish them.

6-12. Given a description, photomicrograph, and/or diagram of *Plasmodium* and/or *Babesia*, correctly:
   A. Identify and/or label the designated characteristic structure(s).
   B. State the purpose of the designated characteristic structure(s).
   C. Identify the parasite by scientific name and morphologic form.
   D. State the common name for the associated conditions and diseases.

6-13. Analyze case studies that include pertinent patient information and laboratory data and:
   A. Identify each responsible *Plasmodium* and *Babesia* organism by scientific name

and morphologic form, with justification.
   B. Identify the associated symptoms, diseases, and conditions (including common names for associated conditions/diseases) associated with the responsible parasite.
   C. Construct a life cycle associated with each *Plasmodium* and *Babesia* parasite present that includes corresponding epidemiology, route of transmission, and infective and diagnostic stages.
   D. Propose each of the following related to stopping and preventing *Plasmodium* and *Babesia* infections:
      1. Treatment options
      2. Prevention and control plan
   E. Determine the specimen of choice, alternate specimen types when appropriate, and appropriate laboratory diagnostic techniques for the recovery of each *Plasmodium* and *Babesia* species
   F. Recognize sources of error, including but not limited to, those involved in specimen collection and processing and specimen testing, and propose solutions to remedy them.
   G. Interpret laboratory data, determine specific follow-up tests to be done, and predict the results of those tests.
   H. Determine additional morphologic forms, where appropriate, that may also be detected in clinical specimens

6-14. Describe the standard, immunologic, and new laboratory approaches for the recovery of *Plasmodium* and *Babesia* species in clinical specimens.

6-15. Given prepared laboratory specimens, and with the assistance of this manual, the learner will be able to:
   A. Differentiate *Plasmodium* and *Babesia* organisms from artifacts.
   B. Differentiate the *Plasmodium* and *Babesia* organisms from each other and from the other appropriate categories of parasites.
   C. Correctly identify each Plasmodium and *Babesia* parasite by its scientific and common names and morphologic form based on its key characteristic structure(s).

CASE STUDY 6-1 **UNDER THE MICROSCOPE**

Bruno, a 48-year-old businessman, presents at the emergency room with a 12-day history of headache, myalgia, nausea, and vomiting. Patient history reveals that Bruno is a consulting engineer for the Panama Canal. On his latest trip, he failed to take his prophylaxis for malaria. According to his general physician's records, all his immunizations (e.g., hepatitis, flu) are up to date. His fever was 103° F (39° C) at the time of initial examination, but alternated with periods of extreme cold and cyanosis. A complete blood count was ordered, along with parasite examination and urinalysis. The thin Giemsa film yielded the morphologic forms noted in the diagram as a, b, and c.

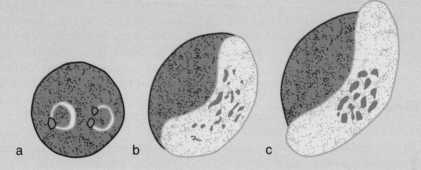

1. What parasite do you suspect? Note the genus and species. (Objective 6-13A)
2. Which factors in these diagrams were important in deciding the species of this organism? (Objective 6-13A)
3. Differentiate the three forms of the parasite shown in the diagram. What are the differences in morphology that allow you to differentiate forms b and c? (Objectives 6-11, 6-13A)
4. Given that the organism is the one you have identified, what other morphologic forms are likely to be seen in the peripheral blood of this patient? What additional forms might be seen if a different species in this genus were involved? (Objective 6-13H)
5. State the common name of the disease usually caused by this organism. (Objective 6-13B)
6. How did Bruno contract this parasitic infection? (Objective 6-13C)
7. Dark red, cleft-shaped dots are seen in the red blood cells of this patient. What are these dots called? Other species in this genus show light pink, stippling-like dots when infecting red blood cells. What are these dots called? (Objectives 6-11)

FOCUSING IN

Malaria and babesiosis refer to disease processes resulting from infections of parasites belonging to the phylum Apicomplexa. Their respective genera are *Plasmodium* and *Babesia*. Both genera of parasites belong to the class of parasites that have no obvious structures for the purpose of motility, known as **sporozoa**. Of approximately 200 known species of *Plasmodium*, only 10 have demonstrated the ability to cause infection in humans.

There are over 100 known species of *Babesia* and, of these species, four have been shown to cause human disease. With one exception, this chapter is limited to a discussion of the most common clinical isolates in these genera. The most clinically relevant organisms belonging to the genera of Plasmodium and Babesia, and the ones included in this discussion are *Plasmodium vivax*, *Plasmodium ovale*, *Plasmodium malariae*, *Plasmodium falciparum*, *Plasmodium knowlesi*, *Babesia microti*, and *Babesia divergens*.

The typical life history of each of these organisms involves more than 24 morphologic forms. However, for the purposes of this text, only the most commonly encountered forms in human specimens will be discussed. These are listed as follows (in chronologic order): ring form (also known as the early trophozoite), developing trophozoite, immature schizont, mature schizont, microgametocyte, and macrogametocyte. All these morphologic forms occur following the invasion of red blood cells (RBCs). This chapter is organized into two main sections, a discussion of *Plasmodium* species and then *Babesia* species.

PLASMODIUM SPECIES

As noted, there are five species of *Plasmodium* known to be of concern regarding transmission to humans. General information, including a historical perspective and generic description of the six most commonly encountered morphologic forms, is followed by a discussion of each of these species in detail.

Historical Perspective

Historical accounts of events leading to the formation of the United States have cited malaria as being of significance on several occasions. Malaria-infected individuals from southwest England apparently transported *Plasmodium* spp. parasites as they migrated to the New World. Malaria quickly spread throughout the colonies, resulting in a shortage of healthy workers. The demand for replacement workers played a significant role in the emergence of the African slave trade. Interestingly, many of those from West Africa who were brought to America to work did not contract malaria. It has since been determined that they were genetically protected from select species of malaria-causing *Plasmodium* spp. parasites.

Malaria was considered endemic in many of the colonies during the Revolutionary War, particularly in areas with significant water sources in which mosquito vectors thrived and soldiers often camped. A group of British soldiers, under the direction of General Charles Cornwallis, was no exception. After several exposures in areas in which malaria was rampant, almost all the British soldiers contracted malaria and were unable to continue fighting. Ultimately, General Cornwallis surrendered, resulting in a successful end to the war.

By some accounts, malaria was first described by a French army doctor, Charles Louis Alphonse Laveran, in 1880. In 1907, he received the Nobel Prize for Physiology or Medicine for his work on malaria. Since then, numerous physicians and scientists have studied the diseases caused by members of the genera *Plasmodium* and have made great strides toward our understanding of these diseases. Today, malaria lethally affects almost 2.5 million people worldwide. Although North America was declared malaria free in 1970, travel and immigration bring it back to the continent regularly.

Morphology and Life Cycle Notes

Ring Forms (Early Trophozoites). The **ring form**, as the name implies, refers to a ringlike appearance of the malarial parasite following invasion into a previously healthy RBC. The typical ring, when stained with Giemsa stain, consists of a blue cytoplasmic circle connected with or to, depending on the species, a red chromatin dot, also referred to in some texts as a nucleus. The space inside the ring is known as a vacuole.

Developing Trophozoites. The appearance of the **developing trophozoite** varies among the *Plasmodium* species. There are numerous growing stages in this category for each organism. However, remnants of the cytoplasmic circle and chromatin dot, which are in some cases both still intact until late in development, are present in the developing trophozoite form. Pigment, primarily brown in color, is often visible. In general, because the parasite is actively growing during this stage, the amount of RBC space invaded is significantly more than that of the ring form. A representative developing trophozoite will be described in more detail under the discussion of each malarial parasite.

Immature Schizonts. Although still unorganized, evidence of active chromatin replication is seen in the typical **immature schizont.** Visible cytoplasmic material surrounds the growing chromatin. Pigment granules, often brown in color, are also commonly seen. As the parasite continues to multiply, it expands and occupies more space within the RBC.

Mature Schizonts. Mature schizonts are characterized by the emergence of the fully developed stage of the asexual sporozoa trophozoite known as **merozoites.** The number and arrangement of these merozoites vary and are described in detail under the discussion of each malarial species. With the exception of *Plasmodium vivax*, cytoplasmic material is not visible and is presumed to be absent.

Microgametocytes. With the exception of *P. falciparum*, which is crescent-shaped, the typical **microgametocyte** is roundish in shape. This morphologic form consists of a large diffuse chromatin mass that stains pink to purple and is surrounded by a colorless to pale halo. Pigment is usually visible; its distribution and color vary by species.

Macrogametocytes. Macrogametocytes range in shape from round to oval, with the exception of *P. falciparum*, which is crescent-shaped. The compact chromatin mass is partially to completely surrounded by cytoplasmic material. Pigment is also present, and its color and distribution in this morphologic form vary by individual *Plasmodium* species. Specific details are described under the discussion of each species.

Life Cycle Notes. Members of the mosquito genus *Anopheles* are responsible for the transmission of malaria to humans via a blood meal. This vector transfers the infective stage of the parasite known as **sporozoites** from its salivary gland into the human bite wound. Following entrance into the body, the sporozoites are carried through the peripheral blood to the parenchymal cells of the liver. It is here that **schizogony** (asexual multiplication) occurs. This **exoerythrocytic cycle,** which literally means reproduction

outside of red blood cells (in this case in human liver cells), of growth and reproduction lasts from 8 to 25 days, depending on the specific *Plasmodium* species involved. The infected liver cells eventually rupture and introduce merozoites into the circulating blood. These migrating merozoites target age- and size-specific RBCs to invade and thereby initiate the phase of reproduction involving red blood cells known as the **erythrocytic cycle** of growth. These RBC specifics vary among each species and are described under the life cycle notes of each species. It is in this asexual phase that the plasmodia feed on hemoglobin and pass through the numerous stages of growth, including their six morphologic forms.

On formation of the merozoites, one of three paths may be taken. Some of the RBCs infected with merozoites rupture, releasing these forms to target and infect new RBCs, and this part of the cycle repeats itself. A number of erythrocytic cycles may occur. However, other infected RBCs containing merozoites develop into microgametocytes and macrogametocytes, and still others are destroyed by the immune system of an otherwise healthy individual. Although never demonstrated in human infection, it is presumed that **hypnozoites** (dormant *Plasmodium*-infected liver cells) may form during infection with *P. vivax* or *P. ovale*. These forms, also known as sleeping forms, may be dormant for months to years after the initial infection. The mechanism behind the reactivation of such cells was not well described in any of the references used to prepare this chapter. However, once stimulated, the hypnozoites rupture and introduce merozoites into the circulating blood, thus initiating the erythrocytic cycle and a relapse infection, or **recrudescence.**

Transmission of the parasite back into the vector occurs when the mosquito ingests mature male (micro) and female (macro) sex cells called **gametocytes** during a blood meal, thus initiating the sexual cycle of growth. Male and female gametocytes unite in the mosquito's stomach and form a fertilized cell called a **zygote** (also known as an **ookinete**). The zygote becomes encysted and matures into an **oocyst.** On complete maturation, the oocyst ruptures and releases numerous sporozoites, which migrate into the salivary gland of the mosquito and are ready to infect another unsuspecting human. Thus, the cycle repeats itself.

In addition to contracting malaria via an *Anopheles* mosquito bite, there are several other modes of transmission for *Plasmodium* species. Transfusion malaria, as the name implies, occurs when uninfected patients receive blood tainted with malaria collected from an infected donor. Malaria may also be spread through the sharing of needles and syringes, a common practice among intravenous drug users; this type of infection is referred to as mainline malaria. Although rarely documented, congenital malaria, which is the passing of the parasite from mother to child, may also occur.

Quick Quiz! 6-1

The infective stage of *Plasmodium* is (are) the: (Objective 6-6)
A. Merozoites
B. Oocyst
C. Sporozoites
D. Gametocytes

Laboratory Diagnosis

Giemsa-stained peripheral blood films are the specimens of choice for the laboratory diagnosis of malaria. Wright's stain may also be used and will result in an accurate diagnosis. However, because Giemsa is the recommended stain for all blood films submitted for parasite study, the specific morphologic discussion of each *Plasmodium* species is based on the use of this stain. Both thick and thin blood films should be made and examined. Thick blood smears serve as screening slides, whereas thin blood smears are used in differentiating the *Plasmodium* species. All blood films should be studied under oil immersion. It is important to note that mixed *Plasmodium* infections may occur, with the most frequently encountered being *P. vivax* and *P. falciparum*.

Careful and thorough screening of all smears is crucial to ensure the correct identification, reporting, and ultimately the proper treatment of all *Plasmodium* organisms present.

The timing of blood collection for the study of malaria is crucial to success in retrieving the malarial parasites. The various morphologic forms of parasites visible at any given time depend on the stage of organism development at the time of specimen collection. For example, when the infected RBCs rupture, merozoites are present in the circulating blood. This stage, when found, is difficult to serve as a species identifier. However, gametocytes may be present at this point in time and they are readily discernible. The greatest number of parasites is present in the blood in between characteristic bouts of fever and chills resulting from the release of merozoites and toxic waste products from infected RBCs, known as **paroxysms**. Thus, this is the optimal time to collect peripheral blood samples to determine the presence of *Plasmodium* spp. parasites (Table 6-1).

It is important to note that multiple sets of blood films, which, as noted, consist of thick and thin smears, are necessary to rule out malarial infections. It is recommended that blood be collected every 6 to 12 hours for up to 48 hours before considering a patient to be free of *Plasmodium* spp. parasites.

In addition to blood films, serologic tests and polymerase chain reaction (PCR) techniques for malaria are available. These tests are not that helpful in regard to the actual treatment of malarial infections. However, one benefit of

TABLE 6-1	Occurrence of Cyclic Paroxysms in Common *Plasmodium* Species	
Plasmodium Species	**Timing of Cyclic Paroxysms**
P. vivax	Every 48 hr
P. ovale	Every 48 hr
P. malariae	Every 72 hr
P. falciparum	Every 36-48 hr

serologic testing is that this methodology does appear to help rule out malaria in patients suffering from a fever of unknown origin, and PCR techniques can confirm the malarial speciation, but is usually not necessary. Representative laboratory diagnostic methodologies are presented in Chapter 2, as well as in each individual parasite discussion, as appropriate.

Quick Quiz! 6-2

The best time to collect blood for *Plasmodium* parasites is: (Objective 6-10)
A. Between paroxysms
B. During paroxysms
C. Morning
D. Evening

Pathogenesis and Clinical Symptoms

The typical patient remains asymptomatic following the initial mosquito bite and exoerythrocytic cycle of malarial infection. However, once the erythrocytic phase is initiated and large numbers of rupturing RBCs simultaneously occur, the resulting merozoites and toxic waste byproducts in the blood system produce the first clinical symptom, a paroxysm. Considered in part as an allergic response of the body to the development of the **schizonts** and to the circulating parasitic antigens following the release of merozoites, a paroxysm is characterized by chills (also known as **rigor**), typically lasting for 10 to 15 minutes or longer, followed by 2 to 6 hours or more of a fever. As the fever subsides and returns to normal, the patient experiences profuse sweating and extreme fatigue. The periodicity of paroxysms varies and is defined under the discussion of each *Plasmodium* species; periodicity often accounts for one of the common names associated with each *Plasmodium* species as well. Patients may experience these clinical symptoms as a result of having a recrudescence. A recurrence, or true relapse, occurs when patients become reinfected with rupturing hypnozoites

months to years after the initial infection, as is often the case with *P. vivax* and *P. ovale* infections.

Additional malarial symptoms may include headache, lethargy, anorexia, **ischemia** (insufficient blood supply in other body tissues caused by blockage of the capillaries and blood sinuses), nausea, vomiting, and diarrhea. Anemia, central nervous system (CNS) involvement, and nephrotic syndrome may occur in all *Plasmodium* infections. It is interesting to note that malaria may mimic a number of other diseases, including meningitis, pneumonia, gastroenteritis, encephalitis, or hepatitis. Specific clinical symptoms are described under the discussion of each individual organism.

Furthermore, persons exhibiting erythrocyte structural abnormalities such as heterozygous (Gd^{A-}/Gd^{B}) glucose-6-phosphate dehydrogenase (G6PD) deficiency and certain hemoglobinopathies (S, C, E, and thalassemia) tend to have a greater resistance to malarial infections than those who do not possess the abnormalities. Similarly, those individuals who are Duffy blood group–negative also tend to show a greater resistance than those who are positive for the antigens on their red blood cells.

Quick Quiz! 6-3

A paroxysm is: (Objective 6-1)
A. An allergic reaction
B. A periodic episode characterized by fever, chills, sweats, and fatigue
C. Both A and B are correct.
D. None of the above

Classification

Malaria belongs to the phylum Apicomplexa, class Aconoidasida, order Haemosporida, family Plasmodiidae, genus *Plasmodium*. All five of the *Plasmodium* species discussed in this chapter are found in the blood, as indicated in Figure 6-1.

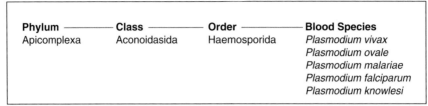

FIGURE 6-1 Parasite classification—*Plasmodium* species.

Plasmodium vivax
(Plaz-mo 'dee-um/vye' vacks)

Common associated disease and condition names: Benign tertian malaria, vivax malaria.

Morphology

■ **Ring Forms.** The cytoplasmic ring of the typical *P. vivax* ring form measures approximately one third the diameter of the red blood cell in which it resides (Figs. 6-2 and 6-3; and Table 6-2). A single chromatin dot serves as the connecting point of this delicate ring. A vacuole is visible inside the ring. The parasite may first be visible as a crescent-shaped mass at the outer edge of the red blood cell, a location known as **accolé** or **appliqué**.

■ **Developing Trophozoites.** Although remnants of the cytoplasmic ring may be visible, the parasite takes on more of an irregularly shaped ameboid appearance (Figs. 6-2 and 6-3; and Table 6-2). A single, large chromatin dot is present among the cytoplasmic material. The vacuole remains visible and basically intact until the late stage of development. The presence of **hemozoin** (a remnant of the parasite feeding on RBC hemoglobin visible as a brown pigment) becomes apparent in the cytoplasm of the parasite in this stage and increases in amount and visibility as the parasites mature.

■ **Immature Schizonts.** The immature schizont form of *P. vivax* is characterized by the presence of multiple chromatin bodies that emerge from progressive chromatin division (Figs. 6-2 and 6-3; and Table 6-2). Cytoplasmic material is present and often contains clumps of hemozoin.

TABLE 6-2	*Plasmodium vivax*: Typical Characteristics at a Glance
Relative age of infected RBCs	Only young and immature cells
Appearance of infected RBCs	Enlarged, distorted
Morphologic Form*	**Typical Characteristics (Based on Giemsa Staining)**
Ring form	Delicate cytoplasmic ring measuring one third of RBC diameter Single chromatin dot Ring surrounds a vacuole Accolé forms possible
Developing trophozoite	Irregular ameboid appearance Ring remnants common Brown pigment becomes apparent, increases in number and visibility as parasites mature
Immature schizont	Multiple chromatin bodies Often contains clumps of brown pigment
Mature schizont	12 to 24 merozoites occupy most of infected red blood cell Merozoites surrounded by cytoplasmic material Brown pigment may be present
Microgametocyte	Large pink to purple chromatin mass surrounded by colorless to pale halo Brown pigment common
Macrogametocyte	Round to oval cytoplasm Eccentric chromatin mass Delicate light-brown pigment—may be visible throughout cell

*All morphologic forms may also contain Schüffner's dots.

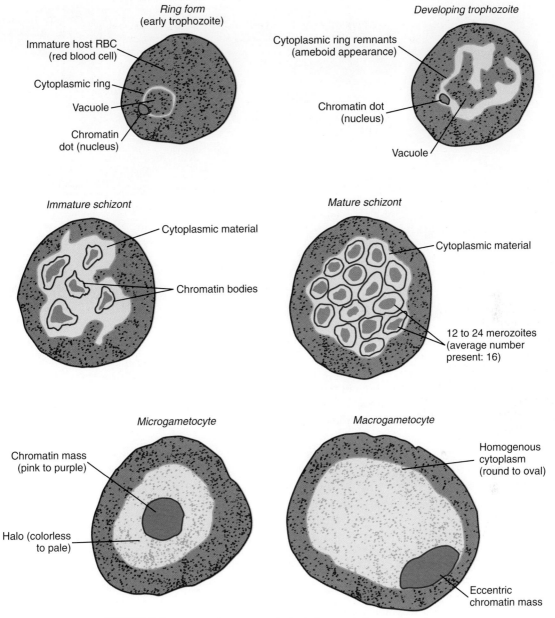

FIGURE 6-2 Commonly seen morphologic forms of *Plasmodium vivax*.

Mature Schizonts. The continuing division of chromatin results in 12 to 24 (average, 16) merozoites. These merozoites, surrounded by cytoplasmic material, occupy most of the RBCs. In some cases, the RBCs can hardly be detected. Brown pigment may also be present.

Microgametocytes. The typical *P. vivax* microgametocyte consists of a large pink to purple chromatin mass, when Giemsa-stained, which is surrounded by a colorless to pale halo. Evenly distributed cytoplasmic hemozoin is usually visible.

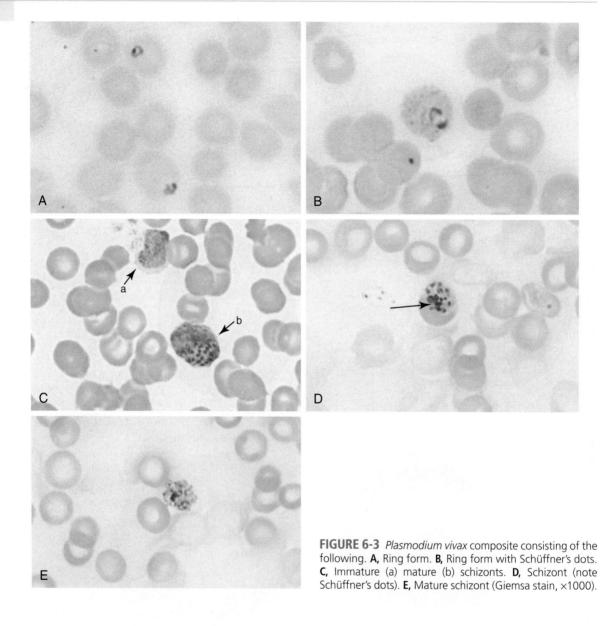

FIGURE 6-3 *Plasmodium vivax* composite consisting of the following. **A,** Ring form. **B,** Ring form with Schüffner's dots. **C,** Immature (a) mature (b) schizonts. **D,** Schizont (note Schüffner's dots). **E,** Mature schizont (Giemsa stain, ×1000).

◪ **Macrogametocytes.** The average *P. vivax* macrogametocyte is characterized by round to oval homogeneous cytoplasm and an eccentric chromatin mass, often located against the edge of the parasite. Diffuse, delicate, light brown pigment may be visible throughout the parasite.

◪ **Other Morphologic Characteristics.** Red blood cells infected with *P. vivax* tend to become enlarged and distorted in response to the presence of the growing parasites. The morphologic forms of *P. vivax*, with the exception of early ring forms that are less than 8 to 10 hours postinfection, may contain tiny granules in the cytoplasm known as **Schüffner's dots** (also referred to as eosinophilic stippling). This characteristic is also typically seen in RBCs infected with *P. ovale*. Although their presence may not be of help in speciating these two *Plasmodium* species, Schüffner's dots may prove to be helpful in preliminarily ruling out the species that do not contain them, *P. malariae* and *P. falciparum*.

Laboratory Diagnosis

All morphologic stages of *P. vivax* may be seen on thick and thin peripheral blood films. However, thin blood films are of the most benefit in species diagnosis. Although the best time to observe numerous infected RBCs is halfway between paroxysms, blood samples may be taken at any time during the illness. The morphologic forms present at a given time reflect the developmental stage occurring at that point in time.

Life Cycle Notes

P. vivax characteristically tends to invade young RBCs. These immature cells are the primary target of invasion because they are typically pliable. This feature allows the RBCs to respond to the presence of the replicating parasite by increasing in size. Thus, distortion of the RBCs occurs.

Epidemiology

P. vivax is the most widely distributed malarial organism. Infections occur worldwide in both the tropics and subtropics. In addition, unlike the other *Plasmodium* species, *P. vivax* is also seen in temperate regions.

Clinical Symptoms

❯❯ **Benign Tertian Malaria.** Patients infected with *P. vivax* typically begin to develop the symptoms of **benign tertian malaria** following a 10- to 17-day incubation period postexposure. These vague symptoms mimic those usually seen in cases of the flu, including nausea, vomiting, headache, muscle pains, and photophobia.

As infected RBCs begin to rupture, the resulting merozoites, hemoglobin, and toxic cellular waste products initiate the first in a series of paroxysms. These paroxysms typically occur every 48 hours (thus, the name tertian malaria). Untreated patients may experience and withstand numerous attacks over several years. However, infections that become chronic in nature may result in serious damage to the brain, liver, and kidney. Blockage of these organs occurs when toxic cellular waste products and hemoglobin, as well as clumps of RBCs, accumulate in the corresponding capillary veins, resulting in ischemia or tissue hypoxia. Dormant hypnozoites may cause relapses months to years following the initial infection.

Treatment

Choosing the appropriate treatment for malaria is, relatively speaking, a bit more complex than selecting chemotherapy for other parasitic infections. It is for this reason that malarial treatment will be discussed for the *Plasmodium* species as a group in this section.

There are numerous antimalarial drugs on the market (not all are available in the United States), including quinine, quinidine, chloroquine, amodiaquine, primaquine, pyrimethamine, sulfadoxine, dapsone, mefloquine, tetracycline, doxycycline, halofantrine, atovaquone, proguanil, ginghaosu, artemisinin, artemether, artesunate, pyronaridine, Fenozan B07, trioxanes, nonane endoperoxides, azithromycin, and WRZ38605. It is important to note that these available malarial medications affect the parasite in different ways, depending on the specific morphologic life cycle stages present at the time of administration. In addition, specific *Plasmodium* species respond differently to the presence of these treatments. Drug-resistant malaria has emerged over recent years, and the threat of a continuing increase in these strains remains a concern in the medical community. Physicians must take the known medication information into account, including the possibility of potential drug toxicity, when selecting the course of treatment for individuals suffering from malaria, as well as the patient's G6PD status.

Prevention and Control

Prevention and control measures designed to halt the spread of *P. vivax* (as well as the other *Plasmodium* species) include personal protection such as netting, screening, protective clothing, and repellents for persons entering known endemic areas. In certain cases, prophylactic treatment may be used based on the geographic location and length of exposure, as well as other factors. Ideally, although difficult to accomplish, mosquito control, or better yet total eradication, would definitely break the organism life cycle in addition to promptly treating infected persons. The avoidance of sharing intravenous needles, as well as thorough screening of donor blood, are additional measures aimed at eliminating the risk of nonmosquito *Plasmodium* species transmission.

A number of studies have focused on developing potential malaria vaccines for *P. vivax* as well as the other *Plasmodium* species. Just as consideration of the specific malarial species and multiple morphologic forms in each organism life cycle is necessary for selecting proper treatment, this information is also important when designing vaccines. Unfortunately, questions have arisen regarding the effectiveness of such a control measure. Additional research is crucial to answer these questions. Although not currently available, the prospects are hopeful that long-awaited and much needed viable vaccines will be developed in the future.

Notes of Interest and New Trends

Methods using recombinant DNA probes and ribosomal RNA probes have been developed and experimentally tested for the diagnosis of malaria. Although they are presently inadequate for diagnostic purposes, they can be useful for screening donor blood and performing epidemiologic studies.

An effective means of preventing the spread of transfusion-acquired malaria has been the implementation of deferring the use of blood donors, including military personnel, who have traveled to known endemic areas, such as Panama and Vietnam. An immunofluorescent test, designed to screen donor units of blood for malaria, has been developed and is available for use.

It has been documented that 131 United States military personnel returned from service in Operation Restore Hope in Somalia infected with mosquito-acquired malaria. Experts agree that the probability of contracting malaria in such conditions has decreased dramatically over the past years because of the increased awareness of proper personal precautions, disease symptoms, and prompt treatment. It is interesting to note that *P. falciparum*, the deadliest *Plasmodium* species, was responsible for 94% of these 131 cases.

> *Quick Quiz! 6-4*
>
> Which morphologic characteristic may help in distinguishing *P. vivax* from *P. falciparum*? (Objective 6-11)
> A. Hemozoin
> B. Schüffner's dots
> C. 72-hour paroxysm
> D. None of the above

> *Quick Quiz! 6-5*
>
> *P. vivax* characteristically invades: (Objective 6-7A)
> A. Immature RBCs
> B. Senescent RBCs
> C. All RBCs
> D. Lymphocytes

> *Quick Quiz! 6-6*
>
> The incubation period for *P. vivax* is generally: (Objective 6-8)
> A. 6 to 8 days
> B. 7 to 10 days
> C. 12 to 24 days
> D. 10 to 17 days

Plasmodium ovale
(plaz-mo' dee-um/ovay'lee)

Common associated disease and condition names: Benign tertian malaria, ovale malaria.

Morphology

▓ **Ring Forms.** The typical *P. ovale* ring form is similar in most respects to that of *P. vivax* (Fig. 6-4; Table 6-3). There are only two notable differences. First, the *P. ovale* ring is larger than *P. vivax*. Second, the *P. ovale* ring is thicker and often more ameboid in appearance than the ring of *P. vivax*.

TABLE 6-3	*Plasmodium ovale*: Typical Characteristics at a Glance
Relative age of infected RBCs	Only young and immature cells
Appearance of infected RBCs	Oval and enlarged, distorted with ragged cell walls
Morphologic Form[*]	**Typical Characteristics (Based on Giemsa Staining)**
Ring form	Resembles that of *P. vivax* Ring larger in size than *P. vivax* Ring thick and often somewhat ameboid in appearance
Developing trophozoite	Ring appearance usually maintained until late in development Ameboid tendencies not as evident as in *P. vivax*
Immature schizont	Progressive dividing chromatin surrounded by cytoplasmic material—often maintains circular shape early in development
Mature schizont	Parasites occupy 75% of RBCs. Rosette arrangement of merozoites (average of eight merozoites typically present)
Microgametocyte, macrogametocyte	Similar to *P. vivax*, only smaller in size

[*]All forms typically contain Schüffner's dots.

▓ **Developing Trophozoites.** The *P. ovale* developing trophozoite maintains its ring appearance as it matures (Fig. 6-4; Table 6-3). The ameboid tendencies common in this stage of *P. ovale* are much less evident than those of *P. vivax*.

▓ **Immature Schizonts.** The typical *P. ovale* immature schizont consists of progressively dividing chromatin material surrounded by cytoplasmic material, which in its earliest stages often maintains a circular shape (Fig. 6-4; Table 6-3).

▓ **Mature Schizonts.** The *P. ovale* mature schizont is characterized by a rosette arrangement of merozoites (eight on average) (Fig. 6-4; Table 6-3). Late in its development, as much as 75% of the cell is occupied by the parasite.

▓ **Microgametocytes.** The *P. ovale* microgametocyte resembles *P. vivax*, only smaller (Fig. 6-4; Table 6-3).

▓ **Macrogametocytes.** As with the microgametocyte, the macrogametocyte of *P. ovale* is similar in appearance to *P. vivax*, only smaller. In Figure 6-4, the *P. ovale* microgametocyte and macrogametocyte are drawn closer in size to those of *P. vivax* to show the similarities in detail of both organisms (Fig. 6-4; Table 6-3).

▓ **Other Morphologic Characteristics.** In addition to becoming enlarged and distorted, RBCs infected with *P. ovale* often develop ragged cell walls in response to the growing parasite. All morphologic forms of *P. ovale*, including very young ring forms, typically contain Schüffner's dots. These dots are often larger and darker than those seen in *P. vivax*.

Laboratory Diagnosis

All developmental stages of *P. ovale* may be seen in blood film preparations. As with the other *Plasmodium* species, thick and thin blood smears are generally examined, using the thick smears to identify the presence of malarial organisms and the thin smears to speciate them. Because all stages of development may be seen, as in *P. vivax* infections, the *P. ovale* morphologic forms present at a given time represent the specific life cycle phase occurring at the sample collection time.

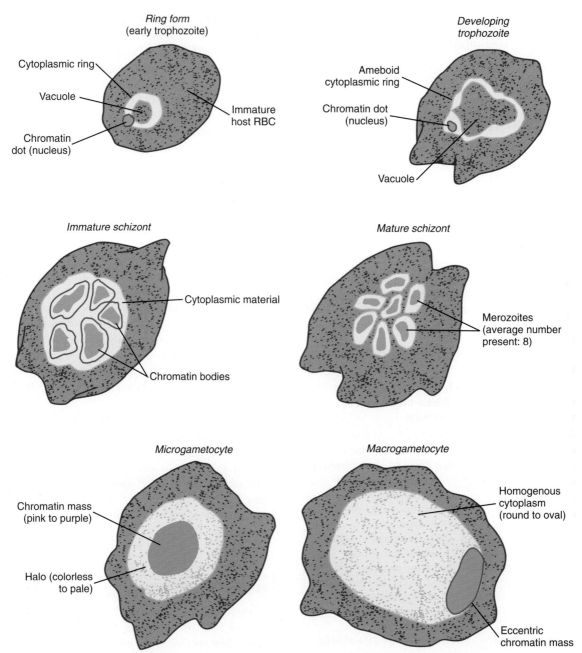

*Ring form
(early trophozoite)*

Cytoplasmic ring

Vacuole

Chromatin
dot (nucleus)

Immature
host RBC

*Developing
trophozoite*

Ameboid
cytoplasmic ring

Chromatin dot
(nucleus)

Vacuole

Immature schizont

Cytoplasmic material

Chromatin bodies

Mature schizont

Merozoites
(average number
present: 8)

Microgametocyte

Chromatin mass
(pink to purple)

Halo (colorless
to pale)

Macrogametocyte

Homogenous
cytoplasm
(round to oval)

Eccentric
chromatin mass

FIGURE 6-4 Commonly seen morphologic forms of *Plasmodium ovale*.

It is important to note that the ring forms, microgametocytes, and macrogametocytes of *P. vivax* and *P. ovale,* are usually difficult to distinguish because of their remarkable similarities. The mature schizont may ultimately be the morphologic form of choice for examination. Because there are definite differences in this form among the two species, the prospects of proper specific identification are much more promising.

Life Cycle Notes

Like *P. vivax*, *P. ovale* targets and subsequently infects young RBCs. These cells have the ability to adapt to the growing parasites by enlarging and assuming an oval shape. This distortion is enhanced by the development of a ragged cell wall.

Epidemiology

P. ovale is primarily found in tropical Africa, where it apparently has surpassed *P. vivax* in frequency of occurrence, as well as in Asia and South America.

Clinical Symptoms

 Benign Tertian Malaria and Ovale Malaria. The clinical scenario of *P. ovale*, including initial infection symptoms, time of typical paroxysm cycle (every 48 hours), and relapses caused by the reactivation of hypnozoites, resembles that of *P. vivax*. A notable difference between the two species is that untreated patients with *P. ovale* typically experience infections that last approximately 1 year, whereas similar patients with *P. vivax* may remain infected for several years. In addition, *P. ovale* relapse infections, when they occur, usually result in spontaneous recovery, a characteristic not typically associated with those of *P. vivax*.

Treatment

The known measures for treating infections with *P. ovale* are the same as those discussed in detail for *P. vivax*.

Prevention and Control

The known measures of preventing and controlling *P. ovale* are the same as those discussed in detail for *P. vivax*. These include adequate personal protection, prophylactic therapy when indicated, prompt treatment of infected persons, mosquito control, screening donor blood, and the avoidance of sharing intravenous drug needles.

> **Quick Quiz! 6-7**
>
> Which morphologic form would be the best choice for distinguishing between *P. vivax* and *P. ovale*? (Objective 6-11)
> A. Mature schizont
> B. Ring form
> C. Early trophozoite
> D. Immature schizont

> **Quick Quiz! 6-8**
>
> In which geographic regions would the laboratorian most likely suspect *P. ovale* as the infecting agent? (Objective 6-2)
> A. Tropical Africa
> B. Asia
> C. South America
> D. All of the above

> **Quick Quiz! 6-9**
>
> Which of the following is considered an antimalarial medication? (Objective 6-9A)
> A. Amoxicillin
> B. Erythromycin
> C. Chloroquine
> D. Dicyclomine

Plasmodium malariae
(plaz-mo′ dee-um/ma-lair′ ee-ee)

Common associated disease and condition names: Quartan malaria, malarial malaria.

Morphology

 Ring Forms. The typical *P. malariae* ring occupies approximately one sixth of the infected RBC (Fig. 6-5; Table 6-4). It is usually smaller than that of *P. vivax* and is connected

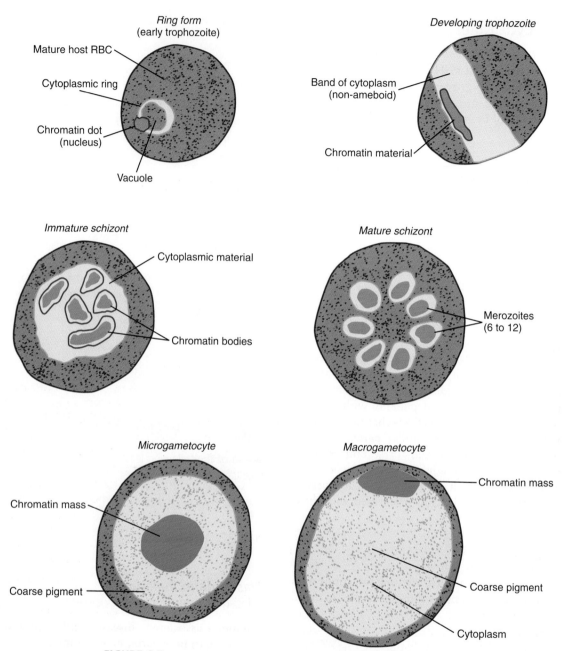

FIGURE 6-5 Commonly seen morphologic forms of *Plasmodium malariae*.

by a heavy chromatin dot. The vacuole may at times appear filled in. Pigment characteristically forms early.

◗ **Developing Trophozoites.** The key characteristic of this morphologic form that distinguishes

it from the other *Plasmodium* species is the formation of a nonameboid solid cytoplasm potentially assuming a band, bar, oval, or roundish shape (Fig. 6-5; Table 6-4). The cytoplasm consists of coarse dark brown pigment often masking

TABLE 6-4	*Plasmodium malariae*: Typical Characteristics at a Glance	
Relative age of infected RBCs	Only mature cells	
Appearance of infected RBCs	Normal size, no distortion	
Morphologic Form*	**Typical Characteristics (Based on Giemsa Stain)**	
Ring form	Smaller than *P. vivax* Occupies one sixth of the RBC Heavy chromatin dot Vacuole may appear filled in Pigment characteristically forms early	
Developing trophozoite	Nonameboid solid cytoplasm that may assume roundish, oval, band, or bar shape Cytoplasm contains coarse dark brown pigment; may mask chromatin material Vacuoles absent in mature stages	
Immature schizont	Similar to that of *P. vivax*, only smaller; may contain large and dark peripheral or central granules	
Mature schizont	Typically contains 6 to 12 merozoites arranged in rosettes or irregular clusters Central arrangement of brown-green pigment may be visible Infected RBC may not be seen because developing parasites often fill the cell completely.	
Microgametocyte, macrogametocyte	Similar to *P. vivax*, only smaller in size; pigment usually darker and coarser Older forms assume an oval shape.	

*The cytoplasm of heavily stained *P. malariae* may contain Ziemann's dots.

the chromatin material. Vacuoles are absent in the mature forms of this stage.

Immature Schizonts. The typical *P. malariae* immature schizont is similar to that of *P. vivax*, with two exceptions (Fig. 6-5; Table 6-4). *P. malariae* immature schizonts are characteristically smaller than those of *P. vivax*. In addition, larger and darker peripheral or central granules may be seen in *P. malariae* immature schizonts.

Mature Schizonts. The mature schizont of *P. malariae* typically contains 6 to 12 merozoites, usually arranged in rosettes or irregular clusters (Fig. 6-5; Table 6-4). A central arrangement of brown-green pigment may often be visible in this stage. In the case of normal-sized RBCs, the cell itself may not be seen because the parasites tend to fill the cell completely. Figure 6-4 shows infection of a larger than normal-sized red blood cell.

Microgametocytes. The average *P. malariae* microgametocyte is similar to that of *P. vivax*, with only one notable exception—the pigment is darker and coarser than the pigment of *P. vivax* (Fig. 6-5; Table 6-4). Older forms of the *P. malariae* microgametocytes are typically oval in shape.

Macrogametocytes. The *P. malariae* macrogametocyte resembles that of *P. vivax*. As with the *P. malariae* microgametocyte, the macrogametocyte pigment is darker and coarser than the pigment seen in *P. vivax*. Older forms of this stage also tend to assume an oval shape.

Other Morphologic Characteristics. *P. malariae* multiplies within the confines of mature RBCs. Enlargement and distortion of these cells does not occur because the mature RBC cell wall is no longer pliable. Unlike both *P. vivax* and *P. ovale*, *P. malariae* does not contain Schüffner's dots. The lack of this feature is important to note when speciating the *Plasmodium* organisms. However, the cytoplasm of heavily stained *P. malariae* may contain fine dustlike dots known as **Ziemann's dots.**

Laboratory Diagnosis

Because *P. malariae* passes through the ring stage quickly, this stage is not commonly seen. The most frequently encountered growth stages of *P.*

malariae seen are the developing trophozoite and the immature and mature schizonts. Although gametocytes may occasionally be seen, they are not readily distinguishable from those of *P. vivax* and thus are of little help in diagnosing *P. malariae* infections. Searching thick and thin Giemsa-stained peripheral blood films will reveal these morphologic forms in patients infected with *P. malariae*. As with the other *Plasmodium* species, detection of infection may be accomplished by reviewing thick blood smears, but the speciation is best determined with the use of thin blood smears.

Life Cycle Notes

P. malariae primarily infects mature RBCs. This particular group of RBCs has well-established cell walls that are not conducive to expansion. Infection with the parasite, therefore, does not result in cell distortion or enlargement. The parasite responds by forming bands and other shapes as necessary to maintain itself.

Epidemiology

P. malariae is found in subtropic and temperate regions of the world. These infections appear to occur less frequently than those with both *P. vivax* and *P. falciparum*.

Clinical Symptoms

Quartan or Malarial Malaria. Patients suffering from **quartan malaria** (also known as **malarial malaria**) infections caused by the presence of *P. malariae* typically experience an incubation period of 18 to 40 days followed by the onset of flulike symptoms. Cyclic paroxysms occur every 72 hours (thus, the name quartan malaria). Spontaneous recovery may result after the initial infection. There are no known relapses because dormant hypnozoites are not associated with *P. malariae* infections. However, repeated attacks may occur for 20 years or more and may be moderate to severe in nature.

Treatment

The known measures for treating infections with *P. malariae* are the same as those discussed for *P. vivax*.

Prevention and Control

The prevention and control measures necessary to eradicate *P. malariae* are similar to those of *P. vivax*. Prophylactic therapy, when appropriate, proper clothing, netting, and screening, as well as the use of insect repellents, offer protection to humans entering known endemic areas. The control of mosquito breeding areas and thorough screening of donor blood units and the avoidance of sharing intravenous drug needles are all essential measures required to halt the spread of *P. malariae*.

Quick Quiz! 6-10

Which morphologic form is not typically seen in infections of *P. malariae*? (Objective 6-7B)
A. Mature schizont
B. Ring form
C. Immature schizont
D. Macrogametocyte

Quick Quiz! 6-11

Which of the following are morphologic features of *P. malariae*? (Objective 6-12A)
A. Schüffner's dots
B. Ziemann's dots
C. Maurer's dots
D. None of the above

Quick Quiz! 6-12

Which of the following is not a prevention and control measure for malaria? (Objective 6-9B)
A. Wearing the hair up
B. Following prophylactic therapy when traveling to malaria-endemic areas
C. Bed netting
D. Proper clothing, such as long-sleeved shirt and long pants

Plasmodium falciparum
(plaz-mo'dee-um/fal-sip'uh-rum)

Common associated disease and condition names: Black water fever, malignant tertian malaria, aestivoautumnal malaria, subtertian malaria, falciparum malaria.

Morphology

Ring Forms. The typical small, delicate ring form of *P. falciparum* consists of scanty cytoplasm connected to one (circle configuration) or two (headphone configuration) small chromatin dots (Figs. 6-6 and 6-7; Table 6-5). A small vacuole is usually visible. Multiple rings in an RBC are frequently seen. *P. falciparum* has the ability to produce accolé (appliqué) forms as well as slender variations.

Developing Trophozoites. The *P. falciparum* developing trophozoite typically consists of one or two rings that each possess a heavy cytoplasmic ring—that is, the cytoplasm is thicker than in the preceding ring form stage (Figs. 6-6 and 6-7; Table 6-5). Fine pigment granules may also be visible. Mature stages of this form are not routinely seen in the peripheral blood.

Immature Schizonts. The immature schizont phase of *P. falciparum* is not routinely seen in the peripheral blood (Figs. 6-6 and 6-7; Table 6-5). This form is characterized by multiple chromatin bodies surrounded by cytoplasm and is only visible in those with severe infections.

Mature Schizonts. As with the immature schizont, the mature schizont is only visible in the peripheral blood of patients with severe *P. falciparum* infection (Figs. 6-6 and 6-7; Table 6-5). Although the typical mature schizont contains 24 merozoites, 8 to 36 merozoites in a cluster arrangement may be present in this stage.

Microgametocytes. The typical *P. falciparum* microgametocyte assumes a characteristic sausage or crescent shape (Figs. 6-6 and 6-7; Table 6-5). Dispersed central chromatin and nearby black chromatin are usually visible.

Macrogametocytes. The macrogametocyte of *P. falciparum* is typically sausage- or crescent-shaped, just like the corresponding

TABLE 6-5	*Plasmodium falciparum*: Typical Characteristics at a Glance
Relative age of infected RBCs*	May infect cells of all ages
Appearance of infected RBCs	Normal size, no distortion
Morphologic Form	**Typical Characteristics (Based on Giemsa Stain)**
Ring form	Circle configuration (one chromatin dot) or headphone configuration (two chromatin dots) Scanty cytoplasm Small vacuole usually visible Multiple rings common Accolé forms possible
Developing trophozoite	Heavy rings common Fine pigment granules Mature forms only seen in severe infections
Immature schizont	Multiple chromatin bodies surrounded by cytoplasm Only detected in severe infections
Mature schizont	Typically consists of 8-36 merozoites (average, 24) in cluster arrangement Only detected in severe infections
Microgametocyte	Sausage- or crescent-shaped Dispersed central chromatin with nearby black pigment usually visible
Macrogametocyte	Sausage- or crescent-shaped Compact chromatin Black pigment surrounding chromatin may be visible

*The cytoplasm of red blood cells infected with *P. falciparum* may contain Maurer's dots.

microgametocyte form described earlier (Figs. 6-6 and 6-7; Table 6-5). Because of this similarity in shape, it is difficult to distinguish the macrogametocyte from the microgametocyte. The macrogametocyte chromatin is usually more compact than the chromatin of the microgametocyte.

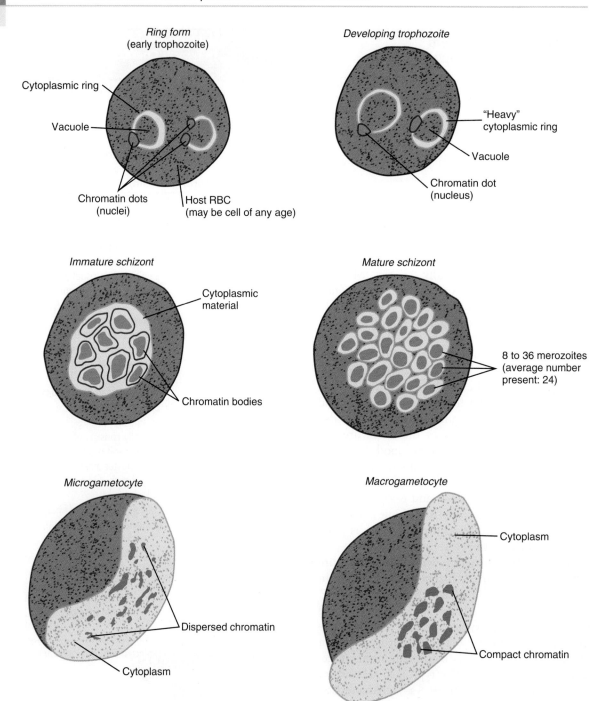

FIGURE 6-6 Commonly seen morphologic forms of *Plasmodium falciparum.*

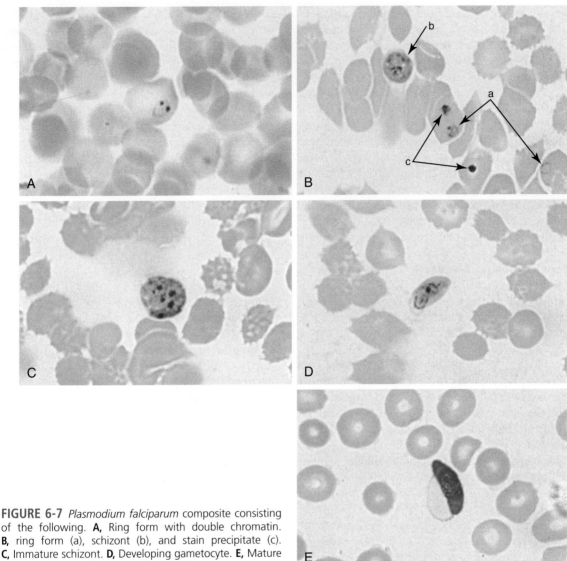

FIGURE 6-7 *Plasmodium falciparum* composite consisting of the following. **A,** Ring form with double chromatin. **B,** ring form (a), schizont (b), and stain precipitate (c). **C,** Immature schizont. **D,** Developing gametocyte. **E,** Mature macrogametocyte (Giemsa stain, ×1000).

Black pigment surrounding the chromatin may also be visible.

Other Morphologic Characteristics. *P. falciparum* may infect RBCs at any age. However, young infected cells do not enlarge and become distorted, as they do when infected with *P. vivax* or *P. ovale*. The morphologic forms of *P. falciparum* do not contain Schüffner's dots or Ziemann's dots. Rather, these growth stages may contain dark-staining, irregular to comma-shaped cytoplasmic dots called **Maurer's dots,** a feature that when present, may be helpful in differentiating the specific malarial species.

Laboratory Diagnosis

Peripheral blood smears from patients suffering with a mild to moderate *P. falciparum* infection typically reveal only the ring forms and gametocyte forms. The trophozoites and schizonts are usually only visible in the peripheral blood of patients with severe infection. Thick smears primarily serve as screening slides, whereas thin smears are used for the speciation of *P. falciparum*.

Because *P. falciparum* may infect RBCs at any age, severe infections and multiple infections may result. Although *P. falciparum* may invade young pliable RBCs, these cells usually do not appear enlarged or distorted, as is the case with *P. vivax* and *P. ovale* infections. Unlike the other *Plasmodium* species, the development of all growth stages of *P. falciparum*, after the formation of the ring form, occurs in the capillaries of the viscera. It is for this reason that typically only the young ring forms and gametocytes are seen in the peripheral blood. Hypnozoites are not produced in the liver of patients with *P. falciparum* infections, and relapses are not known to occur. However, recrudescence may occur, and these attacks may ultimately prove fatal.

Life Cycle Notes

Plasmodium falciparum invades red blood cells of any age and may infect up to 50% of the red blood cell population at any one time throughout the course of the infection. Schizogony generally occurs in the capillaries and blood sinuses of internal organs during infection with this parasite.

Furthermore, infections with *P. falciparum* generally tend to occur in the warmer months of late summer and early autumn—thus, the name **aestivoautumnal malaria**. *P. falciparum* needs the warmer months for reproduction within the *Anopheles* mosquito, which explains this seasonal factor.

Epidemiology

The geographic distribution of *P. falciparum* appears to be limited to the tropical and subtropical regions of the world.

Clinical Symptoms

◤ **Black Water Fever and Malignant Tertian Malaria.** Following a relatively short incubation period of 7 to 10 days, as compared with infections caused by the other *Plasmodium* species, which may last for months to years, patients infected with *P. falciparum* exhibit early flulike symptoms. Daily episodes of chills and fever, as well as severe diarrhea, nausea, and vomiting, rapidly develop followed by cyclic paroxysms, which occur every 36 to 48 hours. A fulminating disease results and the intestinal symptoms (nausea, vomiting, and diarrhea) mimic those seen in malignant infections—hence, the name **malignant tertian malaria**.

P. falciparum typically produces the most deadly form of malaria in untreated patients. This is in part because all ages of RBCs may be infected, thus producing large amounts of toxic cellular debris and capillary plugs consisting of massed red cells, platelets, malarial pigments, and leukocytes. *P. falciparum* may enter the kidney, brain, and/or liver. Kidney involvement, known as **black water fever**, usually results in marked **hemoglobinuria** (the presence of hemoglobin in the urine) caused by *P. falciparum*-induced red cell destruction. Acute renal failure, tubular necrosis, nephrotic syndrome, and death may result. The brain frequently becomes involved when plugs form in the associated capillaries. Patients often slip into a coma, followed by death. Abdominal pain, the vomiting of bile, rapid dehydration, and severe diarrhea are typically noted during *P. falciparum* liver involvement.

Treatment

The known measures for treating infections with *P. falciparum* are the same as those discussed for *P. vivax*. It is important to note that the malaria should be treated first and then the secondary complicating health problems caused by the malaria.

Prevention and Control

Because of the potential severity of infections with *P. falciparum*, prompt treatment of known infected individuals is crucial to halt the spread of the disease. Other prevention and control measures include prophylactic therapy, when appropriate, proper personal protection when entering known endemic areas, mosquito control by chemically destroying their breeding areas, thorough screening of donor blood units, and the avoidance of sharing intravenous drug needles.

The quest to develop a vaccine targeted against malaria has been underway since the mid 1980s. A collaborative effort of the following entities recently resulted in the development of a vaccine against malignant tertian malaria known as RTS,S/AS01: GlaxoSmithKline Biologicals', a global program known as the PATH Malaria Vaccine Initiative (VMI), research organizations in Africa and elsewhere, and the Bill and Melinda Gates foundation which provides funding support. Clinical trials in children ages 5 to 17 months in areas of Africa using other effective malaria prevention and treatment interventions to date show remarkable success. Children who received the vaccine had approximately half the number of clinical outbreaks versus those who did not receive the vaccine. The next phase of clinical trials to be conducted is slated to occur in children 6 to 12 weeks of age.

Notes of Interest and New Trends

Numerous serologic studies that have focused on the detection of antigens and antibodies in specimens of patients with *P. falciparum* have been conducted in recent years. Tests using human serum and plasma, identification reagents, cultures of *P. falciparum*, and urine samples have all been developed. Although serologic tests are presently available for *P. falciparum*, they are hard to obtain and thus are not useful for monitoring therapy in a patient. However, they are useful in ruling out malaria in a patient with fever of unknown origin.

Methodology has been developed and tested to identify high and low numbers of *P. falciparum* by DNA hybridization. It is primarily used as an epidemiologic tool at the present time, but this technology may also prove to be of benefit in the future for diagnostic purposes and screening donor blood supplies.

Quick Quiz! 6-13

What age of red blood cell does *P. falciparum* typically invade? (Objective 6-7A)
A. Mature red blood cells
B. Immature red blood cells
C. All red blood cells, regardless of age
D. Does not invade red blood cells

Quick Quiz! 6-14

P. falciparum is commonly found in the United States. (Objective 6-2)
A. True
B. False

Quick Quiz! 6-15

Black water fever can be described by which of the following: (Objective 6-1)
A. Marked hemoglobinuria
B. Kidney involvement in *P. falciparum* infections
C. Caused by *P. falciparum*–induced red blood cell destruction
D. All of the above

Plasmodium knowlesi
(plaz-mo'dee-um/)

Once thought to be solely a parasite of Old World Monkeys, *P. knowlesi* has recently been identified in humans suffering from malaria in Malaysia and other parts of Southeast Asia. On more than one occasion the infection proved fatal. Although there is still much to learn about *P. knowlesi*, the incidence of corresponding life-threatening malarial illness is predicted to rise and as such it is worthy of brief discussion in this chapter.

P. knowlesi morphologically resembles *P. malariae* to the extent that there is documented evidence that misdiagnosis by microscopic methods has occurred. Depending on the morphologic forms present, *P. knowlesi* may resemble *P. falciparum*. DNA extraction and nested-PCR examination of samples have been known to reveal the differences between the two *Plasmodium* species. On the contrary, cross-reactivity with *P. vivax* appears to interfere with PCR testing. Clinical features of infected individuals range from respiratory distress, acute renal or multi-organ failure, to shock. Treatments vary depending on disease severity. Infected patients with no complications have been treated with quinine, chloroquine or artemether-lumefantrine. Inraveous quinine, artesunate or a combination of chloroquine-primiquine have proven to be effective treatments for patients with severe disease. Artemisinin has shown be quite effective when used as treatment for both mild and severe forms of malaria due to *P. knowlesi*.

BABESIA SPECIES

As noted, there are numerous species of *Babesia* and, of those, four are known to be of concern regarding transmission to humans. Following an introduction to *Babesia* species that includes a historical perspective and descriptions of the most commonly found morphologic forms, two of the most commonly encountered *Babesia* parasites will be discussed.

Historical Perspective

Apicomplexan parasites belonging to the genus *Babesia* are often seen infecting animals, wild and domestic. Babesial organisms were first described in the 1880s as being responsible for **Texas cattle fever** or **red water fever**; this parasitic infection almost decimated the cattle production industry. However, in recent years, several species have demonstrated an ability to cause illness in humans, who are usually considered as an accidental host. The two babesial organisms most commonly isolated from clinical specimens are *B. microti* (*Theileria microti*) and *B. divergens*; other species have demonstrated an ability to cause disease, but are a rarer occurrence. It is important to point out here that some sources suggest that due to ribosomal RNA comparisons *B. microi* fits more into a related genus known as *Theileria* and thus now call it *Theileria microti*. Until this change is universally accepted in the parasitology community, the current name of *B. microti* will be used in this text.

TABLE 6-6	*Babesia* Species Trophozoite: Typical Characteristics at a Glance
Parameter	**Description**
Appearance	Resembles a ring form Does not contain Schüffner's, Ziemann's, or Maurer's dots
Ring characteristics when stained with Giemsa	Blue cytoplasmic circle connected with or to red chromatin dot Vacuole usually present

TABLE 6-7	*Babesia* Species Merozoite: Typical Characteristics at a Glance
Parameter	**Description**
Appearance	Resembles four trophozoites attached by their respective chromatin dots in the shape of a Maltese cross

Morphology and Life Cycle Notes

The typical life history of each of these organisms involves several morphologic forms. However, for the purposes of this text, only the two forms most commonly encountered in human specimens will be discussed, the trophozoite and merozoite. Other morphologic forms are responsible for invading the RBCs, but are generally never seen at the point of laboratory diagnosis.

◗ **Trophozoite.** The trophozoite (Table 6-6) develops after the sporozoite infects the red blood cell. This form resembles the ring form of *Plasmodium* infections. The typical ring, when stained with Giemsa, consists of a blue cytoplasmic circle connected with or to a red chromatin dot, also referred to by some as a nucleus. The space inside the ring is known as a vacuole. The ring form is the most commonly seen diagnostic feature of babesiosis and can be differentiated from malarial organisms by the absence of malarial pigments (hemozoin) and of Schüffner's, Ziemann's, or Maurer's dots (Table 6-7).

◗ **Merozoite.** The merozoite develops within the red blood cell as the trophozoite matures. The merozoite resembles four trophozoites attached together by their respective chromatin dots in the shape of a cross, often referred to as resembling a Maltese cross. Merozoites undergo binary fission in the human host to produce more sporozoites.

Babesiosis has a sexual and asexual phase in its life cycle. The sexual phase occurs within its vector, the tick, and the asexual phase occurs within its host (e.g., mice, deer, cattle, dogs, humans). It is generally transmitted through the bite of an infected tick of the genus *Ixodes*. The uninfected host must be in contact with the tick's saliva for 12 hours or longer before this parasite can be transmitted. The infected tick transmits sporozoites into the uninfected host. The sporozoites invade the red blood cells and develop into trophozoites. Multiple sporozoites can infect a RBC, so multiple trophozoites can be seen within the infected RBC. The trophozoites continue to develop into merozoites. The merozoites mature and develop into gametocytes inside their normal animal host, but are not generally seen in the accidental human host. In the human host, the merozoites undergo binary fission to produce more sporozoites; when the number of sporozoites exceeds the red blood cell's capacity, it ruptures, releasing sporozoites to infect more red blood cells. An ixodid tick bites an infected host and the gametocytes travel to the gut, where they unite to form an ookinete. The ookinete travels to the salivary glands where **sporogony**—the process of spore and sporozoite production via sexual reproduction—takes place, resulting in numerous sporozoites that can be transmitted to a new host.

Quick Quiz! 6-16

Humans are an accidental host of *Babesia* species. (Objective 6-6)
A. True
B. False

Laboratory Diagnosis

Giemsa-stained peripheral blood films are the specimens of choice for the laboratory diagnosis of babesiosis. Wright's stain may also be used and will result in an accurate diagnosis. However, because Giemsa is the recommended stain for all blood films submitted for parasite study, the specific morphologic discussion of *Babesia* is based on the use of this stain. Thick and thin blood films should be made and examined. Thick blood smears serve as screening slides; thin blood smears are used for differentiating *Babesia* from *Plasmodium* spp. All blood films should be studied under oil immersion. Careful and thorough screening of all smears is crucial to ensure the correct identification, reporting, and ultimately the proper treatment of the organisms present. The timing of blood collection for the study of *Babesia* is not crucial to success in retrieving the *Babesia* parasites; they have not shown periodicity, as have the malarial organisms.

In addition to blood films, serologic tests and PCR techniques for babesiosis are available. These tests are generally best used for diagnosing patients with a low parasitemia or in donor blood supply screening and epidemiologic studies. Serologic and PCR testing are also valuable for the speciation of *Babesia*, because this is a limitation of blood film tests. Representative laboratory diagnostic methodologies are described in Chapter 2 as well as within each individual parasite discussion, as appropriate.

Quick Quiz! 6-17

The specimen of choice for the recovery of *Babesia* is: (Objective 6-10)
A. Tissue
B. Cerebral spinal fluid (CSF)
C. Stool
D. Blood

Pathogenesis and Clinical Symptoms of *Babesia*

The typical patient presenting with babesiosis was exposed 1 to 4 weeks prior to the onset of symptoms. Babesiosis is generally a self-limiting infection. Its onset is usually gradual and characterized by prodrome-like symptoms—fever, headache, chills, sweating, arthralgias, myalgias, fatigue, and weakness. The fever shows no periodicity. Hepatosplenomegaly and mild to severe hemolytic anemia have been recorded. Elevated bilirubin and transaminase levels have also been demonstrated.

Babesiosis tends to be worse for the splenectomized and immunocompromised patient. Rare asymptomatic infections have also been recorded. Infections tend to present in late summer to early fall and generally correlate with the breeding cycle of the ixodid tick. It is also not uncommon to see a patient coinfected with Lyme disease and/or human granulocytic ehrlichiosis.

Quick Quiz! 6-18

Babesiosis is characterized by all the following except: (Objective 6-8)
A. Trophozoites resembling the ring form seen in *Plasmodium* infections
B. A mild to severe hemolytic anemia
C. Fever periodicity
D. None of the above

Babesia Classification

Babesia species belongs to the phylum Apicomplexa, class Aconoidasida, order Piroplasmida, family Babesiidae. The *Babesia* species discussed in this chapter occur in the blood, as indicated in Figure 6-8.

Babesia microti
(baa"beez-ee'yuh/my"crō-tee)

Common associated disease and condition names: Presently, no common name exists.

Babesia divergens
(baa"beez-ee'yuh/di"vər-jənz)

Common associated disease and condition names: Presently, no common name exists.

Morphology

The morphologic features of *B. microti* and *B. divergens* are described in the general notes concerning babesiosis.

Laboratory Diagnosis

The laboratory diagnostic procedures for identifying *B. microti* and *B. divergens* are described in the general notes concerning babesiosis.

Life Cycle Notes

The life cycle of *B. microti* and *B. divergens* are described in the general notes concerning babesiosis.

Epidemiology

B. microti is commonly found in areas of southern New England, such as Nantucket, Martha's Vineyard, Shelter Island, Long Island, and Connecticut. It has also been isolated in clinical specimens in patients in New Jersey, Wisconsin, Missouri, Georgia, North Carolina, and Mexico. The vector most commonly associated with the transmission of *B. microti* is *Ixodes dammini*. The principal reservoir host for this infection is the white-footed mouse, *Peromyscus leucopus*.

B. divergens is commonly found in European countries, particularly those in the former Yugoslavia, Russia, Ireland, and Scotland. The vector most commonly associated with the transmission

Phylum	Class	Order	Blood Species
Apicomplexa	Aconoidasida	Piroplasmida	*Babesia microti*
			Babesia divergens

FIGURE 6-8 Parasite classification—*Babesia* species.

of *B. divergens* is *Ixodes ricinus*. The principal reservoir hosts are cattle and rabbits. *B. divergens* has also been described in the Nantucket area, primarily in the rabbits and birds of the region.

Babesiosis has also been demonstrated to be a transfusion-transmissible disease and has the potential to be transmitted congenitally and by the sharing of intravenous drug needles.

Clinical Symptoms

The clinical symptoms for *B. microti* and *B. divergens* infections have been described earlier ("Pathogenesis and Clinical Symptoms"). *B. divergens* tends to be the more severe of the two parasitic infections and is frequently fatal if left untreated. *B. microti* tends to be rather benign and self-limiting. Disease with either of these organisms is often more severe for older adult, immunosuppressed, and/or splenectomized patients.

Treatment

The treatment of babesiosis often involves a combination of drugs. The most common combinations are clindamycin and quinine or atovaquone and azithromycin. Diminazene and pentamidine, in combination or singly, and pyrimethamine and quinine, in combination or singly, have also shown promise, but the side effects of some of these medications may be less than desirable. Patient age, immune status, G6PD status, and other clinical symptoms will play a role in the physician's choice as to which therapy is best for the patient.

Prevention and Control

The best prevention measure is to avoid tick-infested areas. However, examining the body for ticks immediately after leaving such an area and rapid removal of the tick are crucial. The tick must feed for at least 12 hours before it is able to transmit the parasite. Using insect repellents and eradicating the tick population are also helpful for disease prevention and control.

Quick Quiz! 6-19

Which of the following are laboratory diagnostic procedures is recommended for specifically identifying *T. microti*? (Objective 6-10)
A. Thick and thin blood films
B. Serologic testing
C. PCR techniques
D. Both B and C are correct.
E. None of the above

Quick Quiz! 6-20

Which of the following is not a location known for infection by *T. microti*? (Objective 6-2)
A. California
B. North Carolina
C. Mexico
D. Nantucket

Quick Quiz! 6-21

For which patient would babesiosis be more severe? (Objective 6-8)
A. The splenectomized
B. The patient with *Babesia divergens*
C. Older adults
D. All of the above

LOOKING BACK

As with all parasites, the proper identification of malaria and babesiosis is crucial to ensure that the patient is adequately treated when necessary. *Plasmodium* and *Babesia* spp. have morphologic forms that may look similar. However, because not all species typically show all the morphologic forms in the peripheral blood, coupled with the fact that other morphologic forms look different (e.g., mature schizonts, gametocytes) and whether pigment is produced, allow accurate speciation of the malarial organism and differentiation of malaria from babesiosis. Thorough screening of all smears is essential; this practice ensures that even low numbers of organisms will be detected.

It is also important to note that processing and studying multiple sets of smears are generally required to rule out the presence of a malarial infection. A composite drawing of the six morphologic forms of each of the four *Plasmodium* spp.—*P. vivax*, *P. ovale*, *P. malariae*, and *P. falciparum*—are provided at the end of the chapter as a comparative reference.

TEST YOUR KNOWLEDGE!

6-1. The infective stage of the *Plasmodium* parasite and the *Babesia* parasite for humans is the: (Objective 6-6)
A. Merozoite
B. Trophozoite
C. Gametocyte
D. Sporozoite

6-2. What is the name of the dormant parasite form found in patients with *Plasmodium ovale* and *Plasmodium vivax* infections? (Objective 6-1)
A. Trophozoites
B. Sporozoites
C. Hypnozoites
D. Gametocytes

6-3. The species of mosquito most commonly known to serve as a vector for the genus *Plasmodium* is: (Objective 6-6)
A. *Ixodes*
B. *Anopheles*
C. *Culex*
D. *Glossina*

6-4. Which of the following is a self-limiting infection characterized by a gradual onset of headache, chills, sweating, and fatigue that demonstrates no periodicity? (Objective 6-8)
A. *Ehrlichia phagocytophila*
B. *Babesia microti*
C. *Plasmodium vivax*
D. *Plasmodium ovale*

6-5. Giemsa-stained blood smears demonstrate normal-sized red blood cells containing ring form trophozoites in pairs and tetrads, without pigment or stippling. Which parasite listed best fits this description? (Objective 6-12C)
A. *Babesia divergens*
B. *Plasmodium falciparum*
C. *Plasmodium vivax*
D. *Plasmodium malariae*

6-6. Sexual reproduction of *Babesia* species takes place in the: (Objective 6-6)
A. Human gut
B. Red blood cells
C. Tick
D. Parenchymal cells of the liver

6-7. Which species of *Plasmodium* is characterized by a rosette arrangement of merozoites and the presence of Schüffner's dots in the red blood cells? (Objective 6-12C)
A. *Plasmodium vivax*
B. *Plasmodium ovale*
C. *Plasmodium falciparum*
D. *Plasmodium malariae*

6-8. *Babesia* spp. undergo an exoerythrocytic cycle. (Objective 6-6)
A. True
B. False

6-9. Ziemann's dots, band form trophozoites, and 72-hour periodicity of paroxysms is indicative of infection with which *Plasmodium* species? (Objective 6-8)
A. *Plasmodium vivax*
B. *Plasmodium ovale*
C. *Plasmodium falciparum*
D. *Plasmodium malariae*

6-10. Which of the following would be an advised drug therapy for an uncomplicated case of babesiosis? (Objective 6-9A)
A. Clindamycin-quinine
B. Atovaquone-proguanil
C. Penicillin-aspirin
D. Erythromycin-chloroquine

CASE STUDY 6-2 UNDER THE MICROSCOPE

Cindy, a 20-year old woman, developed a febrile illness 10 days after returning from a weekend hiking expedition in the New England countryside. She complained of headache, muscle aches, chills, sweating, and fatigue at the college infirmary. Laboratory studies included Giemsa-stained thick and thin blood smears. Ring and Maltese cross forms were detected within the red blood cells.

1. What is the diagnosis of Cindy's infection? (Objectives 6-2, 6-6, 6-13A)
2. How is speciation of the organism causing this infection best achieved? (Objectives 6-13C)
3. How is this infection transmitted? (Objective 6-13C)
4. What other disease(s) is (are) transmitted by this vector? (Objective 6-8)

COMPARISON DRAWINGS
Malarial Organisms

| *Plasmodium vivax* | *Plasmodium ovale* | *Plasmodium malariae* | *Plasmodium falciparum* |

Ring Form (early trophozoite)

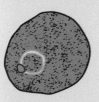 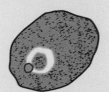 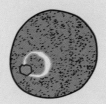 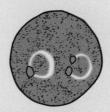

Developing Trophozoite

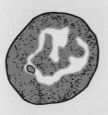 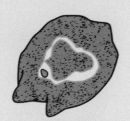 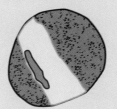 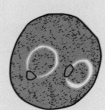

Immature Schizont

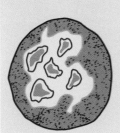 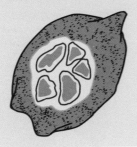 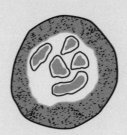 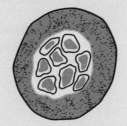

Continued

COMPARISON DRAWINGS
Malarial Organisms—cont'd

Mature Schizont

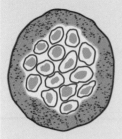
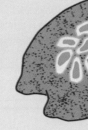
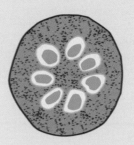
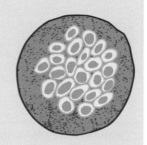

Microgametocyte

| Plasmodium vivax | Plasmodium ovale | Plasmodium malariae | Plasmodium falciparum |

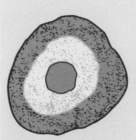
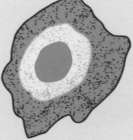
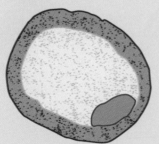
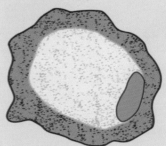

Macrogametocyte

Plasmodium vivax   Plasmodium ovale

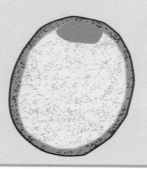
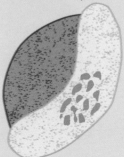

Plasmodium malariae   Plasmodium falciparum

Miscellaneous Protozoa

Jill Dennis and Elizabeth Zeibig

WHAT'S AHEAD

Focusing In
Miscellaneous Protozoa
  Classification
    Balantidium coli
    Isospora belli

Sarcocystis species
Cryptosporidium parvum
Blastocystis hominis
Cyclospora cayetanensis
Microsporidia

Toxoplasma gondii
Pneumocystis jiroveci
  (Pneumocystis carinii)
Looking Back

LEARNING OBJECTIVES

*On completion of this chapter and review of
its figures and corresponding photomicrographs,
the successful learner will be able to:*

7-1. Define the following key terms:
  Bradyzoite (*pl.*, bradyzoites)
  Cilia
  Ciliate (*pl.*, ciliates)
  Coccidia
  Gametogony
  Macronucleus
  Micronucleus
  Sporoblast (*pl.*, sporoblasts)
  Sporocyst (*pl.*, sporocysts)
  Tachyzoite (*pl.*, tachyzoites)

7-2. State the geographic distribution of each of
the protozoa discussed.

7-3. Given a list of parasites, select the
organism(s) belonging to the class Ciliata,
Sporozoa, or Blastocystea. Discuss any
controversy surrounding classification, if
applicable.

7-4. Classify each of these protozoa as intestinal
or extraintestinal.

7-5. Briefly summarize the life cycle of each
organism discussed.

7-6. Identify and describe the populations prone
to contracting symptoms and clinically

significant disease processes associated with
each of the pathogenic organisms discussed.

7-7. Identify and describe each of the following
as they relate to the organisms discussed:
  A. Disease, condition, and prognosis
  B. Treatment options
  C. Prevention and control measures

7-8. Select the specimen(s) of choice, collection
and processing protocol(s), and laboratory
diagnostic technique for the recovery of
each of the miscellaneous Protozoa.

7-9. Given a description, photomicrograph,
and/or diagram of one of the organisms
described, correctly:
  A. Identify and/or label the designated
characteristic structure(s).
  B. State the purpose of the designated
characteristic structure(s).
  C. Identify the parasite by scientific name
and morphologic form.
  D. State the common name for associated
conditions and diseases, if applicable.

7-10. Analyze case studies that include pertinent
information and laboratory data and do the
following:
  A. Identify and differentiate each
responsible organism by scientific name,

common name, and morphologic form, with justification.

B. Identify the diseases and conditions associated with the responsible parasite

C. Construct a life cycle associated with each organism present that includes corresponding epidemiology, route of transmission, infective stage, and diagnostic stage.

D. Propose each of the following related to stopping and preventing further parasite infections:
1. Treatment options
2. Prevention and control plan

E. Determine the specimen(s) of choice and alternative specimen types, when appropriate, as well as appropriate laboratory diagnostic techniques for the recovery of each responsible parasite.

F. Recognize sources of error including but not limited to those involved in specimen collection, processing, and testing and propose solutions to remedy them.

G. Interpret laboratory data, determine specific follow-up tests to be done, and predict the results of those identified tests.

H. Determine additional morphologic forms, where appropriate, that may also be detected in clinical specimens.

7-11 Identify, compare, and contrast the similarities and differences among the parasites discussed in this and the other chapters in this text.

7-12. Describe standard, immunologic, and new laboratory diagnostic approaches for the recovery of the miscellaneous Protozoa in clinical specimens.

7-13. Given prepared laboratory specimens, and with the assistance of this manual, the learner will be able to:

A. Differentiate the protozoan organisms from artifacts and other parasites.

B. Correctly name each protozoan parasite based on its key characteristic structure(s).

CASE STUDY 7-1 | UNDER THE MICROSCOPE

Joseph, a 29-year old man, went to a local health clinic with complaints of intermittent diarrhea for a few months and trouble sleeping. A stool specimen was collected and preserved in 10% formalin and PVA. An O&P examination was performed, along with a permanent trichrome stain. The stain revealed the organism shown below that measured 10 μm in diameter, with a large, centrally located vacuole and small red nuclei within the peripheral ring of cytoplasm.

Questions and Issues for Consideration

1. What parasite do you suspect, and why? (Objectives 7-10A)

2. Why do false-negative results sometime occur with this organism? (Objective 7-10F)

3. How does the organism reproduce? (Objective 7-10C)

4. Describe the controversy surrounding the classification of this organism. (Objective 7-3)

5. Discuss treatment and prevention measures. (Objective 7-10D)

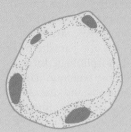

Size range: 5-32 μm
Average size: 7-10 μm

FOCUSING IN

The remaining protozoa of human clinical significance are described in this chapter. This group of organisms is similar in that each of its members is unicellular. However, the specific morphologic forms, methods of laboratory diagnosis, life cycle notes, epidemiology, clinical symptoms treatment protocols, and prevention and control measures vary among the organisms in this group. Because of these variations, the specific information associated with each of the protozoa is described on an individual basis. In addition to the laboratory diagnosis information in this chapter, representative diagnostic methodologies are discussed in Chapter 2.

In addition to a concise yet comprehensive discussion of the well-known miscellaneous protozoa, two relatively new genera, *Cyclospora* and *Microsporidia*, are briefly mentioned in this chapter. These organisms are known to produce human intestinal disease. Because of their relatively recent discovery and the fact that much is still to be learned about these genera of protozoan organisms, their exact classification has not been well described.

MISCELLANEOUS PROTOZOA CLASSIFICATION

The remaining members of the protozoa are classified in four groups. The first group, the **ciliates**, parasites that move by means of hairlike cytoplasmic extensions called **cilia**, contains one human pathogen known as *Balantidium coli* (Fig. 7-1). The second group consists of select sporozoa (Fig. 7-2), excluding *Plasmodium* and *Babesis* spp., which are discussed in Chapter 6. These parasites, which are intestinal and tissue-dwelling in nature, belong to the subclass **Coccidia**, a group of protozoal parasites in which asexual replication occurs outside a human host and sexual replication occurs inside a human host, and are often referred to as coccidian protozoans. *Blastocystis hominis* (Fig. 7-3), initially considered as a yeast, makes up the third group and is now classified as a Protozoa. This organism is the sole member of the class Blastocystea.

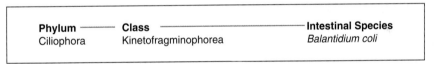

FIGURE 7-1 Parasite Classification: The Cilliates.

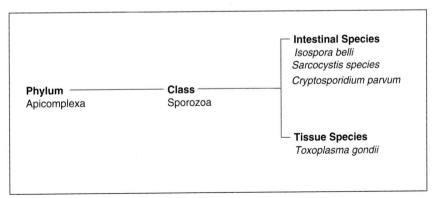

FIGURE 7-2 Parasite Classification: The Sporozoa.

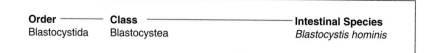

Order ——— Class ———————————— Intestinal Species
Blastocystida   Blastocystea   *Blastocystis hominis*

FIGURE 7-3 Parasite Classification: *Blastocystis hominis.*

Now classified as a fungus ————————— *Pneumocystis jiroveci*

FIGURE 7-4 Parasite Classification: *Pneumocystis jirvoeci.*

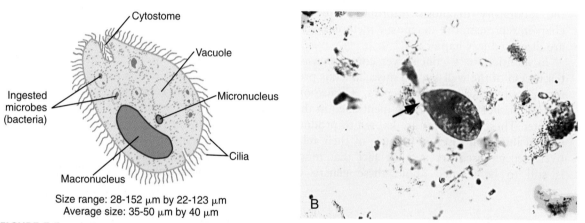

A
Size range: 28-152 μm by 22-123 μm
Average size: 35-50 μm by 40 μm

B

FIGURE 7-5 A, *Balantidium coli* trophozoite. **B,** *Balantidium coli* trophozoite. **(B,** from Mahon CR, Lehmann DC, Manuselis G: Textbook of diagnostic microbiology, ed 4, St Louis, 2011, Saunders.)

Pneumocystis jiroveci (formerly known as *Pneumocystis carinii)* is the only member of the fourth group (Fig. 7-4). This organism was traditionally included with the Protozoa, even though it has been recently reclassified as a fungus.

Balantidium coli
(bal′an-tid′ee-um/ko′ly)

Common associated disease and condition names: Balantidiasis.

Morphology

◢ **Trophozoites.** Considered as the largest protozoan known to humans, the typical *Balantidium coli* trophozoite may measure from 28 to 152 μm in length, with an average length of 35 to 50 μm (Fig. 7-5; Table 7-1). The average trophozoite width is approximately 40 μm but may range from 22 to 123 μm. The ovoid to sacshaped *B. coli* trophozoite tapers at the anterior end. The organism typically exhibits rotary,

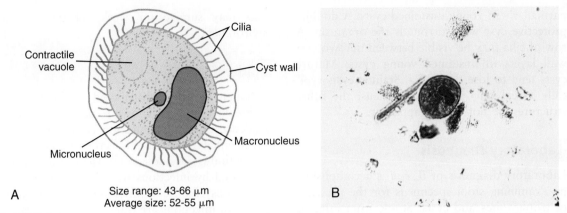

FIGURE 7-6 **A,** *Balantidium coli* cyst. **B,** *Balantidium coli* cyst. **(B,** *from Mahon CR, Lehmann DC, Manuselis G: Textbook of diagnostic microbiology, ed 4, St Louis, 2011, Saunders.)*

TABLE 7-1	*Balantidium coli* Trophozoite: Typical Characteristics at a Glance
Parameter	**Description**
Size range	28-152 µm in length, 22-123 µm wide
Motility	Rotary, boring
Number of nuclei	Two Kidney-shaped macronucleus Small spherical micronucleus
Other features	One or two visible contractile vacuoles Cytoplasm may contain food vacuoles and/or bacteria Small cytostome present Layer of cilia around organism

TABLE 7-2	*Balantidium coli* Cyst: Typical Characteristics at a Glance*
Parameter	**Description**
Size range	43-66 µm
Number and appearance of nuclei	Two Kidney-shaped macronucleus usually present Small spherical micrcnucleus; may not be observable
Other features	One or two visible contractile vacuoles in young cysts Double cyst wall Row of cilia visible in between cyst wall layers of young cysts

*Mature cysts typically only reveal macronucleus on examination. The other structures are usually not apparent.

boring motility. The trophozoite contains two nuclei.

A small dotlike nucleus (**micronucleus**) is located adjacent to a large, often kidney bean–shaped nucleus known as a **macronucleus.** The micronucleus is often not readily visible, even in stained preparations, whereas the macronucleus may often appear as a hyaline mass, especially in unstained preparations. Two contractile vacuoles are located in the granular cytoplasm, although sometimes only one is readily visible, as in Figure 7-5A. In addition, the cytoplasm may also contain food vacuoles, as well as ingested microbes

(bacteria). The trophozoite is equipped with a small cytostome. A layer of cilia surrounds the organism, which serves as its means of locomotion.

■ **Cysts.** Averaging in size from 52 to 55 µm, the subspherical to oval *B. coli* cyst may measure from 43 to 66 µm (Fig. 7-6; Table 7-2). Although the cyst technically contains the macronucleus and micronucleus, the micronucleus may not be observed in wet or permanent preparations. One or two contractile vacuoles may be visible, particularly in young unstained cysts. A double-protective cyst wall surrounds the organism. A row of cilia may be visible between the two cyst wall layers in unstained young cysts. Mature cysts tend to lose their cilia. Stained cysts typically reveal only the macronucleus; the other structures are not usually apparent.

Laboratory Diagnosis

Laboratory diagnosis of *B. coli* is accomplished by examining stool specimens for the presence of trophozoites and cysts. Stools from infected patients experiencing diarrhea are more likely to contain *B. coli* trophozoites. Although it does not occur frequently, suspicious formed stools may contain cysts. Sigmoidoscopy material may also reveal *B. coli* organisms when collected from patients suffering from sigmoidorectal infection. As with any sample submitted for parasitic study, thorough screening of the wet preparations and the permanent stain is crucial to ensure an accurate laboratory test report. In addition, the study of multiple samples may be required to determine the presence or absence of the parasite correctly.

Life Cycle Notes

The *B. coli* life cycle is similar to that of *Entamoeba histolytica*. Human infection with *B. coli* is initiated on ingestion of infective cysts in contaminated food or water. Unlike that of *E. histolytica*, multiplication of the *B. coli* nuclei does not occur in the cyst phase. Following excystation in the small intestine, the resulting trophozoites take up residence and feed primarily in the cecal region and terminal portion of the ileum, as well as in the lumen, mucosa, and submucosa of the large intestine. The multiplication of each trophozoite occurs by transverse binary fission, from which two young trophozoites emerge. The *B. coli* trophozoites are delicate and do not survive in the outside environment. Encystation occurs in the lumen. The resulting cysts mature and ultimately become the infective form for transmission into a new host. These cysts may survive for weeks in the outside environment.

Epidemiology

Although *B. coli* is distributed worldwide and outbreaks have been known to occur, the typical incidence of human infection is very low. The documented frequency of infections in the general population is considered rare. However, epidemics caused by infections with *B. coli* have been noted in psychiatric facilities in the United States.

B. coli infections are transmitted by ingesting contaminated food and water by the oral-fecal as well as person-to-person routes. Recently, it has been presumed that water contaminated with feces (the oral-fecal route) from a pig, which is a known reservoir host, may be a significant source of infection. There is now considerable evidence to support the theory that the pig may not be the primary infection source, because the documented incidence of infection among humans with high pig contact is relatively low. Infected food handlers appear to be the culprit in person-to-person spread of the disease.

Clinical Symptoms

◢ **Asymptomatic Carrier State.** Similar to that seen in certain patients infected with *E. histolytica*, some patients are just carriers of *B. coli* and remain asymptomatic.

◢ **Balantidiasis.** Symptomatic patients may experience a variety of discomforts, ranging from mild colitis and diarrhea to full-blown clinical balantidiasis, which may often resemble amebic dysentery. In this case, abscesses and ulcers may form in the mucosa and submucosa of the large intestine, followed by secondary bacterial infection. Acute infections are characterized by up to 15 liquid stools daily containing pus, mucus, and blood. Patients who suffer from chronic infections may develop a tender colon, anemia, cachexia, and occasional diarrhea, alternating with constipation. *B. coli* has been known to invade areas other than the intestine, such as the liver, lungs, pleura, mesenteric nodes, and urogenital tract. However, the incidence of such extraintestinal infections is rare.

Treatment

Two factors play an important role in determining the prognosis of patients infected with *B. coli*, the severity of the infection and the patient's response to treatment. Asymptomatic patients and those suffering from chronic disease typically have a good chance of recovery. There are two medication choices for the effective treatment of *B. coli* infections, oxytetracycline (Terramycin) and iodoquinol. Metronidazole (Flagyl) may also be used to treat infected patients.

Prevention and Control

Personal hygiene and proper sanitary conditions are effective measures for *B. coli* prevention and control. Until the questions surrounding the pig's role in transmitting *B. coli* are completely understood, the pig should be considered as a possible source of infection and proper precautions should be exercised when handling and dealing with pigs and their feces.

Notes of Interest and New Trends

The *B. coli* trophozoite is often referred to as resembling a sac in shape. As a reflection of this shape, the organism was named *Balantidium*, which means "little bag."

It is estimated that 63% to 91% of pigs harbor *B. coli*. In addition, pigs also carry *Balantidium suis*, a parasite that is morphologically identical to *B. coli* but does not appear to cause human infections. Unsuccessful attempts have been made to infect humans purposely with *B. suis*.

Because the incidence of *B. coli* is low in the population as a whole and in those who have regular contact with pigs, it has been suggested that humans have a relatively high natural resistance to this organism.

Quick Quiz! 7-2

Which structure is always visible in the stained cyst and troph of *Balantidium coli*? (Objective 7-9A)
A. Macronucleus
B. Micronucleus
C. Cilia
D. Ingested bacteria

Quick Quiz! 7-3

The life cycle of *Balantidium coli* and clinical symptoms are similar to that of which of the following? (Objectives 7-11)
A. *Isospora belli*
B. *Entamoeba histolytica*
C. *Crytosporidium parvum*
D. *Giardia intestinalis*

Quick Quiz! 7-4

Which two factors play an important role in the prognosis of a *Balantidum coli* infection? (Objective 7-7A)
A. How infection occurred and duration of the infection
B. Presence of coinfection and duration of the infection
C. Severity of infection and response to treatment
D. Immunocompetent status and severity of infection

Isospora belli
(eye″sos′puh-ruh/bell-eye)

Common associated disease and condition names: Isosporiasis.

Morphology

 Oocysts. The oval transparent oocyst of *Isospora belli* ranges in size from 25 to 35 μm long by 10 to 15 μm wide, with an average of 30 by 12 μm (Fig. 7-7; Table 7-3). The developing

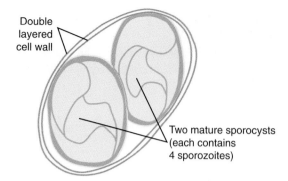

Double layered cell wall

Two mature sporocysts (each contains 4 sporozoites)

Size range: 25-35 μm by 10-15 μm
Average size: 30 μm by 12 μm

FIGURE 7-7 *Isospora belli* oocyst.

TABLE 7-3	*Isospora belli* Oocyst: Typical Characteristics at a Glance
Parameter	**Description**
Size range	25-35 μm long, 10-15 μm wide
Appearance	Transparent
Shape	Oval
Cell wall	Two layered, colorless and smooth
Developing sporoblast	Unicellular with granular cytoplasm
Young oocyst	Two sporoblasts
Mature oocyst	Two sporocysts, each containing four sausage-shaped sporozoites

morphologic form within the oocyst, known as a **sporoblast,** consists of a roundish immature sac that contains a small discrete nucleus and granular cytoplasm. As it matures, the young oocyst divides into two sporoblasts. Each sporoblast continues to mature and eventually becomes a **sporocyst,** which consists of a mature roundish sac containing four sausage-shaped sporozoites. This stage is known as the mature oocyst (Fig. 7-7). Throughout its development, the sporoblast and sporocysts are surrounded by a smooth, colorless, two-layered cell wall.

Laboratory Diagnosis

The specimens of choice for recovery of the *I. belli* oocysts are fresh feces and duodenal contents. Stool samples may contain oocysts that are immature, partially mature, and/or fully mature. In addition, material collected via an Enterotest may also be used to obtain the oocysts. Intestinal biopsies collected from infected patients may reveal the intracellular morphologic stages of the organism. It is interesting to note that a biopsy from an infected patient may contain *I. belli* oocysts, whereas a stool specimen from the same patient may be free of the parasites. This occurs particularly in patients who have only small numbers of organisms present.

I. belli oocysts may be visible in direct wet preparations and in those made following the concentration or flotation procedures. Promising results have been obtained on stool specimens processed using the Sheather's sugar flotation procedure. It is important to note that *I. belli* oocysts appear transparent and may be difficult to recognize when present in saline wet preparations. The oocysts are more readily discernible in iodine preparations. It is therefore important to include an iodine wet preparation in the standard processing of samples for parasite study, particularly those in which *I. belli* is suspected. In addition, a decreased microscope light level and proper contrast are necessary when screening suspicious slides to achieve the most favorable conditions for parasite recovery. This is particularly true when screening samples that have been tested by the zinc sulfate technique or another concentration procedure following polyvinyl alcohol (PVA) preservation.

A tentative diagnosis may be made following preparation and examination of an auramine-rhodamine permanent stain. However, the recommended permanent stain for successful *I. belli* oocyst confirmatory identification is a modified acid-fast stain. This clearly shows the organism's characteristics, as well as those of *Cryptosporidium* oocysts, another important member of the sporozoa (see later). Wet preparations for *Isospora* may also serve as adequate confirmatory tests when necessary.

Life Cycle Notes

I. belli was initially thought to be a typical coccidial parasite. Pigs and cattle appeared to be intermediate hosts for this organism. It has now been determined that *I. belli* is the only known coccidial parasite that does not have intermediate hosts. Humans serve as the definitive host, in whom both sexual and asexual reproduction take place.

It is presumed that infection with *I. belli* is initiated following the ingestion of infective mature (also known as sporulated) oocysts in contaminated food or water. The sporozoites emerge after excystation of the oocyst in the small intestine. Asexual reproduction (schizogony), resulting in merozoites, occurs in the cells of the intestinal mucosa. The formation of macrogametocytes and microgametocytes (**gametogony**) takes place in the same intestinal area. The resulting gametocytes develop and ultimately unite to form oocysts, the form that is excreted in the stool. Immature oocysts typically complete their development in the outside environment. It is the mature sporulated oocyst that is capable of initiating another infection. When this occurs, the life cycle repeats itself. There is evidence suggesting that *I. belli* may also be transmitted through oral-anal sexual contact.

Epidemiology

The frequency of contracting *I. belli* has traditionally been considered rare, even though the organism has worldwide geographic distribution. The difficulty often experienced in organism recognition may have led to potentially false-negative results, which thus may have been the major contributing factor to the documented rare frequency of infection. An increase in reported cases began to occur during and following World War II. Specifically, cases were reported in Africa, Southeast Asia, and Central America. In addition, countries in South America, particularly in Chile, have reported *I. belli* infections. An increase in frequency was particularly noted in patients suffering from AIDS. Unprotected oral-anal sexual contact has been suggested as the mode of parasite transmission in these patients. The resulting infections with *I. belli* are now considered opportunistic.

Clinical Symptoms

▶ **Asymptomatic.** A number of infected individuals remain asymptomatic. In such cases, the infection is self-limited.

▶ **Isosporiasis.** Infected patients may complain of a number of symptoms, ranging from mild gastrointestinal discomfort to severe dysentery. The more commonly noted clinical symptoms include weight loss, chronic diarrhea, abdominal pain, anorexia, weakness, and malaise. In addition, eosinophilia may occur in asymptomatic and symptomatic patients. Charcot-Leyden crystals (Chapter 12) may form in response to the eosinophilia and may be visible in corresponding stool samples. Patients experiencing severe infection typically develop a malabsorption syndrome. In these cases, patients produce foul-smelling stools that are pale yellow and of a loose consistency. Fecal fat levels of these stool samples may be increased. Infected patients may shed oocysts in their stools for as long as 120 days. Death may result from such severe infections.

Treatment

The treatment of choice for asymptomatic or mild infections consists of consuming a bland diet and obtaining plenty of rest. Patients suffering from more severe infections respond best to chemotherapy, consisting of a combination of trimethoprim and sulfamethoxazole or pyrimethamine and sulfadiazine. It is interesting to note that chemotherapy at a lower dosage for a longer period may be necessary for AIDS patients infected with *I. belli*.

Prevention and Control

The prevention and control measures for *I. belli* are similar to those of *E. histolytica*. They include proper personal hygiene, adequate sanitation practices, and avoidance of unprotected sex, particularly among homosexual men.

Quick Quiz! 7-5

All the following are highly recommended when processing samples for the identification of *Isospora belli* to ensure identification except: (Objective 7-8)
A. Iodine wet prep
B. Decreased microscope light level
C. Modified acid-fast stain
D. Saline wet prep

Quick Quiz! 7-6

Which stage of reproduction is considered capable of initiating another infection of *Isospora belli*? (Objectives 7-5)
A. Sporozoites
B. Immature oocysts
C. Merozoites
D. Mature oocysts

Quick Quiz! 7-7

Which of the following patients would be more likely to contract an infection with *Isospora belli*? (Objective 7-6)
A. HIV-positive man
B. Female leukemia patient
C. Pig farmer
D. Nursing home resident

Sarcocystis species
(sahr″ko-sis-tis)

Common associated disease and condition names: *Sarcocystis* infection.

There are a number of species of parasites that fall within the group known as *Sarcocystis*. Cattle may harbor *Sarcocystis hovihominis*, also known as *Sarcocystis hominis*. Similarly, *Sarcocystis suihominis* may be found in pigs. In addition to these typical farm animals, a variety of wild animals may also harbor members of the *Sarcocystis* group. *Sarcocystis lindemanni* has been designated as the umbrella term for those organisms that may potentially parasitize humans.

Morphology

Mature Oocysts. Members of the genus *Sarcocystis* were originally classified and considered as members of the genus *Isospora*, in part because of the striking morphologic similarities of these parasites (Fig. 7-8; Table 7-4). The oval transparent organism consists of two mature sporocysts that each average from 10 to 18 μm in length. Each sporocyst is equipped with four sausage-shaped sporozoites. A double-layered clear and colorless cell wall surrounds the sporocysts.

Laboratory Diagnosis

Stool is the specimen of choice for the recovery of *Sarcocystis* organisms. The oocysts are usually passed into the feces fully developed. When present, these mature oocysts are typically seen

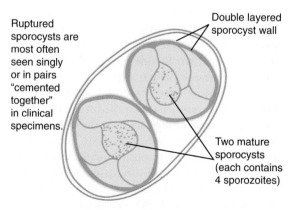

Ruptured sporocysts are most often seen singly or in pairs "cemented together" in clinical specimens.

Double layered sporocyst wall

Two mature sporocysts (each contains 4 sporozoites)

Average sporocyst length: 10-18 μm

FIGURE 7-8 *Sarcocystis species* oocyst.

TABLE 7-4	*Sarcocystis* spp. Mature Oocyst: Typical Characteristics at a Glance*	
Parameter	**Description**	
Shape	Oval	
Appearance	Transparent	
Number of sporocysts	Two	
Size of each sporocyst	10-18 µm long	
Contents of each sporocyst	Four sausage-shaped sporozoites	
Oocyst cell wall appearance	Clear, colorless, double layered	

*In many cases, only single or double sporocysts cemented together may be visible in stool samples.

in wet preparations. However, in many cases, the oocysts have already ruptured and only the sporocysts are visible on examination of the stool specimen. The sporocysts may be seen singly or in pairs that appear to be cemented together. Routine histologic methods may be used to identify the *Sarcocystis* cyst stage, known as the sarcocyst, from human muscle samples. An in-depth discussion of these histologic methods is beyond the scope of this text.

Life Cycle Notes

Although the morphology of the oocysts of *Sarcocystis* resembles that of *Isospora*, the life cycles of these two genera are different—hence, the current organism classification. Asexual reproduction of *Sarcocystis* occurs in the intermediate host. Human infection of *Sarcocystis* species may be initiated in one of two ways. The first transmission route occurs when uncooked pig or cattle meat infected with *Sarcocystis* sarcocysts is ingested. Humans are the definitive host. Gametogony usually occurs in the human intestinal cells. The development of oocysts and subsequent release of sporocysts thus follow. This sets the stage for continuation of the life cycle in a new intermediate host. The second transmission route occurs when humans accidentally swallow oocysts from stool sources of animals other than cattle or pigs. In this case, the ingested sarcocysts

take up residence in human striated muscle. Under these circumstances, the human serves as the intermediate host. It is interesting to note that *Sarcocystis* oocysts do not infect the host of their origin.

Epidemiology

The frequency of *Sarcocystis* infections is relatively low, even though its distribution is worldwide. In addition to its presence in cattle and pigs, *Sarcocystis* spp. may also be found in a variety of wild animals.

Clinical Symptoms

Sarcocystis Infection. There have only been a few documented symptomatic cases of *Sarcocystis* infections in compromised patients. These persons experienced fever, severe diarrhea, weight loss, and abdominal pain. It is presumed that patients suffering from muscle tenderness and other local symptoms are exhibiting symptoms caused by *Sarcocystis* invasion of the striated muscle.

Treatment

The treatment protocol for infections with *Sarcocystis* spp. when humans are the definitive host is similar to that for *Isospora belli*. The combined medications of trimethoprim plus sulfamethoxazole or pyrimethamine plus sulfadiazine are typically given to treat these infections. There is no known specific chemotherapy to treat *Sarcocystis* infections of the striated muscle when humans are the intermediate host.

Prevention and Control

The primary prevention and control measures of *Sarcocystis* infections in which humans are the definitive host consist of adequate cooking of beef and pork. Prevention of those infections in which humans are the intermediate host includes the proper care and disposal of animal stool that may be potentially infected with *Sarcocystis*.

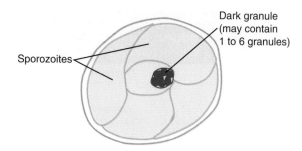

Average size: 4-6 μm

FIGURE 7-9 *Cryptosporidium parvum* oocyst.

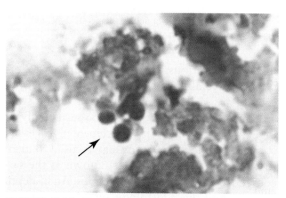

FIGURE 7-10 Modified acid-fast stain, ×1000). Arrows indicate *Cryptosporidium* oocysts, each containing four undefined sporozoites. Note dark-staining granules.

TABLE 7-5	*Cryptosporidium parvum* Oocyst: Typical Characteristics at a Glance
Parameter	**Description**
Size	4-6 μm
Shape	Roundish
Number of sporocysts	None
Number of sporozoites	Four (small)
Other features	Thick cell wall
	One to six dark granules may be visible

Cryptosporidium parvum
(krip″toe-spor-i'dee-um/par-voom)

Common associated disease and condition names: Cryptosporidosis.

Morphology

▶ **Oocysts.** Measuring only 4 to 6 μm, the roundish *Cryptosporidium* oocysts are often confused with yeast (Figs. 7-9 and 7-10; Table 7-5). Although not always visible, the mature oocyst consists of four small sporozoites surrounded by a thick cell wall. Contrary to other members of the sporozoa, such as *Isospora*, *Cryptosporidium* oocysts do not contain sporocysts. One to six dark granules may also be seen.

Schizonts and Gametocytes. The other morphologic forms required to complete the life cycle of *Cryptosporidium* include schizonts containing four to eight merozoites, microgametocytes, and macrogametocytes. The average size of these forms is a mere 2 to 4 μm. It is important to note that these morphologic forms are not routinely seen in patient samples.

Laboratory Diagnosis

The specimen of choice for the recovery of *Cryptosporidium* oocysts is stool. Several methods have been found to identify these organisms successfully. The oocysts may be seen using iodine or modified acid-fast stain. In addition, formalin-fixed smears stained with Giemsa may also yield the desired oocysts. As noted, it is important to distinguish yeast (Chapter 12) from true oocysts. Oocysts have also been detected using the following methods: the Enterotest, enzyme-linked immunosorbent assay (ELISA), and indirect immunofluorescence. Concentration via modified zinc sulfate flotation or by Sheather's sugar flotation have also proven successful, especially when the treated sample is examined under phase contrast microscopy. It is important to note that merozoites and gametocytes are usually only recovered in intestinal biopsy material.

Life Cycle Notes

Cryptosporidium infection typically occurs following ingestion of the mature oocyst. Sporozoites emerge after excystation in the upper gastrointestinal tract, where they take up residence in the cell membrane of epithelial cells. Asexual and sexual multiplication may then occur. Sporozoites rupture from the resulting oocysts and are capable of initiating an autoinfection by invading new epithelial cells. A number of the resulting oocysts remain intact, pass through the feces, and serve as the infective stage for a new host.

It is interesting to note that two forms of oocysts are believed to be involved in the *Cryptosporidium* life cycle. The thin-shelled version is most likely responsible for autoinfections because it always seems to rupture while still inside the host. The thick-shelled oocyst usually remains intact and is passed out of the body. This form is believed to initiate autoinfections only occasionally.

Epidemiology

Cryptosporidium has worldwide distribution. Of the 20 species known to exist, only *C. parvum* is known to infect humans. Infection appears to primarily occur by water or food contaminated with infected feces, as well as by person-to-person transmission. Immunocompromised persons, such as those infected with the AIDS virus, are at risk of contracting this parasite. Other populations potentially at risk include immunocompetent children in tropical areas, children in day care centers, animal handlers, and those who travel abroad.

Clinical Symptoms

Cryptosporidiosis. Otherwise healthy persons infected with *Cryptosporidium* typically complain of diarrhea, which is self-limiting and lasts approximately 2 weeks. Episodes of diarrhea lasting 1 to 4 weeks have been reported in some day care centers. Fever, nausea, vomiting, weight loss, and abdominal pain may also be present. When fluid loss is great because of the diarrhea and/or severe vomiting, this condition may be fatal, particularly in young children.

Infected immunocompromised individuals, particularly AIDS patients, usually suffer from severe diarrhea and one or more of the symptoms described earlier. Malabsorption may also accompany infection in these patients. In addition, infection may migrate to other body areas, such as the stomach and respiratory tract. A debilitating condition that leads to death may result in these patients. Estimated infection rates in AIDS patients range from 3 to 20% in the United States and 50 to 60% in Africa and Haiti. *Cryptosporidium* infection is considered to be a cause of morbidity and mortality.

Treatment

Numerous experiments to treat *Cryptosporidium* using a wide variety of medications have been conducted. Unfortunately, most of these potential treatments have proven ineffective. However, the use of spiramycin, even though still in the experimental stage, has preliminarily proven helpful in ridding the host of *Cryptosporidium*. More research on this treatment and on the newer antiparasitic medications are necessary to develop effective medications.

Prevention and Control

Proper treatment of water supplies, handling known infected material by using gloves and wearing a gown (when appropriate), proper hand washing, and properly disinfecting potentially infected equipment with full-strength commercial bleach or 5% to 10% household ammonia are crucial to the prevention and control of *Cryptosporidium*. In addition, enteric precautions should be observed when working with known infected persons.

Notes of Interest and New Trends

Cryptosporidium spp. were first associated with poultry and cattle. *C. parvum* is now recognized as the agent responsible for neonatal diarrhea in calves and lambs, a life-threatening condition.

Human *Cryptosporidium* infection was first reported in 1976. The first cases were isolated from persons with compromised immune systems and were considered infrequent in occurrence.

Several outbreaks in the public water supply were attributed to contamination of *Cryptosporidium* oocysts. This occurred in Carroll County, Georgia in 1987. More recently in June 2011, and Indiana fire station reported gastrointestinal illness in a substantial percentage of their workers who had extinguished a barn fire on a nearby Michigan farm. An investigation by the Michigan Department of Community Health revealed that the firefighters used local hydrant water and on site swimming pond water to extinguish the fire. The pond water was discovered to be contaminated with **Cryptosporidium** from calf feces.

A modification of the standard stool processing technique (see Chapter 2), which includes layering and flotation of the sample over a hypertonic sodium chloride solution, has successfully separated *Cryptosporidium* oocysts from fecal debris.

Quick Quiz! 7-11

Which stage of reproduction is considered capable of autoinfection of *Cryptosporidium*? (Objectives 7-5)
A. Intact oocysts
B. Merozoites
C. Gametocytes
D. Sporozoites

Quick Quiz! 7-12

The permanent stain of choice for the recovery of *Cryptosporidium parvum* is: (Objective 7-8)
A. Iron hematoxylin
B. Modifed acid-fast
C. Gram
D. Trichrome

Quick Quiz! 7-13

All the following are recommended to prevent and control an outbreak of *Cryptosporidium* except: (Objective 7-7C)
A. Proper treatment of water supplies
B. Sterilize equipment using high heat.
C. Sterilize equipment using full-strength bleach.
D. Sterilize equipment using 5% to 10% household ammonia.

Blastocystis hominis
(blas'toe-sis-tis/hom'i-nis)

Common associated disease and condition names: *Blastocystis hominis* infection.

Morphology

Although a number of different morphologic forms of *B. hominis* are known to exist, the most

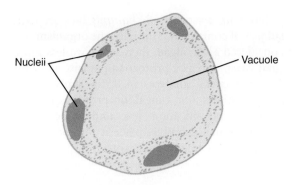

Size range: 5-32 μm
Average size: 7-10 μm

FIGURE 7-11 *Blastocystis hominis* vacuolated form.

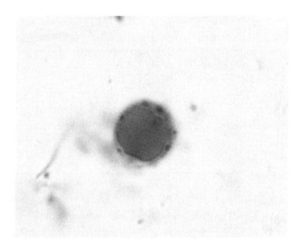

FIGURE 7-12 Trichrome stain, 1000×. Typical *Blastocystis hominis* vacuolated form.

common form seen and the easiest to recognize is the vacuolated form. Therefore, only this form will be described here.

▧ **Vacuolated Forms.** Although the vacuolated form of *B. hominis* may range in size from 5 to 32 μm, the average form measures only 7 to 10 μm (Figs. 7-11 and 7-12; Table 7-6). This morphologic form is characterized by a large, central, fluid-filled vacuole that consumes almost 90% of the cell. The remaining 10% assumes the periphery of the organism; it consists of a ring of cytoplasm in which two to four nuclei are typically present.

TABLE 7-6	*Blastocystis hominis* Vacuolated Form: Typical Characteristics at a Glance
Parameter	**Description**
Size	5-32 μm
Vacuole	Centrally located
	Fluid-filled structure
	Consumes almost 90% of organism
Cytoplasm	Appears as ring around periphery of organism
Nuclei	Two to four located in cytoplasm

Laboratory Diagnosis

Stool is the specimen of choice for the recovery of *Blastocystis*. In iodine wet preparations, the peripheral cytoplasm containing one or more nuclei appears a light yellow in color, whereas the central vacuole does not stain and appears clear and transparent. In permanent stain preparations, the central vacuole may vary in its ability to stain from not at all to very apparent. The nuclei located in the peripheral cytoplasm in these preparations typically stain dark. It is important to note here that saline, like water, usually lyses this organism and may lead to a false-negative result. Therefore, it is important to screen suspicious samples with an iodine wet preparation and to use a permanent stain to confirm the presence of the parasite.

Life Cycle Notes

B. hominis reproduces by sporulation or binary fission. The organism passes through a number of morphologic forms during these processes. *B. hominis* participates in sexual and asexual reproduction, and exhibits pseudopod extension and retraction. A detailed discussion of the *B. hominis* life cycle has not been widely presented.

Epidemiology

Early nonscientific documentation of *B. hominis* infections indicated that they occurred as epidemics in subtropical countries. Select articles on *B. hominis* over the past 10 to 25 years or so suggest that this organism may be found in a number of climates worldwide, ranging from Saudi Arabia to British Columbia. The results of one study conducted in Saudi Arabia were inconclusive regarding whether travel is a risk factor in contracting this parasite. Infection of *B. hominis* is initiated by ingestion of fecally contaminated food or water.

Clinical Symptoms

 Blastocystis hominis Infection. The pathogenicity of *B. hominis* is not totally clear, although the symptoms have been defined. Patients who suffer from infection with *B. hominis* in the absence of other intestinal pathogens (including parasites, bacteria, and viruses) may experience diarrhea, vomiting, nausea, and fever, as well as abdominal pain and cramping. Thus, *B. hominis* might be considered a pathogen. However, it has also been suggested that these patients may have an additional undetected pathogen that is ultimately responsible for the discomfort.

In persons infected with *B. hominis* in addition to another pathogenic organism (e.g., *E. histolytica, Giardia intestinalis*), it is this underlying agent that is thought to be the pathogen. These patients usually experience severe symptoms, as described earlier.

Treatment

Iodoquinol or metronidazole is recommended for the treatment of *B. hominis*. This has been suggested for patients infected with *Blastocystis* who have no other obvious reason for their diarrhea.

Prevention and Control

Proper treatment of fecal material, thorough hand washing, and subsequent proper handling of food and water are critical to halt the spread of *Blastocystis*.

Notes of Interest and New Trends

Blastocystis hominis was given its current name in 1912 by Emile Brumpt.

Since its discovery, *B. hominis* has been the subject of controversy. Initially, the organism was considered as an algae, then as a harmless intestinal yeast, and as a protozoan parasite since the 1970s. Genetic analyses in 1996 showed that Blastocystis is not fungal or protozoan. Since then, its classification has undergone major reviews which definitely place it into Stramenopiles, a major line of eukaryotes.

Quick Quiz! 7-14

Which is the best screening method for the identification of *Blastocystis hominis*? (Objective 7-8)
A. Saline wet prep
B. Modified acid-fast stain
C. Iodine wet prep
D. Iron hematoxylin stain

Quick Quiz! 7-15

Blastocystis hominis is always considered as being responsible for clinical symptoms when present in human samples. (Objective 7-6)
A. True
B. False

Quick Quiz! 7-16

Which of the following measures that when taken can prevent the spread of *Blastocystis hominis*? (Objective 7-7C)
A. Avoid swimming in potentially contaminated water.
B. Proper sewage treatment
C. Use insect repellent.
D. Avoid unprotected sex.

Cyclospora cayetanensis
(si'klō-spor-uh)

Common associated disease and condition names: *Cyclospora cayetanensis* infection.

Morphology

 Oocysts. *Cyclospora cayetanensis* infection is similar to cryptosporidiosis (Table 7-7). It is an

TABLE 7-7	*Cyclospora cayetanensis* Mature Oocyst: Typical Characteristics at a Glance
Parameter	**Description**
Size	7-10 μm in diameter
Number of sporocysts	Two
Contents of sporocysts	Each sporocyst contains two sporozoites

intestinal coccidial organism. Infected patients shed oocysts that measure 7 to 10 μm in diameter and, on maturation, form two sporocysts, each containing only two sporozoites.

Laboratory Diagnosis

Diagnosis of *C. cayetanensis* may be accomplished when stool samples are concentrated nontraditionally without the use of formalin fixative. *C. cayetanensis* oocysts sporulate best at room temperature. The addition of 5% potassium dichromate allows the sporocysts to become visible. Flotation methods followed by examination using the preferred phase contrast or bright field microscopy have also proven successful in isolating *C. cayetanensis*. Modified acid-fast stain may also be used to detect the oocysts. Oocysts autofluoresce under ultraviolet light microscopy.

Life Cycle Notes

The life-cycle of *C. cayetanensis*, like that of *Isospora*, begins with ingestion of an oocyst. The oocyst contains two sporocysts, each enclosing two sporozoites. Once inside a human host, cells in the small intestine provide a suitable environment for the emergence of sporozoites. The sporozoites undergo asexual reproduction, producing numerous merozoites, as well as sexual development, resulting in macrogametocyte and microgametocyte production. Male and female gametocytes unite and form oocysts. Infected humans pass immature oocysts in the stool. Under optimal conditions, these oocyts continue to develop and mature outside the human body,

a process that may take 1 or more weeks to complete. Once the maturation process is complete, the resultant oocysts are capable of initiating a new cycle. No animal reservoir exists.

Epidemiology

C. cayetanensis infections are known to occur in many countries, including the United States and Canada. Furthermore, cases of infection caused by *C. cayetanensisa* have been reported in children living in unsanitary conditions in Lima, Peru, as well as in travelers and foreigners residing in Nepal and parts of Asia. Contaminated water in Chicago presumably was the source of a minioutbreak in 1990 that occurred in a physician's dormitory. Contaminated lettuce and fresh fruit (raspberries have been known to be a source of infection), often imported, have also been associated with *C. cayetanensis* infections.

Clinical Symptoms

▰ *Cyclospora cayetanensis* Infection. The clinical symptoms associated with *C. cayetanensis* infections in children are similar to those seen in cases of cryptosporidiosis. The notable difference among infections caused by these two organisms in adults is that *C. cayetanensis* produces a longer duration of diarrhea. There is no known connection between *C. cayetanensis* infection and immunocompromised patients.

Prevention and Control

Prevention and control measures associated with *C. cayetanensis* consist of properly treating water prior to use and only using treated water when handling and processing food.

Notes of Interest and New Trends

It appears that this parasite may not be recovered using standard or traditional specimen processing techniques. The alternative techniques discussed in the laboratory diagnosis section may be necessary for samples suspected of containing *C. cayetanensis* in the future.

Microsporidia
(mi'kro-spor-i'dee-uh)

Common associated disease and condition names: Microsporidia infection, microsporidial infection.

Although it is classified as a protozoal disease by the World Health Organization, Microsporidia's phylogenetic placement has been resolved within the Fungi as a result of DNA testing. There are a number of genera and species of parasites that are members of the phylum Microsporidia. Three of the five genera known to cause

human disease have been reported in patients suffering from AIDS. The most well-known member is *Enterocytozoon bieneusi,* which causes enteritis in these patients. Species of *Encephulitozoon* and *Pleistophora* have also been described as infecting AIDS patients and causing severe tissue infections. Of the remaining two genera, *Microsporidium* is noted for corneal infections, as well as *Nosema.* In addition, *Nosema* produced a fatal infection in a severely immunocompromised infant.

Morphology

◼ **Spores.** Although it has been documented that there are a number of different morphologic forms, spores are the only ones that have been well described (Table 7-8). These spores are very small, ranging in size from 1 to 5 μm. Unlike the other protozoa, Microsporidia spores are characteristically equipped with extruding polar filaments (tubules), which initiate infection by injecting sporoplasm (infectious material) into a host cell.

Laboratory Diagnosis

Diagnosis of the different species of Microsporidia varies. Serologic tests are available for the detection of some species. In addition, some species will grow in cell culture. A number of stains may be used to detect all or part of the spore microscopically. Thin smears stained with trichrome or acid-fast stain may show the desired spores. Microsporidia stain gram-positive and show partial positive staining when treated with acid-fast stain or the histologic

TABLE 7-8	*Microsporidia* Spore: Typical Characteristics at a Glance	
Parameter	**Description**	
Size	1-5 μm	
Other features	Equipped with extruding polar filaments (or tubules) that initiate infection by injecting sporoplasm (infectious material) into host cell	

stain periodic acid-Schiff (PAS). Giemsa-stained biopsy material and fecal concentrate specimens readily show the spores. It is important to note that speciation of the Microsporidia requires the use of transmission electron microscopy. Molecular diagnostic methods are being developed.

Life Cycle Notes

Transmission of Microsporidia may be direct or may involve an intermediate host. On entering the host, human infection is initiated when the infective spores inject sporoplasm into a host cell. A complex reproductive process occurs, new spores emerge, and additional cells typically become infected. Spores are dispersed into the outside environment in the direct transmission cycle in the feces or urine, or by the death of the host. In addition, the spores may be ingested by a carnivorous animal.

Epidemiology

Cases of *E. bieneusi* infection have been reported in AIDS patients from Haiti, Zambia, Uganda, the United Kingdom, the United States, and the Netherlands. Although most documented infections of Microsporidia parasites have occurred in AIDS patients, cases in persons with normal immune systems have also been described.

Clinical Symptoms

 Microsporidial Infection. Patients suffering from infections with Microsporidia have been known to develop enteritis, keratoconjunctivitis, and myositis. Infections involving peritonitis and hepatitis have rarely occurred.

Treatment

Albendazole is recommended for the treatment of *E. bieneusi*; oral fumagillin is recommended as an alternative treatment. Albendazole plus fumagillin eye drops are recommended for the treatment of *Nosema* infection.

Notes of Interest and New Trends

Persons infected with *C. cayetanensis* in addition to Microsporidia have been reported and are considered somewhat common.

In recent years, the United States Environmental Protection Agency (EPA) has listed Microsporidia in the EPA Candidate Contaminate List, deeming it an emerging water-borne pathogen needing monitorial attention.

Although Microsporidia infection in humans mostly occurs in immunocompromised patients, the further spread of AIDS worldwide increases our need to understand and manage Microsporidia for the near future.

Quick Quiz! 7-20

How do *Microsporidia* spores differ from other protozoan spores? (Objective 7-11)
A. Double outer wall
B. Extruding polar filaments
C. Cilia
D. Pseudopods

Quick Quiz! 7-21

Of the following, which laboratory technique is required for species identification of Microsporidia? (Objective 7-8)
A. Giemsa-stained biopsy material
B. Electron microscopy
C. Fecal concentration
D. PAS stain

Quick Quiz! 7-22

The life cycle of Microsporidia is a complex process in which both the infective and diagnostic stages are spores. (Objective 7-5)
A. True
B. False

Toxoplasma gondii
(tock"so-plaz'muh/gon'dee-eye)

Common associated disease and condition names: Toxoplasmosis, congenital toxoplasmosis, cerebral toxoplasmosis.

Morphology

There are only two morphologic forms of tro-phozoites seen in humans, tachyzoites and brady-zoites. The infective form for humans is the oocyst. This form may be encountered on occa-sion, especially where veterinary parasitologic techniques are performed. Thus, all three of these morphologic forms are discussed in this section.

■ **Oocyst.** The typical infective form of *Toxo-plasma gondii*, the oocyst, is similar in appear-ance to that of *Isospora belli*. The most notable difference between the two organisms is that *T. gondii* is smaller. The round to slightly oval form measures 10 to 15 μm long by 8 to 12 μm wide. The transparent oocyst contains two sporocysts, each with four sporozoites. The organism is bor-dered by a clear, colorless, two-layered cell wall.

■ **Tachyzoites.** The actively multiplying, cres-cent-shaped tachyzoites range in size from 3 to 7 μm by 2 to 4 μm (Fig. 7-13; Table 7-9). One end of the organism often appears more rounded than the other end. Each tachyzoite is equipped with a single centrally located nucleus, sur-rounded by a cell membrane. A variety of other organelles are present, including a mitochon-drion and Golgi apparatus; however, these struc-tures are not readily visible.

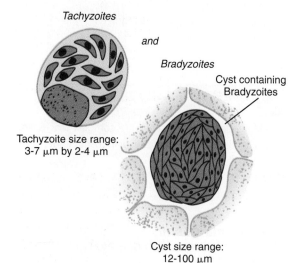

Tachyzoite size range:
3-7 μm by 2-4 μm

Cyst size range:
12-100 μm

FIGURE 7-13 *Toxoplasma gondii* tachyzoites and bradyzoites.

■ **Bradyzoites.** Although there is evidence to support an antigenic difference, the typical bradyzoite basically has the same physical appearance as the tachyzoite, only smaller (see Fig. 7-13; Table 7-10). These slow-growing viable forms gather in clusters inside a host cell, develop a surrounding membrane, and form a cyst in a variety of host tissues and muscles outside the intestinal tract. Such cysts may contain as few as 50 and up to as many as several thousand bradyzoites. A typical cyst measures from 12 to 100 μm in diameter.

Laboratory Diagnosis

The primary means of diagnosing *T. gondii* infec-tions is analyzing blood samples using serologic

TABLE 7-9	*Toxoplasma gondii* Tachyzoites: Typical Characteristics at a Glance
Parameter	**Description**
General comment	Actively multiplying morphologic form
Size	3-7 × 2-4 μm
Shape	Crescent-shaped, often more rounded on one end
Number of nuclei	One
Other features	Contains a variety of organelles that are not readily visible

TABLE 7-10	*Toxoplasma gondii* Bradyzoites: Typical Characteristics at a Glance
Parameter	**Description**
General comment	Slow-growing morphologic form
Size	Smaller than tachyzoites
Physical appearance	Similar to that of the tachyzoites
Other features	Hundreds to thousands of bradyzoites enclose themselves to form a cyst that may measure 12-100 μm in diameter

test methods. The recommended test for the determination of immunoglobulin M (IgM) antibodies present in congenital infections is the double-sandwich ELISA method. Both IgM and IgG levels may be determined using the indirect fluorescent antibody (IFA) test. Additional serologic tests for the IgG antibody include the indirect hemagglutination (IHA) test and ELISA. The actual demonstration of *T. gondii* trophozoites (tachyzoites) and cysts (filled with bradyzoites) involves tedious microscopic examination of infected human tissue samples or the inoculation of laboratory animals. The time and effort to perform such testing is, in most cases, not practical.

Life Cycle Notes

Although the natural life cycle of *T. gondii* is relatively simple, the accidental cycle may involve a number of animals and humans. The definitive host in the *T. gondii* life cycle is the cat (or other felines). On ingestion of *T. gondii* cysts present in the brain or muscle tissue of contaminated mice or rats, the enclosed bradyzoites are released in the cat and quickly transform into tachyzoites. Both sexual and asexual reproduction occur in the gut of the cat. The sexual cycle results in the production of immature oocysts, which are ultimately shed in the stool. The oocysts complete their maturation in the outside environment, a process that typically takes from 1 to 5 days. Rodents, particularly mice and rats, serve as the intermediate hosts, ingesting the infected mature *T. gondii* oocysts while foraging for food. The sporozoites emerge from the mature oocyst and rapidly convert into actively growing tachyzoites in the intestinal epithelium of the rodent. These tachyzoites migrate into the brain or muscle of the intermediate host, where they form cysts filled with bradyzoites. The cat becomes infected on ingestion of a contaminated rodent and the cycle repeats itself.

Human infection of *T. gondii* is accidental and may be initiated in four ways. One route occurs when humans are in contact with infected cat feces and subsequently ingest the mature oocysts present via hand-to-mouth transmission. Cat litter boxes, as well as children's sandboxes, are the primary sources of such infected fecal matter.

The second route involves human ingestion of contaminated undercooked meat from cattle, pigs, or sheep. These animals, as well as a wide variety of other animals, may contract *T. gondii* during feeding by ingesting infective oocysts present in cat feces. The infective sporozoites are released following ingestion and follow the same cycle in these animals as they do in the natural intermediate hosts. The resulting cysts form in the animal muscle and the parasites within them may remain viable for years.

The third means of human *T. gondii* transfer is transplacental infection. This occurs when an asymptomatic infection in a mother is unknowingly transmitted to her unborn fetus. In response to the parasite, the mother produces IgG, which also crosses the placenta and may appear for several months in the circulation of the fetus/newborn. In addition, the mother produces IgM, which does not cross the placenta. However, the infant may demonstrate anti–*T. gondii* IgM from birth to several months old.

Although extremely rare, the fourth route of human infection occurs when contaminated blood is transfused into an uninfected person.

Once inside the human, *T. gondii* tachyzoites emerge from the ingested cyst and begin to grow and divide rapidly. The tachyzoite form is responsible for the tissue damage and initial infection. The tachyzoites migrate to a number of tissues and organs, including the brain, where cysts filled with bradyzoites then form.

Epidemiology

T. gondii is found worldwide, primarily because such a large variety of animals may harbor the organism. It appears from information collected to date that no population is exempt from the possibility of contracting *T. gondii*. One of the most important populations at risk for contracting this parasite is individuals suffering from AIDS.

There are several epidemiologic considerations worth noting. First, it has been documented that *T. gondii* infections occur in 15% to 20% of the population in the United States. Second, infection caused by the consumption of undercooked meat and its juices by women and their children in Paris was reported in 93% (the highest recorded rate) and 50%, respectively, of the local population. Third, there have been an estimated 4000 infants born with transplacentally acquired *T. gondii* infections in the United States each year. Fourth, the *T. gondii* mature oocysts are incredibly hardy and can survive for long periods under less than optimal conditions. In the state of Kansas, it was documented that these oocysts survived up to 18 months in the outside environment, withstanding two winter seasons. Finally, human infections in the United States are usually acquired by hand-to-mouth contamination of infected oocysts in cat feces, ingesting contaminated meat, or transplacentally during pregnancy. As noted, transfusion-acquired *T. gondii* may also occur; however, it is extremely rare.

There are numerous other reports of *T. gondii* infections that have occurred worldwide. However, an in-depth discussion of these epidemiologic findings is beyond the scope of this chapter.

Clinical Symptoms

Asymptomatic. Many patients infected with *T. gondii* remain asymptomatic, especially children who have passed the neonatal stage of their lives. Although well adapted to its surroundings, *T. gondii* appears to only cause disease in humans when one or more of the following conditions have been met: (1) a virulent strain of the organism has entered the body; (2) the host is in a particularly susceptible state (e.g., those suffering from AIDS); and (3) the specific site of the parasite in the human body is such that tissue destruction is likely to occur.

Toxoplasmosis: General Symptoms. Although severe symptoms may be noted, the typical symptoms experienced by individuals infected with *T.*

gondii are mild and mimic those seen in cases of infectious mononucleosis. This acute form of the disease is characterized by fatigue, lymphadenitis, chills, fever, headache, and myalgia. In addition to the symptoms mentioned, chronic disease sufferers may develop a maculopapular rash as well as show evidence of encephalomyelitis, myocarditis, and/or hepatitis. Retinochoroiditis with subsequent blindness has been known to occur on rare occasions.

Congenital Toxoplasmosis. This severe and often fatal condition occurs in approximately one to five of every 1000 pregnancies. Transmission of the disease occurs when the fetus is infected (via transplacental means) unknowingly by its asymptomatic infected mother. The degree of severity of the resulting disease varies and is dependent on two factors: (1) antibody protection from the mother; and (2) the age of the fetus at the time of infection. Mild infections occur occasionally and result in what appears to be a complete recovery. Unfortunately, these patients may develop a subsequent retinochoroiditis years after the initial infection. Typical symptoms in an infected child include hydrocephaly, microcephaly, intracerebral calcification, chorioretinitis, convulsions, and psychomotor disturbances. Most of these infections ultimately result in mental retardation, severe visual impairment, or blindness.

There are a number of important documented statistics regarding the symptoms that infants born with *T. gondii* infection are likely to experience.

It is estimated that 5% to 15% of infected infants will die as a result of toxoplasmosis infection.

Another 10% to 13% of infected infants will most likely develop moderate to severe handicaps.

Severe eye and brain damage will occur in approximately 8% to 10% of infected infants.

The remaining 58% to 72% of infected infants will most likely be asymptomatic at birth.

Although the mechanism of this infection reactivation is unknown, a small percentage of these infants will develop mental retardation or retinochoroiditis later in life, usually as children or young adults.

▨ **Toxoplasmosis in Immunocompromised Patients.** Patients immunosuppressed because of organ transplantation or the presence of neoplastic disease, such as Hodgkin's lymphoma, have long been known to contract toxoplasmosis as an opportunistic infection. It is important to note, particularly in patients needing blood transfusions, the importance of screening potential donor units for toxoplasmosis prior to transfusion.

▨ **Cerebral Toxoplasmosis in AIDS Patients.** A focus of attention has been the association of *T. gondii* and AIDS patients. Since the 1980s, toxoplasmic encephalitis has been considered a significant complication in these individuals. In fact, one of the first apparent clinical symptoms of patients with AIDS may be that of central nervous system (CNS) involvement by *T. gondii*. AIDS patients suffering from infection with *T. gondii* may experience early symptoms of headache, fever, altered mental status (including confusion), and lethargy. Subsequent focal neurologic deficits, brain lesions, and convulsions usually develop.

The *T. gondii* organisms do not spread into other organs of the body but rather stay confined within the CNS. A rise in spinal fluid IgG antibody levels is diagnostic, as is the demonstration of tachyzoites in the cerebrospinal fluid (CSF) on microscopic examination. The serum IgG level in these patients does not respond, nor does that of the CSF. Most infected patients do not have serum levels of IgM antibodies. The lack of serum IgM coupled with the lack of change in serum IgG levels in these patients suggests that their infections occurred because of a reactivation of a chronic latent infection and not because of an acquired primary infection.

Treatment

The treatment of choice for symptomatic cases of *T. gondii* infection consists of a combination of trisulfapyrimidines and pyrimethamine (Daraprim). It is important to note that infected pregnant women should not be given pyrimethamine. An acceptable alternative drug is spiramycin. Spiramycin is used in Europe, Canada, and Mexico but is still considered an experimental drug in the United States. However, it can be obtained by special permission from the FDA for toxoplasmosis in the first trimester of pregnancy. Corticosteroids used as an anti-inflammatory agent may also be of value. Folinic acid (leucovorin) may be administered to infected AIDS patients to counteract the bone marrow suppression caused by pyrimethamine. An effective drug, particularly for the treatment of toxoplasmic encephalitis in patients with AIDS, is atovaquone.

Prevention and Control

There are a number of measures that must be implemented and enforced to prevent the spread of *T. gondii* infections. One is the avoidance of contact with cat feces. This may be accomplished by wearing protective gloves when cleaning out a cat litter box, disinfecting the litter box with boiling water, and thorough hand washing afterward. In addition, placing a protective cover over children's sandboxes when not in use will keep cats from using them as litter boxes.

T. gondii infections may also be prevented by the avoidance of ingesting contaminated meat. This may be accomplished by thorough hand washing after handling contaminated meat, as well as the avoidance of tasting raw meat. In addition, all meat should be thoroughly cooked prior to human consumption. Additional *T. gondii* prevention and control measures include keeping cats away from potentially infective rodents, feeding cats only dry or cooked canned cat food, and/or not having cats at all.

All humans should practice these preventive measures. However, pregnant women should be especially cautious around cat feces and contaminated meat because of the possibility of contracting toxoplasmosis and transferring the disease to their unborn children.

Notes of Interest and New Trends

In 1908, the African rodent *Ctenodactylus gondii* was the first animal discovered with *T.*

gondii—hence, the name. It was not until 1939 that *T. gondii* was recognized as a cause of transplacental infections.

Techniques using the polymerase chain reaction (PCR) assay have been developed. Successful results were achieved when analyzing samples of venous blood from AIDS patients and amniotic fluid from pregnant women.

Research has been conducted designed to detect specific IgE in patients suffering from toxoplasmosis. Known as an immunocapture assay, samples of CSF, fetal blood, umbilical cord blood, sera, and amniotic fluid were used. This technique is easy to perform and may prove to be helpful in diagnosing toxoplasmosis, particularly in pregnant women.

T. gondii tachyzoites, both invasive and intracellular, have been successfully demonstrated in AIDS patients suffering from pulmonary toxoplasmosis. A bronchoalveolar lavage was collected on each patient. Samples were then Giemsa-stained and microscopically examined.

Quick Quiz! 7-23

All the following are morphologic forms in the life cycle of *Toxoplasma gondii* except: (Objectives 7-5)
A. Oocysts
B. Tachyzoites
C. Bradyzoites
D. Sporozoites

Quick Quiz! 7-24

Human infection of *Toxoplasma* is initiated in all the following ways except: (Objectives 7-5)
A. Accidental ingestion of rodent feces
B. Ingestion of contaminated undercooked meat from cattle, pigs, or sheep
C. Transplacental infection
D. Transfusion of contaminated blood

Quick Quiz! 7-25

In which geographic area would you be likely to find *Toxoplasma gondii*? (Objective 7-2)
A. Tropics
B. Africa
C. United States
D. All of the above

Pneumocystis jiroveci (*Pneumocystis carinii*)
(new-moe"sis-tis/kah-reye"nee-eye)

Common associated disease and condition names: Pneumocystosis, atypical interstitial plasma cell pneumonia.

Morphology

Pneumocystis jiroveci, formerly called *Pneumocystis carinii*, is now considered as a fungus. However, its morphologic and biologic characteristics warrant inclusion in the discussion of miscellaneous protozoal parasites.

Trophozoites. The trophozoite or single organism, as it is often referred to, is the most commonly seen form (Fig. 7-14; Table 7-11). It

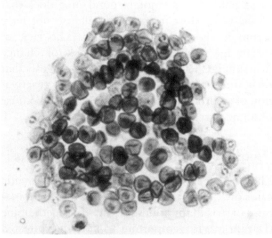

FIGURE 7-14 *Pneumocystis jiroveci,* multiple forms (iron hematoxylin stain, ×1000).

TABLE 7-11	*Pneumocystis jiroveci* Trophozoite: Typical Characteristics at a Glance
Parameter	**Description**
Size	2-4 µm
Shape	Ovoid, ameboid
Number of nuclei	One

TABLE 7-12	*Pneumocystis jiroveci* Cyst: Typical Characteristics at a Glance
Parameter	**Description**
Size	Diameter, 4-12 µm
Shape	Roundish
Number of nuclei	Four to eight; unorganized or arranged in a rosette

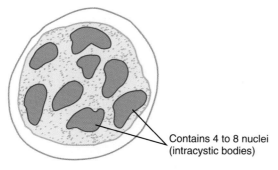

Contains 4 to 8 nuclei (intracystic bodies)

Size range: 4-12 µm in diameter

FIGURE 7-15 *Pneumocystis jiroveci* cyst.

is a simple ovoid and ameboid organism, measuring just 2 to 4 µm, with a single nucleus.

Cysts. The cysts of *P. jiroveci* contain four to eight intracystic bodies, also referred to in some sources as nuclei or trophozoites (Fig. 7-15; Table 7-12; see Fig. 7-14). These nuclei, as they will be called in this text, may be arranged in an organized fashion (in a rosette shape) or unorganized (scattered about the organism). The typical roundish cyst is relatively small, ranging in diameter from 4 to 12 µm.

Laboratory Diagnosis

Although Giemsa and iron hematoxylin stains may be used, successful diagnosis of *P. jiroveci* is usually done using histologic procedures, particularly Gomori's methenamine silver nitrate stain. Details of these histologic methods are beyond the scope of this text. Serologic techniques have been developed but are not yet considered to be appropriate for clinical diagnosis. Techniques such as the monoclonal immunofluorescent stain have also proven helpful in organism identification. Specimens that may be submitted for *P. jiroveci* examination vary and include sputum (usually obtained on individuals who are immunocompromised), bronchoalveolar lavage, tracheal aspirate, bronchial brushings, and lung tissue.

Life Cycle Notes

The life cycle of *P. jiroveci* is still considered as unknown. However, it has been presumed that once inside the host, *P. jiroveci* takes up residence in the alveolar spaces in lung tissue. Mature cysts rupture, producing actively growing, multiplying, and feeding trophozoites. The trophozoites eventually convert into precysts and cysts. The cycle would thus repeat itself. Sites other than lung have been known to harbor *P. jiroveci*, including the spleen, lung, lymph nodes, and bone marrow.

Epidemiology

P. jiroveci is prevalent in many parts of the world. Areas of particular note include the United States, Asia, and Europe. The route of organism transmission is believed to be via the transfer of pulmonary droplets through direct person-to-person contact. The population most at risk for contracting *P. jiroveci* is immunosuppressed patients, particularly those suffering from AIDS. Children, including malnourished infants and those with predisposing conditions such as a malignancy, have also been traditionally considered a high-risk group. *P. jiroveci* has been known to pass through the placenta and to cause infection in the fetus as well as stillbirth.

Clinical Symptoms

 Pneumocystosis: Atypical Interstitial Plasma Cell Pneumonia. In immunosuppressed adults and children, this condition results in a nonproductive cough, fever, rapid respirations, and cyanosis. These symptoms occur only a few days after onset. Interstitial plasma cell pneumonia is the leading cause of death in AIDS patients. It is interesting to note that AIDS persons infected with *P. jiroveci* often also suffer from Kaposi's sarcoma, a malignant skin disease. Infected malnourished infants experience poor feeding, loss of energy, a rapid respiration rate, and cyanosis. Onset is longer, lasting several weeks.

All infected patients typically exhibit an infiltrate on chest x-ray. Breathing difficulties may result in a low PO_2 (arterial oxygen tension) and a normal to low PCO_2 (carbon dioxide tension). Prognosis is usually poor. The lack of proper oxygen and carbon dioxide exchange in the lungs is the primary cause of death.

Treatment

Trimethoprim-sulfamethoxazole (Bactrim) is considered by many to be the first line treatment of infections caused by *P. jiroveci*. Pentamidine isethionate and cotrimoxazole are alternative treatments.

Prevention and Control

Because the life cycle of *Pneumocystis* is considered by some to be uncertain, prevention and control measures are obviously difficult to implement. However, based on the assumption that direct person-to-person contact through pulmonary droplets is the route of infection, personal protection from these droplets is crucial to prevent and control the spread of infection. Protective gear, such as a mask, worn around known infected persons may be one such measure.

 Quick Quiz! 7-26

What is the preferred method of diagnosis for *Pneumocystis jiroveci*? (Objective 7-8)
A. Histologic stain
B. Giemsa stain
C. Iron hematoxylin stain
D. Iodine wet prep

 Quick Quiz! 7-27

Which of the following groups of individuals is considered at highest risk for contracting *Pneumocystis jiroveci*? (Objective 7-6)
A. Veterans
B. Active military personnel
C. Immunosuppressed individuals
D. Newborns

Quick Quiz! 7-28

Pneumocystis jiroveci is believed to be spread via which of the following? (Objective 7-5)
A. Contaminated water
B. Mosquito bite
C. Person-to-person
D. Hand-to-mouth

LOOKING BACK

The miscellaneous protozoa described in this chapter have morphologic similarities (e.g., the oocsts of *Isospora* and *Sarcocystis*) and distinct differences (e.g., *Balantidium coli* versus *Blastocystis hominis*). When screening suspected samples, attention to organism size, shape, and structural details is imperative to identify parasites correctly. Organisms that are intestinal in nature, as well as the atrial protozoa, are pictured next to each other in the comparison drawings at the end of this chapter.

TEST YOUR KNOWLEDGE!

7-1. Match the parasite (column A) with the specimen(s) of choice (column B). (Objective 7-8)

Column A	Column B
___ **A.** *Balantidium coli*	**1.** Duodenal contents
___ **B.** *Isospora belli*	**2.** Stool
___ **C.** *Sarcocystis*	**3.** Blood
___ **D.** *Cryptosporidium parvum*	**4.** Sigmoidoscopy material
___ **E.** *Blastocystis hominis*	
___ **F.** *Cyclospora cayetanensis*	

7-2. List possible invasion areas of *Balantidium coli* other than the intestine. (Objective 7-7A)

7-3. The following animals or vectors are associated with which parasite(s)? (Objective 7-5)
A. Cat
B. Pig
C. Cow

7-4. A saline wet prep is not recommended for which two parasites? (Objective 7-8)

7-5. Lung biopsies can aid in the identification of which parasites? (Objective 7-8)

7-6. Which of the following sporozoan oocysts do not contain sporocysts? (Objective 7-11)
A. *Isospora*
B. *Cryptosporidium*
C. *Sarcocystis*
D. *Blastocystis*

7-7. The scientific name for sexual reproduction that occurs in select miscellaneous protozoa is: (Objective 7-1)
A. Sporogony
B. Erthyrocytic cycle
C. Gametogony
D. Binary fission

7-8. This parasite is recognizable because of the presence of two nuclei. Name that parasite! (Objective 7-9C)
A. *Isospora belli*
B. *Balantidium coli*
C. *Sarcocystis spp.*
D. *Pneumocystis jiroveci*

7-9. The presence of cilia sets this parasite apart from the other members of the miscellaneous protozoa. (Objective 7-11)
A. *Cryptosporidium*
B. *Microsporidium*
C. *Cyclospora*
D. *Balatidium*

7-10. This member of the other protozoa group is typically identified via serologic test methods. (Objective 7-8)
A. *Blastocystis*
B. *Toxoplasma*
C. *Sarcocystis*
D. *Pneumocystis*

CASE STUDY 7-2 | UNDER THE MICROSCOPE

Alette, a 17-year-old Haitian woman, presented to a women's clinic complaining of watery and foamy bowel movements 5 to 10 times a day. She had also experienced abdominal cramps and a low-grade fever. The physician ordered a stool sample for routine O&P as well as for culture and sensitivity tests.

The culture and sensitivity tests were reported as negative for enteric pathogens. The laboratory technician performed a routine O&P examination, including a permanent trichrome stain. No parasites were observed.

Two days later, a repeat O&P was ordered. The patient was now diagnosed as HIV-positive. The repeat sample was again examined for ova and parasites by routine laboratory procedures. This time, the technologist noted oval forms of the wet preps that were highly refractile and suggestive of fungal cells, but no budding was seen. The trichrome

Continued

CASE STUDY 7-2   UNDER THE MICROSCOPE—cont'd

permanent stain did not confirm the laboratory technician's suspicions. Not satisfied that the sample was negative, the laboratory technician performed an alternative permanent stain. The organisms seen on this stain are illustrated in the diagram. These organisms were noted as 5 μm in size with one to six dark granules within their cytoplasm.

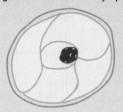

Average size: 4-6 μm

Questions and Issues for Consideration*

1. What organism did the laboratory technician suspect, and why? What morphologic form is seen in this diagram? (Objective 7-10A)
2. What was the alternative permanent stain, and how would these parasites appear following this stain procedure? (Objective 7-10E, 7-12)
3. What fungal elements might appear similar to this organism? How would they stain with the alternative stain? (Objective 7-10H, 7-12)

*Please see Chapter 2 for assistance in answering questions relating to parasite appearance after staining.

COMPARISON DRAWINGS
Intestinal Miscellaneous Protozoa

FIGURE 7-5A. *Balantidium coli* trophozoite

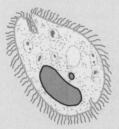

Size range: 28-152 μm by 22-123 μm
Average size: 35-50 μm by 40 μm

FIGURE 7-6A. *Balantidium coli* cyst

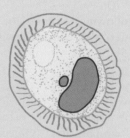

Size range: 43-66 μm
Average size: 52-55 μm

FIGURE 7-7. *Isospora belli* oocyst

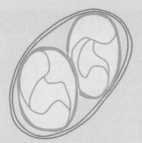

Size range: 25-35 μm by 10-15 μm
Average size: 30 μm by 12 μm

FIGURE 7-8. *Sarcocystis* oocyst

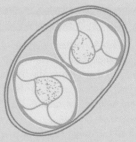

Average sporocyst length: 10-18 μm

COMPARISON DRAWINGS
Intestinal Miscellaneous Protozoa—cont'd

FIGURE 7-9. *Cryptosporidium parvum* oocyst

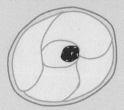

Average size: 4-6 μm

FIGURE 7-11. *Blastocystis hominis,* vacuolated form

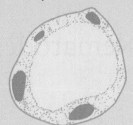

Size range: 5-32 μm
Average size: 7-10 μm

COMPARISON DRAWINGS
Atrial Miscellaneous Protozoa

Tissue

FIGURE 7-13. *Toxoplasma gondii* tachyzoites and bradyzoites

Tachyzoite size range:
3-7 μm by 2-4 μm

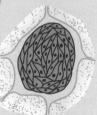

Cyst size range:
12-100 μm

FIGURE 7-15. *Pneumocystis jiroveci* cyst

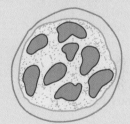

Size range: 4-12 μm in diameter

The Nematodes

Elizabeth Zeibig

WHAT'S AHEAD

Focusing In
Morphology and Life Cycle
  Notes
Laboratory Diagnosis
Pathogenesis and Clinical
  Symptoms

Nematode Classification
  Enterobius vermicularis
  Trichuris trichiura
  Ascaris lumbricoides
Hookworms
  Necator americanus

Ancylostoma duodenale
Strongyloides stercoralis
Trichinella spiralis
Dracunculus medinensis
Looking Back

LEARNING OBJECTIVES

*On completion of this chapter and review of
its figures and corresponding photomicrographs,
the successful learner will be able to:*

8-1. Define the following key terms:
  Autoreinfection
  Buccal capsule
  Buccal cavity
  Chitin
  Copepod (*pl.*, copepods)
  Copulation
  Copulatory bursa
  Corticated
  Cuticle
  Decorticated
  Egg
  Embryonated
  Filariform larva (*pl.*, larvae)
  Genital primordium
  Gravid
  Helminth (*pl.*, helminthes or helminthes)
  Larva (*pl.*, larvae)
  Nematode (Nematoda)
  Parthenogenic
  Retroinfection
  Rhabditiform larva (*pl.*, larvae)
  Unembryonated
  Zoonosis

8-2. State the geographic distribution of the
  nematodes.
8-3. State the common name associated with
  each of the nematodes.
8-4. Given a list of parasites, select those
  belonging to the class *Nematoda*.
8-5. Classify each nematode as intestinal or
  extraintestinal.
8-6. Briefly summarize the life cycle of each of
  the nematodes.
8-7. Identify and describe the populations prone
  to contracting symptoms and clinically
  significant disease processes associated with
  each nematode.
8-8. Identify and describe each of the
  following as they relate to the
  nematodes:
  A. Disease or condition, prognosis
  B. Treatment options
  C. Prevention and control measures
8-9. Select the specimen of choice, collection
  and processing protocol, and laboratory
  diagnostic technique for the recovery of
  each of the nematodes.
8-10. Given a description, photomicrograph, and/
  or diagram of a nematode, correctly do the
  following:

A. Identify and/or label the designated characteristic structure(s).
B. State the purpose of designated characteristic structure(s).
C. Identify the organism by scientific name, common name, and morphologic form.
D. State the common name for associated conditions or diseases, if applicable.

8-11. Analyze case studies that include pertinent patient information and laboratory data and do the following:
A. Identify each responsible nematode organism by scientific name, common name, and morphologic form.
B. Identify the associated diseases and conditions associated with the responsible parasite
C. Construct a life cycle associated with each nematode parasite present that includes corresponding epidemiology, route of transmission, infective stage, and diagnostic stage.
D. Propose each of the following related to stopping and preventing nematode infections:
   1. Treatment options
   2. Prevention and control plan
E. Recognize sources of error, including but not limited to those involved in specimen collection, processing, and testing and propose solutions to remedy them.
F. Interpret laboratory data, determine specific follow-up tests to be done, and predict the results of those identified tests.

8-12. Identify, compare, and contrast the similarities and differences among the parasites discussed in this and other chapters in this text.

8-13. Describe standard and alternative laboratory diagnostic approaches as appropriate for the recovery of nematodes in clinical specimens.

8-14. Given prepared laboratory specimens and with the assistance of this manual, the learner will be able to do the following:
A. Differentiate nematode organisms from artifacts.
B. Differentiate the nematode organisms from each other and from the other appropriate categories of parasites.
C. Correctly identify each nematode parasite by scientific, common name, and morphologic form based on its key characteristic structure(s).

CASE STUDY 8-1   UNDER THE MICROSCOPE

Maria, a 5-year-old girl, presented to a local clinic complaining of diarrhea and gastrointestinal pain and bleeding. Patient history revealed that Maria recently emigrated to the United States from Puerto Rico. The physician on duty ordered a series of stool samples for O&P. Barrel-shaped structures, as noted below, that appeared to have plugs at each end were seen on the direct wet preps, concentrated wet preps after performing a zinc sulfate flotation method, and permanent stains.

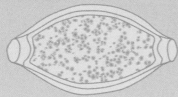

Questions and Issues for Consideration
1. What is the scientific name and morphologic form of the parasite present in Maria's samples? (Objective 8-11A)
2. What is the common name for this parasite? (Objective 8-11 A)
3. How did Maria contract this parasite? (Objective 8-11C)
4. Which disease state is associated with this parasite? (Objective 8-11B)
5. Which morphologic form of this parasite may be visible on microscopic examination of the intestinal mucosa of this patient? (Objective 8-11F)

FOCUSING IN

This chapter begins with the discussion of the **helminths**. These organisms differ from the previously described single-cell protozoa in the fact that they are multicellular and contain internal organ systems. The first group of helminths discussed are the nematodes, commonly known as the intestinal roundworms.

MORPHOLOGY AND LIFE CYCLE NOTES

Members of the class **Nematoda** (multicellular parasites that appear round in cross section) may assume three basic morphologic forms: **eggs** (female sex cells after fertilization), juvenile worms known as **larvae**, and adult worms. The eggs vary in size and shape. In the appropriate environment, developing larvae located inside fertilized eggs emerge and continue to mature. These larvae are typically long and slender. The growing larvae complete the maturation process, resulting in the emergence of adult worms. Sexes are separate. The adult female worms are usually larger than the adult males. The adults are equipped with complete digestive and reproductive systems. Specific features vary with the individual species.

The life cycles of the individual nematodes are similar but organism-specific. An intestinal nematode infection may be initiated in several ways. In the case of pinworms, for example, ingestion of the infected eggs transmits the disease. The hookworm larvae, on the other hand, burrow through the skin of the foot and make way into the intestinal tract. The exact means whereby each organism enters the host and migrates into the intestinal tract varies by species. The eggs or larvae, depending on the species, continue to develop into adulthood. The resulting adult worms reside in the intestine, where they concentrate on obtaining nutrition and reproduction.

Fertilized adult female nematodes lay their eggs in the intestine. These eggs may be passed into the stool. Once outside the body, the larvae located inside the eggs require warm moist soil and 2 to 4 weeks for continued development. The developed egg is then ready for infection into a new host and the cycle is repeated. It is important to note that this description of a nematode life cycle is only basic and general. In two of the nematode life cycles, *Trichinella* and *Dracunculus*, tissue becomes involved, serving as the primary residence of the organisms. It is interesting to note here that in general terms, most members of the nematode group have the ability to exist independent of a host (i.e., they are free-living). The specifics of each nematode organism's life cycle are addressed on an individual basis.

Quick Quiz! 8-1

The junvenile stage of developing nematode worms is referred to as: (Objective 8-1)
A. Eggs
B. Cysts
C. Larvae
D. Adults

LABORATORY DIAGNOSIS

The laboratory diagnosis of nematodes may be accomplished by the recovery of eggs, larvae, and occasional adult worms. The specimens of choice vary by species and include cellophane tape preparations taken around the anal opening, stool samples, tissue biopsies, and infected skin ulcers. In addition, serologic test methods are available for the diagnosis of select nematode organisms. Representative laboratory diagnosis methodologies are located in Chapter 2 as well as in each individual parasite discussion, as appropriate.

Quick Quiz! 8-2

Adult nematodes are never recovered in clinical samples. (Objective 8-6)
A. True
B. False

PATHOGENESIS AND CLINICAL SYMPTOMS

In general terms, three possible factors may contribute to the ultimate severity of a nematode infection: (1) the number of worms present; (2) the length of time the infection persists; and (3) the overall health of the host. Infections with nematodes have been known to last for up to 12 months or longer (some infections may last 10 to 15 years or more), depending on the specific species involved. The occurence of reinfections and/or autoinfections may increase the infection time up to several years and beyond; some infections persist indefinitely. In most cases, an infection of a small number of worms in a relatively healthy individual may remain asymptomatic or cause minimal discomfort. However, patients who have a heavy worm burden, particularly if combined with other health problems, are probably more likely to experience severe symptoms and/or complications.

The life cycle of each of the nematodes involves the intestinal tract. With one exception, all the nematodes may cause intestinal infection symptoms at some point during their invasion of the host. These typically include abdominal pain, diarrhea, nausea, vomiting, fever, and eosinophilia. Skin irritation, the formation of skin blisters, and muscle involvement may also be present.

> ### Quick Quiz! 8-3
>
> These individuals are prone to experiencing severe nematode infections: (Objective 8-7)
> A. Completely healthy individuals with a heavy worm burden
> B. Unhealthy individuals who are asymptomatic
> C. Healthy individuals with a light worm burden
> D. Unhealthy individuals with a heavy worm burden

NEMATODE CLASSIFICATION

The nematodes belong to the phylum Nemathelminthes. Recent investigation of current taxonomy classification terms revealed that the placement of the term Nematoda varies by source, listing it as a phylum, order or class. For the purposes of this text and to maintain taxonomic consistency, Nematoda is considered as a class just like all of the helminth groups covered in this text. The nematode species may be divided into two groups, those primarily involved with the intestinal tract, termed *intestinal species,* and those that migrate into the tissues following initial contact with the intestinal tract, termed *intestina tissue species.* The species discussed in this chapter under each category are listed in Figure 8-1.

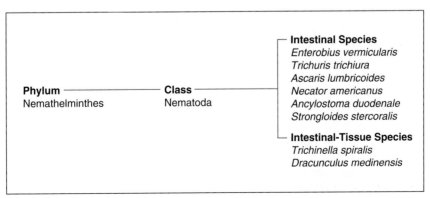

FIGURE 8-1 Parasite classification: The nematodes.

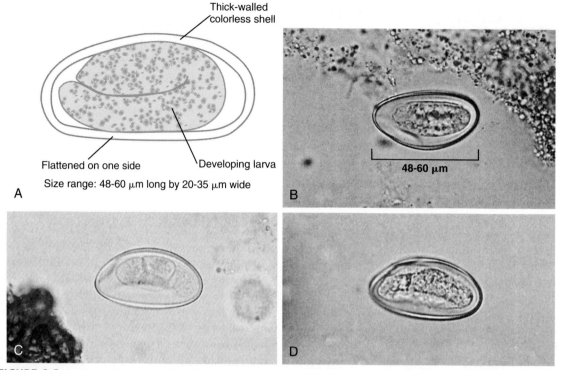

FIGURE 8-2 **A,** *Enterobius vermicularis* egg. **B,** *Enterobius vermicularis* unembryonated egg, ×400. **C,** *Enterobius vermicularis* immature embryonated egg, ×400. **D,** *Enterobius vermicularis* mature embryonated egg, ×400. (**B-D** *courtesy of WARD'S Natural Science Establishment, Rochester, NY.*)

Enterobius vermicularis
(en"tir-o'bee-us/vur-mic-yoo-lair'is)

Common names: Pinworm, seatworm.

Common associated disease and condition names: Enterobiasis, pinworm infection.

Morphology

◗ **Eggs.** The typical *Enterobius vermicularis* egg measures 48 to 60 μm in length by 20 to 35 μm in width (Fig. 8-2; Table 8-1). The somewhat oval egg is characteristically flattened on one side. The egg consists of a developing larva surrounded by a conspicuous double-layered, thick-walled colorless shell. The egg may be seen at various stages of development, as shown in Figure 8-2*B* (unfertilized egg referred to as being **unembryonated**), Figure 8-2*C* (fertilized egg; also known as an **embryonated** egg), and Figure 8-2*D* (mature egg).

TABLE 8-1	*Enterobius vermicularis* Egg: Typical Characteristics at a Glance
Parameter	**Description**
Size	48-60 μm long, 20-35 μm wide
Shape	Oval, one-side flattened
Embryo	Stage of development varies; may be unembryonated, embryonated, mature
Shell	Double-layered, thick, colorless

◗ **Adults.** The adult female *E. vermicularis* worm (Fig. 8-3) measures 7 to 14 mm in length by up to 0.5 mm wide (Table 8-2). The yellowish-white females are equipped with primitive organ systems, including a digestive tract, intestinal tract, and reproductive structures. In addition, the adult female possesses a clear, pointed tail that resembles a pinhead—hence, the

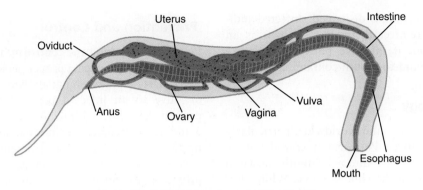

Size range: 7-14 mm long by up to 0.5 mm wide

FIGURE 8-3 Enterobius vermicularis adult female.

TABLE 8-2	*Enterobius vermicularis* Adults: Typical Characteristics at a Glance	
Characteristic	**Adult Female**	**Adult Male***
Length	7-14 mm	2-4 mm
Width	Up to 0.5 mm	≤0.3 mm
Color	Yellowish-white	Yellowish-white
Tail	Pointed; resembles pinhead	

*Adult males are only rarely seen.

common name pinworm. The rarely seen adult male worms are also yellowish-white in color and typically are smaller in size than the females, ranging from 2 to 4 mm long by no more than 0.3 mm wide.

Laboratory Diagnosis

The specimen of choice for the recovery of *E. vermicularis* is a cellophane tape preparation collected from the perianal region of the person suspected of infection. Although eggs are the primary morphologic form seen, adult females may also be present if the sample is collected when the females enter the perianal region to lay their eggs. It is important to note that multiple samples may be required to confirm the presence of a light infection as well as to determine that a patient is free of infection. On rare occasions, eggs and/or adult females may be recovered in stool samples.

Life Cycle Notes

Humans are the only known host of *E. vermicularis*. Pinworm infection, which is usually self-limiting, is initiated following the ingestion of the infective eggs. The eggs migrate through the digestive tract into the small intestine, where they hatch and release young larvae. The resulting larvae continue to grow and mature, ultimately transforming into adult worms. The adult worms reside in the colon. Following mating of select worms (**copulation**), including round-worms, the resulting pregnant (**gravid**) female worm migrates outside the body to the perianal region, where she may deposit up to 15,000 eggs. Following 4 to 6 hours incubation, the developing eggs achieve infective status. These infective eggs may then become dislodged from the body, caused at least in part by intense scratching of the anal area by the infected person. Once apart from the host, the infective eggs may take up residence in a number of locations, including dust, sandboxes, linens, and clothing. In addition, the eggs may become airborne. The infective eggs may survive for a few days up to several weeks under suitable environmental conditions. The ideal surroundings for thriving infective eggs consist of a moderate temperature accompanied by high humidity. Ingestion of these infective eggs initiates a new cycle.

A **retroinfection**, defined in pinworm-specific terms as infective pinworm eggs that migrate back into the host body, develop and reproduce rather than becoming dislodged. Infected individuals may reinfect themselves, known as an **autoreinfection,** if infective pinworm eggs are ingested via hand-to-mouth contamination.

Epidemiology

E. vermicularis is found worldwide, particularly in temperate areas. Pinworm is considered by many to be the most common helminth known to cause infection in the United States. White children appear to be at the greatest risk of contracting this parasite. Transmission of pinworm occurs primarily by hand-to-mouth contamination.

As noted in Chapter 4, it is believed that *E. vermicularis* may be responsible for the transmission of *Dientamoeba fragilis*. This theory suggests that the *D. fragilis* trophozoite may actually take up residence inside the pinworm egg for transmission. Infections with both organisms have been reported.

Clinical Symptoms

 Asymptomatic. Many cases of *E. vermicularis* infection are asymptomatic.

 Enterobiasis: Pinworm Infection. The most common symptoms experienced by individuals infected with pinworm include intense itching and inflammation of the anal and/or vaginal areas. These symptoms may be accompanied by intestinal irritation, mild nausea or vomiting, irritability, and difficulty sleeping. Additional symptoms known to occur with much less frequency consist of minute ulcers as well as mild intestinal inflammation and abdominal pain.

Treatment

The treatment of choice for the eradication of *E. vermicularis* is albendazole, mebendazole, or pyrantel pamoate. It is important to note that in many cases treatment is suggested for the family members of an infected individual because pinworm eggs spread readily into the environment.

Prevention and Control

Pinworm prevention and control measures include the following: practicing proper personal hygiene, particularly hand washing; applying an ointment or salve to an infected perianal area to help prevent egg dispersal into the environment; and avoiding scratching the infected area. Furthermore, thorough cleaning of all potentially infected environmental surfaces, including linens, and providing treatment to all household members are important steps to help prevent future infections. Because of the ease with which this parasite is capable of being transmitted, total eradication of pinworm is highly unlikely in the near future.

Quick Quiz! 8-4

The specimen of choice for the recovery of *Enterobius vermicularis* is: (Objective 8-9)
A. Stool
B. Urine
C. Cellophane tape prep
D. Tissue biopsy

Quick Quiz! 8-5

The most likely individual to contract pinworm infection is(are) a(an): (Objective 8-7)
A. Older adult
B. Child
C. Adult prisoner
D. Military personnel

Quick Quiz! 8-6

The morphologic forms recovered in cases of pinworm infection are which of the following? (Objective 8-6)
A. Eggs and adult females
B. Adult males and females
C. Eggs and larvae
D. Larvae and adult males

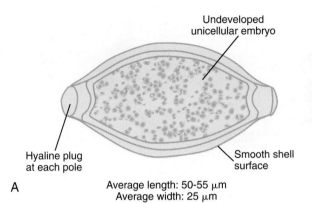

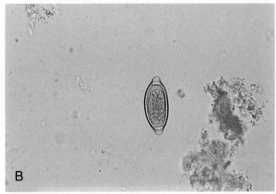

FIGURE 8-4 A, *Trichuris trichiura* egg. **B,** *Trichuris trichiura* egg. (*B from Mahon CR, Lehman DC, Manuselis G: Textbook of diagnostic microbiology, ed 4, St Louis, 2011, Saunders.*)

TABLE 8-3	*Trichuris trichiura* Egg: Typical Characteristics at a Glanee	
Parameter	**Description**	
Size	50-55 by 25 μm	
Shape	Barrel, football; hyaline polar plug at each end	
Embryo	Unicellular; undeveloped	
Shell	Smooth; yellow-brown color because of bile contact	

TABLE 8-4	*Trichuris trichiura* Adults: Typical Characteristics at a Glance	
Parameter	**Description**	
Size	2.5-5 cm long; males usually smaller than females	
Anterior end	Colorless; resembles a whip handle; contains a slender esophagus	
Posterior end	Pinkish-gray; resembles whip itself; contains digestive and reproductive systems; males possess prominent curled tail	

Trichuris trichiura
(trick-yoo′ris/trick″ee-yoo′ruh)

Common name: Whipworm.

Common associated disease and condition names: Trichuriasis, whipworm infection.

Morphology

Eggs. The average barrel-shaped (also considered by some to be football-shaped) *Trichuris trichiura* egg measures 50 to 55 μm by 25 μm (Fig. 8-4; Table 8-3). The undeveloped unicellular embryo is surrounded by a smooth shell that retains a yellow-brown color from its contact with host bile. A prominent hyaline polar plug is visible at each end.

Adults. The typical adult whipworm measures 2.5 to 5 cm in length (Table 8-4). The anterior end of the adult appears colorless and contains a slender esophagus. The posterior end assumes a pinkish-gray color, consisting of the intestine and reproductive systems. The adult male (Fig. 8-5) is usually smaller than the adult female. In addition to a digestive system, intestinal tract, and reproductive organs, the male possesses an easily recognizable curled tail. The posterior end of the adult *T. trichiura* is large and resembles that of a whip handle. The anterior end is much smaller and looks like the whip itself. It is these two morphologic features that are the basis for the name whipworm.

Laboratory Diagnosis

The specimen of choice for the recovery of *T. trichiura* eggs is stool. These eggs are particularly

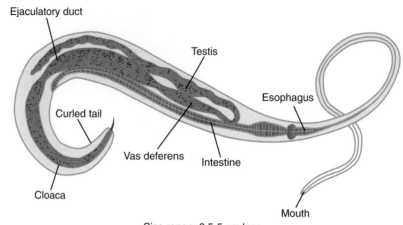

Size range: 2.5-5 cm long

FIGURE 8-5 *Trichuris trichiura,* adult male.

prominent in infected samples processed using the zinc sulfate flotation method (described in more detail in Chapter 2). Adult worms may be visible on macroscopic examination of the intestinal mucosa. Adults may also be seen in areas of the intestinal tract down to and including the rectum in heavy infections. It is important to be aware that samples examined from patients treated for whipworm infection may reveal distorted eggs, showing a variety of unusual shapes.

Life Cycle Notes

Ingestion of infective *T. trichiura* eggs containing larvae initiates human infection. The larvae emerge from the eggs in the small intestine. Growth and development of the larvae occur as they migrate within the intestinal villi. The larvae return to the intestinal lumen and proceed to the cecum, where they complete their maturation. The resulting adults take up residence in the colon, embedding in the mucosa. The life span of the adult worms in untreated infections may be from 4 to 8 years. Following copulation, the adult female lays her undeveloped eggs. It is this stage of egg that is passed into the outside environment via the feces. Following approximately 1 month outside the human body, usually in the soil, the eggs embryonate, become infective, and are ready to initiate a new cycle.

Epidemiology

Considered as the third most common helminth, *T. trichiura* is found primarily in warm climates of the world where poor sanitation practices are common, such as defecating directly into the soil or using human feces as a fertilizer. Areas of the United States that have been known to harbor whipworm include the warm humid South, particularly in rural settings. Persons most at risk for contracting whipworm infections include children as well as those in psychiatric facilities.

Infections with both *Trichuris* and *Ascaris,* another intestinal nematode (covered later in this chapter), are known to occur. This is likely caused at least in part because the human port of entry, which serves as the mode of organism transmission, is identical for both parasites.

Clinical Symptoms

▨ **Asymptomatic.** Patients who suffer from a slight whipworm infection often remain asymptomatic.
▨ **Trichuriasis: Whipworm Infection:** Heavy infections of 500 to 5000 worms produce a wide variety of symptoms. The conditions that a whipworm infection may simulate vary with the age

of the host. Children infected with *T. trichiura* usually present with symptoms resembling those of ulcerative colitis. An infection of as few as 200 worms may cause a child to develop chronic dysentery, severe anemia, and possibly growth retardation. It is interesting to note that in treated children, catch-up growth usually occurs. In addition, increased rectal prolapse and peristalsis are common in infected children. Infected adults experience symptoms that mimic those of inflammatory bowel disease. Common symptoms found in infected persons include abdominal tenderness and pain, weight loss, weakness, and mucoid or bloody diarrhea.

Treatment

Mebendazole or albendazole are considered as the treatment of choice for whipworm infections.

Prevention and Control

The spread of *T. trichiura* infections may be halted by exercising proper sanitation practices, especially avoidance of defecating directly into the soil, using feces as a fertilizer, and placing potentially infective hands into the mouth and prompt and thorough treatment of infected persons, when indicated. Educating children and aiding institutionalized mentally handicapped persons in their personal hygiene and sanitation practices is crucial to eradicate whipworm infections completely.

Quick Quiz! 8-7

Trichuris trichiura eggs are characterized by the presence of which of the following? (Objective 8-10A)
A. Triple-layer cell wall
B. Flattened side
C. Hyaline polar plugs
D. Prominent cytostome

Quick Quiz! 8-8

Of the following choices, the best laboratory diagnosis technique for the recovery of *Trichuris trichiura* eggs is which of the following? (Objective 8-9)
A. Zinc sulfate flotation
B. Modified acid-fast stain
C. Ethyl acetate concentration
D. Wright-Giemsa stain

Quick Quiz! 8-9

Children infected with *Trichuris trichiura* commonly suffer from: (Objective 8-7)
A. Mental confusion
B. Hemoglobinuria
C. Severe anemia
D. Rectal prolapse

Ascaris lumbricoides
(as′kar-is/lum-bri-koy′deez)

Common names: Large intestinal roundworm, roundworm of man.

Common associated disease and condition names: Ascariasis, roundworm infection.

Morphology

▧ **Unfertilized Eggs.** The typical oblong, unfertilized, *Ascaris lumbricoides* egg characteristically measures 85 to 95 μm by 38 to 45 μm (Fig. 8-6; Table 8-5). A thin shell protects the inner amorphous mass of protoplasm. The egg is usually **corticated** (i.e., the egg possesses an outer mammillated, albuminous coating). Variations in shape, size, and cortication may also be seen, as in Figure 8-6B.

▧ **Fertilized Eggs.** The fertilized *A. lumbricoides* egg is more rounded than the unfertilized egg, usually measuring 40 to 75 μm by 30 to 50 μm (Figs. 8-7 and 8-8; Table 8-6). Fertilization of the egg transforms the amorphous mass of protoplasm into an undeveloped unicellular embryo. A thick nitrogen-containing polysaccharide

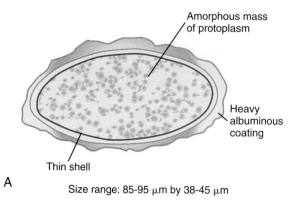

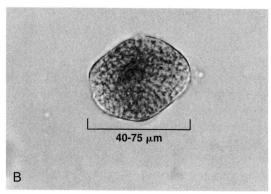

FIGURE 8-6 A, *Ascaris lumbricoides,* unfertilized egg. **B,** *Ascaris lumbricoides,* decorticated unfertilized egg, ×400. *(Courtesy of WARD'S Natural Science Establishment, Rochester, NY.)*

TABLE 8-5	*Ascaris lumbricoides* Unfertilized Egg: Typical Characteristics at a Glance
Parameter	**Description**
Size	85-95 µm by 38-45 µm; size variations possible
Shape	Varies
Embryo	Unembryonated; amorphous mass of protoplasm
Shell	Thin
Other features	Usually corticated

TABLE 8-6	*Ascaris lumbricoides* Fertilized Egg: Typical Characteristics at a Glance
Parameter	**Description**
Size	40-75 µm by 30-50 µm
Shape	Rounder than nonfertilized version
Embryo	Undeveloped unicellular embryo
Shell	Thick chitin
Other features	May be corticated or decorticated

TABLE 8-7	*Ascaris lumbricoides* Adults: Typical Characteristics at a Glance	
Characteristic	**Female Adult**	**Male Adult**
Size (length)	22-35 cm	Up to 30 cm
Color	Creamy white pink tint	Creamy white pink tint
Other features	Pencil lead thickness	Prominent incurved tail

coating called a **chitin,** also known as a shell, is sandwiched in between the embryo and mammillated albuminous material (corticated). Both layers protect the embryo from the outside environment. Eggs lacking an outer mammillated, albuminous coating (refered to as **decorticated**) fertilized eggs (see Fig. 8-8) may also be present. The chitin shell is less evident in corticated eggs than in those that have lost their outer albuminous coating.

Adults. Adult *A. lumbricoides* worms usually assume a creamy white color with a tint of pink Fine striations are visible on the **cuticle** (a surface covering present on adult nematodes). *Ascaris* adult worms are the largest known intestinal nematodes (Table 8-7). The average adult male (Fig. 8-9) is small, seldomly reaching 30 cm in length. The male is characteristically slender and possesses a prominent incurved tail. The adult female (Fig. 8-10) measures 22 to 35 cm in length and resembles a pencil lead in thickness.

Laboratory Diagnosis

The specimen of choice for the recovery of *A. lumbricoides* eggs is stool. Adult worms may be recovered in several specimen types, depending

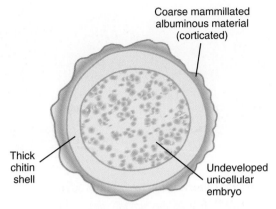

Coarse mammillated
albuminous material
(corticated)

Thick
chitin
shell

Undeveloped
unicellular
embryo

Size range: 40-75 μm by 30-50 μm

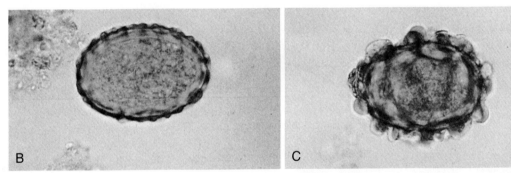

B

C

FIGURE 8-7 **A,** *Ascaris lumbricoides,* mature egg. **B,** *Ascaris lumbricoides,* corticated mature egg, ×400. **C,** *Ascaris lumbricoides,* very corticated mature egg, ×400. **(B, C** *courtesy of WARD'S Natural Science Establishment, Rochester, NY.)*

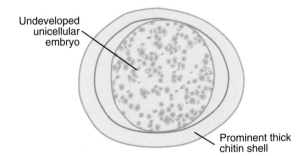

Undeveloped
unicellular
embryo

Prominent thick
chitin shell

Size range: 40-75 μm by 30-50 μm

FIGURE 8-8 *Ascaris lumbricoides,* decorticated egg.

on the severity of infection, including the small intestine, gallbladder, liver, and appendix. In addition, adult worms may be present in the stool, vomited up, or removed from the external nares, where they may attempt to escape. An enzyme-linked immunosorbent assay (ELISA) is also available.

Life Cycle Notes

The life cycle of *A. lumbricoides* is relatively complex compared with the parasites presented thus far. Infection begins following the ingestion of infected eggs that contain viable larvae. Once inside the small intestine, the larvae emerge from the eggs. The larvae then complete a liver-lung migration by first entering the blood via penetration through the intestinal wall. The first stop on this journey is the liver. From there, the larvae continue via the bloodstream to the second stop, the lung. Once inside the lung, the larvae burrow their way through the capillaries into the alveoli. Migration into the bronchioles then follows.

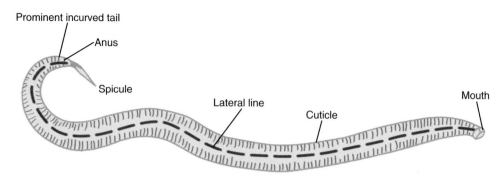

Average size: length is seldom up to 30 cm

FIGURE 8-9 *Ascaris lumbricoides,* adult male.

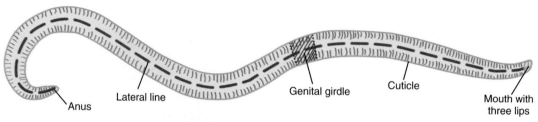

Average size: 22-35 cm long

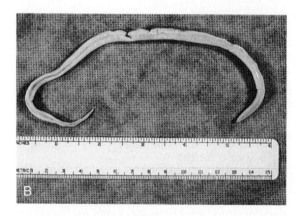

FIGURE 8-10 A, *Ascaris lumbricoides,* adult female. **B,** *Ascaris lumbricoides,* adult female.

From here, the larvae are transferred through coughing into the pharynx, where they are swallowed and returned to the intestine.

Maturation of the larvae occurs, resulting in adult worms, which take up residence in the small intestine. The adults multiply and a number of the resulting undeveloped eggs (up to 250,000/day) are passed in the feces. The outside environment, specifically soil, provides the necessary conditions for the eggs to embryonate. Infective eggs may remain viable in soil, fecal matter, sewage, or water for years. It is important to note that these eggs may even survive in 10% formalin fixative used in stool processing. The longevity of these eggs is partly because they are not easily destroyed by chemicals. The resulting embryonated eggs are the infective stage for a new host and, when consumed by a human host, initiate a new cycle.

Epidemiology

Ascariasis is considered as the most common intestinal helminth infection in the world, affecting approximately 1 billion people. It ranks second in frequency in the United States, the first being pinworm infection. The regions of the world and of the United States most susceptible to harbor *Ascaris* resemble those for *Trichuris*—warm climates and areas of poor sanitation, particularly where human feces is used as a fertilizer and where children defecate directly on the ground. The frequency of *A. lumbricoides* in the United States is highest in the Appalachian Mountains and in the surrounding areas east, west, and south of them.

The population most at risk of contracting *A. lumbricoides* infection is children who place their contaminated hands into their mouths. Sources of contamination range from children's toys to the soil itself. Persons of all ages may become infected where vegetables are grown using contaminated human feces as fertilizer. Although water has been known to be the source of *A. lumbricoides* infection, this occurs only rarely.

As mentioned in Chapter 4, it is suspected that *A. lumbricoides*, in addition to pinworm, may be responsible for the transmission of *Dientamoeba fragilis*. This theory has not yet been proven.

Clinical Symptoms

Asymptomatic. Patients infected with a small number of worms (5 to 10) will often remain asymptomatic. These patients usually ingest only a few eggs. They may only learn of their infection if they happen to notice an adult worm in their freshly passed feces or if they submit a stool for a routine parasite examination.

Ascariasis: Roundworm Infection. Patients who develop symptomatic ascariasis may be infected with only a single worm. Such a worm may produce tissue damage as it migrates through the host. A secondary bacterial infection may also occur following worm perforation out of the intestine.

Patients infected with many worms may exhibit vague abdominal pain, vomiting, fever, and distention. Mature worms may entangle themselves into a mass that may ultimately obstruct the intestine, appendix, liver, or bile duct. Such intestinal complications may result in death. In addition, discomfort from adult worms exiting the body through the anus, mouth, or nose may occur. Heavily infected children who do not practice good eating habits may develop protein malnutrition.

In addition to symptoms relating to the intestinal phase of ascariasis, patients may also experience pulmonary symptoms when the worms migrate through the lungs. During this phase, patients may develop a low-grade fever, cough, eosinophilia, and/or pneumonia. An asthmatic reaction to the presence of the worms, which is allergic in nature, may also occur.

Treatment

The recommended medications for *A. lumbricoides* infections requiring treatment consist of medications designed to rid the body of parasitic worms. These include albendazole and mebenazole.

Prevention and Control

The avoidance of using human feces as fertilizer, as well as exercising proper sanitation and personal hygiene practices, are critical measures for breaking the life cycle of *A. lumbricoides*.

Quick Quiz! 8-10

Individuals contract *Ascaris lumbricoides* via which of the following? (Objective 8-6)
A. Inhalation
B. Insect bite
C. Ingestion
D. Inappropriate sexual practices

Quick Quiz! 8-11

The term that describes the lack of an outer mammillated albuminous coating is called which of the following? (Objective 8-1)
A. Unfertilized
B. Fertilzed
C. Corticated
D. Decorticated

Quick Quiz! 8-12

The specimen of choice for the recovery of *Ascaris lumbricoides* eggs is which of the following? (Objective 8-9)
A. Stool
B. Gallbladder biopsy
C. Urine
D. Sputum

HOOKWORMS

Necator americanus
(ne-kay'tur/ah'merr"i-kay'nus)

Common Name: New World hookworm.

Ancylostoma duodenale
(an"si'ios'tuh'muh/dew"o-de-nay'lee)

Common Name: Old World hookworm.

Common associated disease and condition names: Hookworm infection, ancylostomiasis, necatoriasis.

The term *hookworm* refers to two organisms, *Necator americanus* and *Ancylostoma duodenale*. There are two primary differences between the two organisms. First, the geographic distribution varies slightly with each organism. Second, and more importantly for identification purposes, the adult worms of each have minor morphologic differences. The egg and larva stages, however, are basically indistinguishable.

Morphology

Eggs. Although the only difference between the eggs of *N. americanus* and those of *A. duodenale* is size, differentiation of the two genera is not generally made solely on this characteristic (Fig. 8-11; Table 8-8). The average *N. americanus* egg ranges in length from 60 to 75 μm, whereas the typical *A. duodenale* egg measures 55 to 60 μm. The width of both organisms ranges from 35 to 40 μm. Eggs recovered in

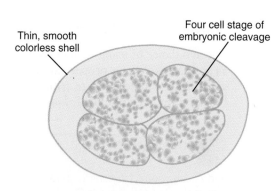

Thin, smooth colorless shell

Four cell stage of embryonic cleavage

Necator size range: 60-75 μm by 35-40 μm
Ancylostoma size range: 55-60 μm by 35-40 μm

A

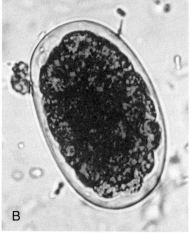

B

FIGURE 8-11 A, Hookworm egg. **B,** Hookworm egg. (**B** *from Forbes BA, Brown I, Sahm DF, Weissfeld AS: Bailey and Scott's diagnostic microbiology, ed 12, St. Louis, 2007, Mosby.*)

freshly passed stool may be unsegmented or show a visible embryonic cleavage, usually at the two-, four-, or eight-cell stage. A thin, smooth, colorless shell provides protection for the developing worm. Because the size ranges of these two organisms are so close and the other characteristics are identical, recovered eggs are considered as indistinguishable and are usually reported as hookworm eggs.

Rhabditiform Larvae. The average immature, newly hatched hookworm rhabditiform larva measures approximately 15 by 270 µm (Fig. 8-12; Table 8-9). The actively feeding larva will, at a minimum, double in length, ranging from 540 to 700 µm, when it is only 5 days old. This morphologic form is characterized by the presence of a long oral cavity known as a **buccal cavity** or **buccal capsule** and a small **genital**

TABLE 8-8	Hookworm Egg: Typical Characteristics at a Glance
Parameter	**Description**
Size	
Length	*Necator,* 60-75 µm; *Ancylostoma,* 55-60 µm
Width	35-40 µm
Embryonic cleavage	Two-, four-, or eight-cell stage
Shell	Smooth, colorless

TABLE 8-9	Hookworm rhabditiform larva: Typical Characteristics at a Glance
Parameter	**Description**
Size	
Newly hatched	270 by 15 µm
5 days old	540-700 µm long
Other features	Long buccal cavity; small genital primordium

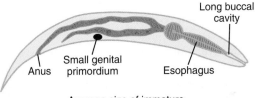

Long buccal cavity

Small genital primordium

Anus

Esophagus

Average size of immature, newly hatched rhabditiform larvae: 270 µm by 15 µm
Size range at 5 days old: 540-700 µm long

A

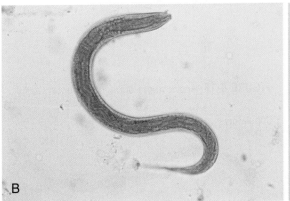

B

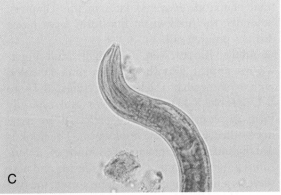

C

FIGURE 8-12 A, Hookworm rhabditiform larva. **B,** Hookworm rhabditiform larva. Note long buccal capsule and lack of prominent genital primordium. **C,** Hookworm rhabditiform, larval form buccal capsule. (***B, C** from Mahon CR, Lehman DC, Manuselis G: Textbook of diagnostic microbiology, ed 4, St Louis, 2011, Saunders.*)

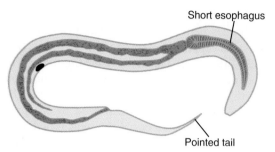

FIGURE 8-13 Hookworm filariform larva.

TABLE 8-10	Hookworm Filariform Larva: Typical Characteristics at a Glance
Parameter	**Description**
Length of esophagus	Short
Tail	Pointed

primordium (i.e., a precursor structure to a reproductive system consisting of a clump of cells in an ovoid formation).

■ **Filariform Larvae.** The infective, nonfeeding filariform larva emerges after the rhabditiform larva completes its second molt (Fig. 8-13; Table 8-10). There are two notable characteristics that aid in identifying this morphologic form. First, this slender larva has a shorter esophagus than that of *Strongyloides stercoralis*, a similar intestinal nematode (covered later in this chapter). Secondly, the hookworm filariform larva has a distinct pointed tail.

■ **Adults.** Rarely seen, the small adult hookworms appear grayish-white to pink in color, with a somewhat thick cuticle (Figs. 8-14 to 8-17; Table 8-11). The anterior end typically forms a conspicuous bend, referred to as a hook—hence, the name hookworm. The hook is usually much more pronounced in the *N. americanus* adult than in that of *A. duodenale* and may serve as a means of distinguishing among the two species by the trained eye.

The average adult female hookworm usually measures about 9 to 12 mm in length by 0.25 to

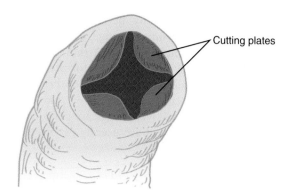

FIGURE 8-14 *Necator americanus,* buccal capsule.

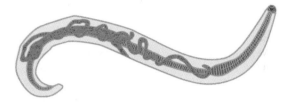

Size range: 9-12 mm long by 0.25-0.5 mm wide
FIGURE 8-15 *Necator americanus,* adult male.

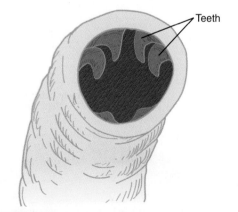

FIGURE 8-16 *Ancylostoma duodenale,* buccal capsule.

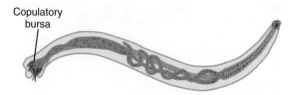

Size range: 5-10 mm long by 0.2-0.4 mm wide
FIGURE 8-17 *Ancylostoma duodenale,* adult female.

TABLE 8-11	Hookworm Adults: Typical Characteristics at a Glance	
General Characteristics		
Color	Grayish-white to pink	
Cuticle	Somewhat thick	
Anterior end	Conspicuous bend, hook	
Characteristic	**Female Adults**	**Male Adults**
Size	9-12 mm long, 0.25-0.50 mm wide	5-10 mm long, 0.2-0.4 mm wide
Other features		Prominent posterior copulatory bursa
Buccal Capsule Characteristics		
Necator	Contains pair of cutting plates	
Ancylostoma	Contains actual teeth	

0.5 mm in width (see Fig. 8-17). Males are typically smaller, ranging in size from 5 to 10 mm by 0.2 to 0.4 mm. The male is equipped with a prominent, posterior, umbrella-like structure that aids in copulation, known as a **copulatory bursa** (see Fig. 8-15).

Differences in the makeup of the buccal capsule distinguish adult *N. americanus* and *A. duodenale* worms. The buccal capsule of *N. americanus* (see Fig. 8-14) contains a pair of cutting plates, whereas that of *A. duodenale* consists of actual teeth (see Fig. 8-16).

Laboratory Diagnosis

The primary means for laboratory diagnosis of hookworm is the recovery of the eggs in stool samples. Larvae may mature and hatch from the eggs in stool that has been allowed to sit at room temperature, without fixative added. Differentiation of these larvae from those of *S. stercoralis* is crucial to ensure proper diagnosis and subsequent treatment (see later). Recovery and examination of the buccal capsule is necessary to determine the specific hookworm organism (i.e., whether it is *A. duodenale* or *N. americanus*).

Life Cycle Notes

Humans contract hookworm when third-stage filariform larvae penetrate through the skin, particularly into areas such as unprotected feet. Once inside the body, the filariform larvae migrate to the lymphatics and blood system. The blood carries the larvae to the lungs, where they penetrate the capillaries and enter the alveoli. Migration of the larvae continues into the bronchioles, where they are coughed up to the pharynx, subsequently swallowed, and deposited into the intestine.

Maturation of the larvae into adult hookworms occurs in the intestine. The resulting adults live and multiply in the small intestine. Adult females lay 10,000 to 20,000 eggs/day. Many of the resulting eggs are passed into the outside environment via the feces. Within 24 to 48 hours and under appropriate conditions—warm, moist soil—first-stage rhabditiform larvae emerge from the eggs. The larvae continue to develop by molting twice. Third-stage infective filariform larvae result and are ready to begin a new cycle.

Epidemiology

It is estimated that almost 25% of the world's population is infected with hookworm. The frequency of hookworm infection is high in warm areas in which the inhabitants practice poor sanitation practices, especially with regard to proper fecal treatment and disposal. Mixed infections with any combination of hookworm, *Trichuris*, and *Ascaris* are possible because all three organisms require the same soil conditions to remain viable. The specific geographic locations for each species of hookworm are presented later. Persons at risk for contracting hookworm in these areas are those who walk barefoot in feces-contaminated soil.

N. americanus is primarily found in North and South America. However, because of spread from international travel, this species is also known to exist in China, India, and Africa.

Although historically a parasite of the Old World, *A. duodenale* has been transported to other areas of the globe via modern world travel. Today, *A. duodenale* may be found in Europe, China, Africa, South America, and the Caribbean.

Clinical Symptoms

▼ **Asymptomatic Hookworm Infection.** Some persons infected with a light hookworm burden do not exhibit clinical symptoms. An adequate diet rich in iron, protein, and other vitamins helps maintain this asymptomatic state.

▼ **Hookworm Disease: Ancylostomiasis, Necatoriasis.** Patients who are repeatedly infected may develop intense allergic itching at the site of hookworm penetration, a condition known as ground itch. A number of symptoms experienced by infected persons are associated with larvae migration into the lungs, including sore throat, bloody sputum, wheezing, headache, and mild pneumonia with cough.

The symptoms associated with the intestinal phase of hookworm disease depend on the number of worms present. Chronic infections, consisting of a light worm burden (defined as <500 eggs/g of feces) are the most common form seen. These patients may experience vague mild gastrointestinal symptoms, slight anemia, and weight loss or weakness.

Patients with acute infections (>5000 eggs/g of feces) may develop a number of symptoms, including diarrhea, anorexia, edema, pain, enteritis, and epigastric discomfort. Furthermore because adult hookworms compete with the human host for nutrients as they feed, infected patients may develop a microcytic hypochromic iron deficiency, weakness, and hypoproteinemia. Mortality may result from the enormous loss of blood.

Treatment

The drugs of choice for treatment of hookworm disease are mebendazole and pyrantel pamoate. When indicated, especially in persons with asymptomatic hookworm infection, only iron replacement and/or other dietary therapy (including proteins, iron, and other vitamins) may be administered.

Prevention and Control

Hookworm prevention and control measures are similar to those for *A. lumbricoides*. Proper sanitation practices, especially appropriate fecal disposal, prompt and thorough treatment of infected persons, and personal protection of persons entering known endemic areas, such as covering bare feet, are measures targeted at breaking the hookworm life cycle.

Notes of Interest and New Trends

The advent of indoor plumbing is said by some to have contributed to a considerable decrease in hookworm infections, and considered by others to have eradicated them, in areas of the United States known to have sandy soil. Infections in those regions were contracted by individuals who walked barefoot to and from the outhouse.

The incidence of hookworm among soldiers during World War II was high. A significant number of them exhibited no clinical symptoms. Their diagnosis was based solely on the presence of hookworm eggs in the stool. These soldiers were unnecessarily hospitalized and given potent medications that resulted in toxic side effects. In those asymptomatic cases, only simple dietary therapy would have been warranted.

Research has been conducted using a reverse enzyme immunoassay for specific immunoglobulin E (IgE) in patients with known hookworm infections. This serodiagnosis methodology has shown favorable results and has been suggested as an alternative means of hookworm infection diagnosis.

There are two other species of hookworms known to infect humans accidentally, although they are primarily a parasite of dogs and cats, *Ancylostoma braziliense*, and of dogs only, *Ancylostoma caninum*. When they infect humans, these organisms are unable to complete their life cycle, infecting the subcutaneous or skeletal tissues. Human infection with either of these organisms may produce a condition known as cutaneous larva migrans. Characteristic symptoms include skin lesions and intense itching, which may lead to a secondary bacterial infection. The lesions resemble creeping worms through the skin. The treatment of choice is thiabendazole; prevention of infection and control of this accidental parasite may be accomplished by avoidance of skin contact with dog and cat feces.

Quick Quiz! 8-13

This adult hookworm is characterized by a buccal cavity that contains teeth. (Objective 8-10A)

A. *Ancylostoma*
B. *Necator*
C. Both *Ancylostoma* and Necator
D. Neither *Ancylostoma* nor *Necator*

Quick Quiz! 8-14

Individuals contract hookworm via which of the following? (Objective 8-6)

A. Contaminated water
B. Skin penetration
C. Insect bite
D. Contaminated food

Quick Quiz! 8-15

Which of the following are appropriate *Ascaris lumbricoides* prevention and control strategies? (Objective 8-8C)

A. Proper water treatment
B. Appropriate food handling
C. Use of insect repellent
D. Proper sanitation practices

Strongyloides stercoralis
(stron"ji-loy'deez/stur"kor-ray'lis)

Common Name: Threadworm.

Common associated disease and condition names: Strongyloidiasis, threadworm infection.

Morphology

Eggs. The eggs of *Strongyloides stercoralis* have historically been considered indistinguishable from those of hookworm (Fig. 8-18; Table 8-12). However, there are two features that when present may help identify the eggs specifically. First, the typical *S. stercoralis* egg measures only slightly smaller than hookworm eggs, averaging 48 by 35 μm. Second, unlike hookworm, well-developed larvae are almost always contained in the *S. stercoralis* eggs. The eggs of both organisms are similar in that when present, the two-,

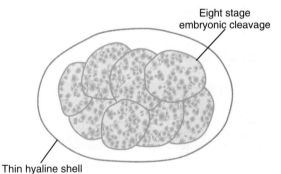

Eight stage embryonic cleavage

Thin hyaline shell

Average size: 48 μm by 35 μm

FIGURE 8-18 *Strongyloides stercoralis* egg.

TABLE 8-12	*Strongyloides stercoralis* Egg: Typical Characteristics at a Glance
Parameter	**Description**
Size	Average, 48 by 35 μm
Typical growth phase	Contains well-developed larvae
Embryonic cleavage	Two-, four-, or eight-cell stage, when present
Shell	Thin, hyaline

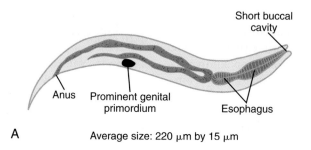

A   Average size: 220 μm by 15 μm

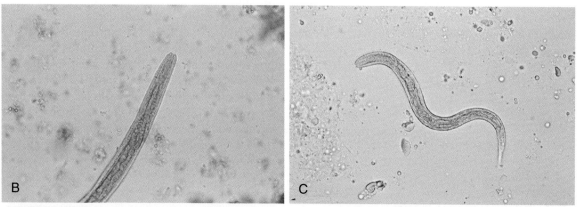

FIGURE 8-19 **A,** *Strongyloides stercoralis,* rhabditiform larva. **B,** *Strongyloides stercoralis,* rhabditiform larva, buccal capsule. **C,** *Strongyloides stercoralis,* rhabditiform larva. Note the short buccal capsule and prominent genital primordium. (**B, C** *from Mahon CR, Lehman DC, Manuselis G: Textbook of diagnostic microbiology, ed 4, St Louis, 2011, Saunders.*)

TABLE 8-13	*Strongyloides stercoralis* Rhabditiform Larva: Typical Characteristics at a Glance
Parameter	**Description**
Average size	220 by 15 μm
Other features	Short buccal cavity; prominent genital primordium

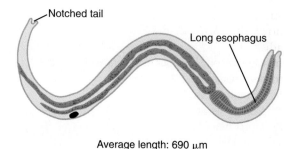

Average length: 690 μm

FIGURE 8-20 *Strongyloides stercoralis,* filariform larva.

four-, or eight-cell stage of embryonic cleavage is surrounded by a thin hyaline shell.

■ **Rhabditiform Larvae.** The actively feeding *S. stercoralis* rhabditiform larva has an average size of 220 by 15 μm (Fig. 8-19; Table 8-13). The larva is equipped with a short buccal cavity and a prominent genital primordium, whereas that of the hookworm contains a long buccal cavity and a relatively small genital primordium.

■ **Filariform Larvae.** The long, slender, nonfeeding filariform larva results from the molting of the rhabditiform form (Fig. 8-20; Table 8-14). The average length for this morphologic form is 690 μm. The *S. stercoralis* filariform larva differs from that of the hookworm in two respects. First, it has a long esophagus, compared with that of the hookworm. Second, the tail of *S. stercoralis* is notched, unlike that of *S. stercoralis* hookworm, which is pointed.

TABLE 8-14	*Strongyloides stercoralis* Filariform Larva: Typical Characteristics at a Glance
Parameter	**Description**
Average length	690 µm
Length of esophagus	Long
Tail	Notched

TABLE 8-15	*Strongyloides stercoralis* Adult Female: Typical Characteristics at a Glance
Parameter	**Description**
Approximate size	2 by 0.4 mm
Other features	Colorless, transparent body; finely striated cuticle; short buccal cavity; Long and slender esophagus

▌ **Adult Female.** Only the female adult *S. stercoralis* has been described (Table 8-15). Measuring approximately 2 by 0.4 mm, this small female worm is equipped with a short buccal cavity as well as a long and slender esophagus. The colorless body appears almost transparent. A finely striated cuticle covers the body. Probably because no adult male *S. stercoralis* is known to exist, the adult female is considered as **parthenogenic,** because there are no obvious morphologic structures to indicate that a male is not required for fertilization.

Laboratory Diagnosis

Laboratory diagnosis of threadworm may be accomplished in several ways. Diagnostic eggs, often indistinguishable from those of the hookworm, may be present in stool samples from patients suffering from severe diarrhea. Stool concentration with zinc sulfate has successfully recovered these eggs. Diagnostic rhabditiform larvae may be recovered in fresh stool samples and duodenal aspirates. It is important to note that careful screening of feces is necessary to distinguish the rhabditiform larvae of the hookworm from those of *S. stercoralis.* Furthermore,

the Enterotest has proven successful in obtaining the desired larvae and the hookworm-like eggs. Sputum samples have also yielded *S. stercoralis* larvae in patients suffering from disseminated disease. It is important to note that threadworm larvae have a typically higher recovery rate in concentrated specimens than those in which a flotation technique has been used. In addition to these methods, several serologic tests, including ELISA, have been developed.

Life Cycle Notes

There are three possible routes threadworms may take in their life cycles—direct, similar in most respects to that of the hookworm, indirect, and autoinfection. Unlike in the hookworm life cycle, in which eggs are the primary morphologic form seen in feces, life cycle rhabditiform larvae in the threadworm are usually passed in the feces. Eggs are only occasionally found in such samples. These rhabditiform larvae develop directly into the third-stage infective filariform larvae in warm, moist soil. The remaining phases of the threadworm life cycle basically mimic those of the hookworm life cycle.

In the indirect cycle, threadworm rhabditiform larvae are passed into the outside environment (soil) and mature into free-living adults that are nonparasitic. These adult females produce eggs that develop into rhabditiform larvae. These larvae mature and transform into the filariform stage, at which time they may initiate a new indirect cycle or become the infective stage for a human host and begin a direct cycle.

Autoinfection occurs when the rhabditiform larvae develop into the filariform stage inside the intestine of the human host. The resulting infective larvae may then enter the lymphatic system or bloodstream and initiate a new cycle of infection.

Epidemiology

Similar to the hookworm, *Strongyloides* is found predominantly in the tropical and subtropical regions of the world. In addition to being present in immigrants to the United States from known endemic areas, this organism has been reported in areas of the South that are mostly rural and in the Appalachian Mountain region. Areas of poor sanitation, in which feces are disposed in the warm moist soil, provide a wonderful atmosphere for the organism to exist, especially when participating in the indirect cycle of reproduction. Those at risk for contracting threadworm are those who come into skin contact with contaminated soil. In addition, persons living in institutions in which sanitation may be poor, such as psychiatric facilities, are also at risk.

Clinical Symptoms

Asymptomatic. Patients suffering from only a light infection often remain asymptomatic.

Strongyloidiasis: Threadworm Infection. The most common symptoms experienced by patients suffering from threadworm infection include diarrhea and abdominal pain. These patients may also exhibit urticaria accompanied by eosinophilia. Additional intestinal symptoms may occur, such as vomiting, constipation, weight loss, and variable anemia. Furthermore, patients with heavy infections may develop malabsorption syndrome. The site of larvae penetration may become itchy and red. Recurring allergic reactions may also occur. When the larvae migrate into the lungs, patients may develop pulmonary symptoms. Immunocompromised persons often suffer from severe autoinfections that may result in the spread of the larvae throughout the body, increased secondary bacterial infections, and possibly death.

Treatment

The treatment for a threadworm infection is ivermectin with albendazole as an alternative.

Prevention and Control

The measures necessary to prevent and control the spread of *S. stercoralis* are similar to those

for hookworm. In addition to proper handling and disposal of fecal material and adequate protection of the skin from contaminated soil, prompt and thorough treatment of infected persons is essential, especially to stop or prevent autoinfections.

Quick Quiz! 8-16

This diagnostic stage of *Strongyloides stercoralis* is best seen in stool using fecal concentration techniques: (Objective 8-9)
A. Eggs
B. Rhabditiform larvae
C. Filariform larvae
D. Adult worms

Quick Quiz! 8-17

The life cycle of *Stronglyoides* most resembles that of which of the following? (Objective 8-12)
A. Pinworm
B. Whipworm
C. Hookworm
D. Threadworm
E. Human roundworm

Quick Quiz! 8-18

The two clinical symptoms most commonly associated with *Trichinella spiralis* are which of the following? (Objective 8-7)
A. Constipation and abdominal pain
B. Vomiting urticaria
C. Diarrhea and vomiting
D. Abdominal pain and diarrhea

Trichinella spiralis
(trick"i-nel'uh/spy'ray'lis)

Common name: Trichina worm.

Common associated disease and condition names: Trichinosis, trichinellosis.

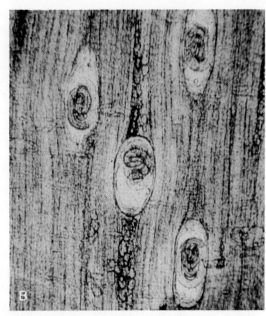

Inflammatory infiltrate

Striated muscle

Coiled larva

Nurse cell

Size range—juvenile: 75-120 μm by 4-7 μm
Fully developed: up to 1 mm long

A

B

FIGURE 8-21 **A,** *Trichinella spiralis,* encysted larva. **B,** *Trichinella spiralis* larvae in muscle press. (***B** from Bowman DD: Georgis' parasitology for veterinarians, ed 9, St. Louis, 2009, Saunders.)*

TABLE 8-16	*Trichinella spiralis* Encysted Larva: Typical Characteristics at a Glance
Parameter	**Description**
Average juvenile size	75-120 μm long, 4-7 μm wide
Average mature size	Up to 1 mm in length
Appearance	Colied
Encysted in	Nurse cells of striated muscle
Notable features	Inflammatory infiltrate present around nurse cell

TABLE 8-17	*Trichinella spiralis* Adults: Typical Characteristics at a Glance	
Characteristic	**Adult Female**	**Adult Male**
Size	4 by 0.5 mm	2 by 0.04 mm
Notable features	Blunt, round posterior end; single ovary with vulva in anterior fifth of body	Curved posterior end with two rounded appendages
Common to Both Adult Males and Females		
Thin anterior end		
Small mouth		
Long slender digestive tract		

Morphology

Encysted Larvae. The average juvenile encysted larvae measures from 75 to 120 μm by 4 to 7 μm (Fig. 8-21; Table 8-16). A fully developed larva may reach up to a length of 1 mm. These larvae settle by coiling up in muscle fibers and becoming encysted. Biopsies of these larvae often reveal a distinctive inflammatory infiltrate (see Fig. 8-21A) in response to the presence of the larvae. A striated muscle cell, known as a nurse cell, surrounds the coiled larva.

Adults. Although the small *T. spiralis* adult worms have rarely been seen, they have been described (Table 8-17). The female measures 4 by 0.5 mm, whereas the male is significantly smaller, measuring 2 by 0.04 mm. The typical male adult characteristically possesses a thin anterior end equipped with a small mouth, long and slender digestive tract, and curved posterior end with two somewhat rounded appendages. The female differs from the male in two respects. The female possesses a blunt, rounded posterior end and a single ovary with a vulva located in the anterior fifth of the body.

Laboratory Diagnosis

Although clinical symptoms and patient history play a vital role in helping diagnose *T. spiralis* infections, laboratory testing is essential to confirm all suspicions. Examination of the affected skeletal muscle is the method of choice for recovery of the encysted larvae. Serologic methods are also available. Other laboratory findings such as eosinophilia and leukocytosis may also serve as indicators for disease. Elevated serum muscle enzyme levels, such as lactate dehydrogenase, aldolase, and creatinine phosphokinase, may also aid in *T. spiralis* diagnosis. It is important to note that several tests may be required to confirm the presence of *T. spiralis*. No known test is completely 100% accurate. This, coupled with the fact that some tests may yield false-negative results in early infections, depending on when the sample is collected, often accounts for the need to perform multiple tests.

Life Cycle Notes

Human infection with *T. spiralis* is the result of accidental human infection with a parasite whose normal host is an animal (**zoonosis**). Infection is initiated after consuming undercooked contaminated meat, primarily striated muscle. Human digestion of the meat releases *T. spiralis* larvae into the intestine. Maturation into adult worms occurs rapidly. Mating occurs and the gravid adult female migrates to the intestinal submucosa to lay her live larvae because there is no egg stage in this life cycle. The infant larvae then enter the bloodstream and travel to striated muscle, where they encyst nurse cells. Over time, a granuloma forms, which becomes calcified around these cells. Because humans are not the traditional hosts, completion of the *T. spiralis* life cycle does not occur and the cycle ceases with the encystation of the larvae.

Epidemiology

With the exception of the tropics, where it is only rarely reported, *T. spiralis* is found worldwide, particularly in members of the meat-eating population. This organism may be found in a number of different animals, including the pig, deer, bear, walrus, and rat. The wide variety of temperature zones in which these animals reside suggests that *T. spiralis* is resistant to colder regions of the world as compared with most parasites studied thus far.

In developed areas, it is presumed that the feeding of contaminated pork scraps to hogs accounts for a major mode of *T. spiralis* transmission. Similarly, other animals contract this parasite from consuming contaminated meat.

Clinical Symptoms

Trichinosis, Trichinellosis. *T. spiralis* is known as the great imitator because infected patients may experience a variety of symptoms that often mimic those of other diseases and conditions. Persons with a light infection typically experience diarrhea and possibly a slight fever, suggestive of the flu. Heavily infected patients complain of symptoms such as vomiting, nausea, abdominal pain, diarrhea, headache, and perhaps a fever during the intestinal phase of infection. As the larvae begin their migration through the body, infected persons experience a number of symptoms, particularly eosinophilia, pain in the pleural area, fever, blurred vision, edema, and cough. Death may also result during this phase. Muscular discomfort, edema, local inflammation, overall fatigue, and weakness usually develop once the larvae settle into the striated muscle and begin the encystation process. The striated muscle of the face and limbs, as well as that of other parts of the body, may become infected.

Treatment

No medications are indicated if the infected person has a non–life-threatening strain of the disease. These patients are instructed to get plenty of rest, supplemented by adequate fluid intake, fever reducers, and pain relievers. Patients with severe infections that may be potentially life-threatening are usually treated with prednisone. Thiabendazole may also be given, even though research to date indicates that the effectiveness of this medication is questionable. Under appropriate conditions, steroids may also be administered.

Prevention and Control

Thorough cooking of meats, especially from animals known to harbor *T. spiralis*, is paramount to the eradication of this parasite. It has been determined that proper storage of these meats, at below-zero temperatures (i.e., –15° C [59° F] for 20 days or –30° C [86° F] for 6 days) will greatly decrease the viability of the organism. Furthermore the avoidance of feeding pork scraps to hogs is also necessary to break the *T. spiralis* life cycle.

Quick Quiz! 8-19

The specimen of choice for the identification of *Trichinella spiralis* is which of the following? (Objective 8-9)
A. Cerebral spinal fluid
B. Stool
C. Skeletal muscle
D. Urine

Quick Quiz! 8-20

The diagnostic stage of *Trichinella spiralis* is which of the following? (Objective 8-6)
A. Encysted larvae
B. Cysts
C. Eggs
D. Adult worms

Quick Quiz! 8-21

Trichinosis is acquired via which of the following? (Objective 8-6)
A. Swimming in contaminated water
B. Consuming contaminated water
C. Ingestion of contaminated food
D. Inhalation of contaminated air droplets

Dracunculus medinensis
(Drah-kung"ku-lus/med"in-en'-sis)

Common name: Guinea worm.

Common associated disease and condition names: Dracunculosis, dracunculiasis, guinea worm infection.

Morphology

Larvae. There are two larval stages (Table 8-18). The diagnostic stage, also known as the first stage or rhabditiform larvae, is relatively small, measuring an average size of 620 by 15 μm. The tail makes up about one third of the body length and culminates in a point. The third-stage larvae, which reside in an intermediate host, have not been well described.

Adults. Considered as one of the largest adult nematodes, the average elongated female *Dracunculus medinensis* measures approximately 840 mm long by 1.5 mm wide (Table 8-19). The female possesses a prominent blunt, rounded anterior end. The rarely seen adult male is smaller than the female, measuring only 21 by 0.4 mm.

TABLE 8-18	*Dracunculus medinensis* First-Stage Larva: Typical Characteristics at a Glance
Parameter	**Description**
Average size	620 by 15 μm
Tail characteristics	Consumes one third of body length; culminates in a point

TABLE 8-19	*Dracunculus medinensis* Adults: Typical Characteristics at a Glance	
Characteristic	**Adult Female**	**Adult Male**
Size	840 by 1.5 mm	21 by 0.4 mm
Other features	Prominent rounded anterior end	Anterior end coils itself at least once

The anterior end of the male characteristically coils on itself a minimum of one time.

Laboratory Diagnosis

Adult *D. medinensis* worms may be recovered by observing infected ulcers for the emergence of the worms. Induced rupture of the infected ulcers by immersing in cool water reveals the first-stage larvae.

Life Cycle Notes

Ingestion of drinking water contaminated with infected **copepods** (freshwater fleas) initiates human infection. These copepods contain infective *D. medinensis* third-stage larvae, which upon human ingestion emerge into the intestine. The larvae mature into adult worms, penetrate the intestinal wall, and proceed to connective tissues or body cavities. Following mating, the gravid female worms migrate into the subcutaneous tissue, especially in the skin of the extremities, where they lay live first-stage larvae. On release of all their larvae, the adult females may escape from the body at the larvae deposit site or migrate back into deeper tissues, where they eventually become absorbed. The fate of the adult males is unknown. An infected ulcer results at the site of the larvae deposit. Under appropriate conditions, such as contact with cool freshwater, the ulcer ruptures and releases the larvae into the water. Copepods living in the water consume the first-stage larvae, serving as its intermediate host. Maturation of the larvae into their third-stage infective form then occurs. Ingestion of the infected copepod begins the cycle again.

Epidemiology

Guinea worm is found in parts of Africa, India, Asia, Pakistan, and the Middle East. Copepods reside in fresh water, located particularly in areas called step wells, from which people obtain drinking water and bathe. First-stage *D. medinensis* larvae escape from the ulcers of infected persons who come into contact with this water. Ponds, human-made water holes, and standing water may also serve as sources of infection. There are a number of known reservoir hosts, including dogs. Like humans, these animals become infected via contaminated drinking water.

Clinical Symptoms

▧ **Guinea Worm Infection: Dracunculosis, Dracunculiasis.** Patients infected with guinea worm typically experience symptoms associated with allergic reactions as migration of the organism occurs. Secondary bacterial infections may also develop, some of which may cause disability or even death. Once the gravid female settles into the subcutaneous tissues and lays her larvae, a painful ulcer develops at the site. Unsuccessful attempts to remove an entire adult female worm may result in a partial worm being left at the site and subsequent toxic reactions in the ulcer. Additional allergic reactions and nodule formation may develop on the death and calcification of an adult worm.

Treatment

Because there are no specific dracunculiasis medicines available, successful treatment typically consists of total worm removal. The process of removal usually takes place in five steps:

Step 1. This step consists of placing the affected body part, in the form of a blister, in cool water.

Contact with the water creates an environment of interest to the underlying adult worm.

Step 2. In this step, the adult worm breaks through the blister and is eager to explore the outside world.

Step 3. It is important at this juncture to clean the resulting wound thoroughly.

Step 4. Manual extraction of the entire worm by winding it around a stick or a similar item that creates tension constitutes this step.

Step 5. Once the worm is removed, this step is performed, which consists of applying topical antibiotics to the wound site as a protective measure against the emergence of secondary bacterial infections.

Prevention and Control

The use of properly treated water for consumption, boiling water suspected of contamination, prohibiting the practice of drinking and bathing in the same water, and ceasing the practice of allowing standing water to be ingested are all logical guinea worm prevention and control measures. One of the simplest means whereby copepods may be removed from suspected water is to filter it using a finely meshed filter. This measure has been introduced into endemic areas. In addition to it being almost impossible to educate the entire population in endemic areas, the religious practices of some people in these areas lead to water contamination. It is highly unlikely that total eradication of guinea worm will occur in the near future.

Notes of Interest and New Trends

The history of *D. medinensis* dates back to biblical times. Guinea worms were suspected of being the "fiery serpents" responsible for a plague that affected the Israelites who lived by the Red Sea. This organism was also described by Egyptian priests, the Greeks, and the Romans.

Quick Quiz! 8-22

The two morphologic stages present in the *Dracunculus medinensis* are which of the following? (Objective 8-6)
A. Eggs and larvae
B. Larvae and adults
C. Eggs and adults
D. None of the above

Quick Quiz! 8-23

The specimen of choice for the recovery of *Dracunculus medinensis* is which of the following? (Objective 8-9)
A. Infected ulcer
B. Skeletal muscle
C. Stool
D. Blood

Quick Quiz! 8-24

When humans contract *Dracunculus medinensis*, the parasite's life cycle ceases to continue. (Objective 8-6)
A. True
B. False
C. Unable to determine

LOOKING BACK

Clinical laboratory scientists must take several considerations into account when identifying suspicious nematode organisms from patient specimens. Notation of the specimen type is crucial to ensure that the correct organism is ultimately identified because nematodes are recovered from specific samples. An accurate measurement of the size and shape of the suspected organism is necessary, not only to speciate the nematode but also to determine the correct morphologic form. Furthermore, careful examination of internal structures must be performed to confirm the presence and identification of a suspected parasite. It is also important that practitioners be cognizant of the specific diagnostic stage(s) of each nematode life cycle.

Several major differences in size, shape, and internal features help distinguish the nematode morphologic forms. These characteristics may best be compared at the end of this chapter in three composite drawings grouped by morphologic form—eggs, larvae, and adults.

TEST YOUR KNOWLEDGE!

8-1. For each nematode listed below (column A), select the corresponding common name (column B). (Objective 8-3)

Column A

A. *Trichinella spiralis*
B. *Trichuris trichiura*
C. *Enterobius vermicularis*
D. *Dracunculus medinensis*
E. *Necator americanus*

Column B

1. Hookworm
2. Guinea worm
3. Trichina worm
4. Pinworm
5. Roundworm of man
6. Whipworm
7. Threadworm

8-2. The eggs of which group of nematodes are indistinguishable? (Objective 8-12)
  A. Whipworm and trichina worm
  B. Hookworm and threadworm
  C. Guinea worm and roundworm of man
  D. Pinworm and whipworm

8-3. Once inside a human, these two nematodes take up residence outside the intestinal tract. (Objective 8-12)
  A. *Enterobius vermicularis* and *Strongyloides stercoralis*
  B. *Necator americanus* and *Ancylostoma duodenale*
  C. *Dracunculus medinensis* and *Trichinella spiralis*
  D. *Trichuris trichiura* and *Ascaris lumbricoides*

8-4. Match each nematode (column A) with the name of its corresponding common disease or condition (column B). (Objective 8-7)

Column A

A. Roundworm of man
B. Whipworm
C. Hookworm
D. Pinworm
E. Guinea worm

Column B

1. Ascariasis
2. Trichina worm
3. Trichuriasis
4. Ancylostomiasis
5. Enterobiasis
6. Dracunculosis

8-5. These two nematodes are similar in that they are both suspected of being transport hosts of *Dientamoeba fragilis*. (Objective 8-12)
  A. *Trichinella* and *Dracunculus*
  B. *Necator* and *Trichuris*
  C. *Strongyloides* and *Ancylostoma*
  D. *Ascaris* and *Enterobius*

8-6. The eggs of these two nematodes are never to rarely seen in stool samples. (Objective 8-12)
  A. Trichina and threadworm
  B. Whipworm and roundworm of man
  C. Guinea worm and pinworm
  D. Threadworm roundworm and hookworm

8-7. Match each nematode (column A) with its key distinguishing characteristic in the egg morphologic form (column B). (Objective 8-10)

Column A

A. *Ascaris*
B. *Anyclostoma*
C. *Enterobius*
D. *Trichuris*

Column B

1. Flattened on one side
2. Obvious albuminous coating
3. Surrounded by a nurse cell
4. Thin shell surrounding embryonic cleavage
5. Polar plug on each end

8-8. Differences in which of the following morphologic forms serve as criteria necessary to speciate the hookworms? (Objective 8-12)
  A. Eggs
  B. Rhabditiform larvae
  C. Encysted larvae
  D. Adult worms

8-9. Match the term (column A) with its key word or phrase definition (column B). (Objective 8-1)

Column A
A. Gravid

B. Embryonated
C. Cuticle

Column B
1. Presence of an outer albuminous coating
2. Surface covering
3. Fertilized

Column A
D. Parthenogenic

E. Decorticated

Column B
4. Absence of an outer albuminous coating
5. Pregnant
6. Unfertilized
7. Formation without fertilization

8-10. Which of these parasites are contracted via skin penetration? (Objective 8-6)
  A. *Enterobius, Necator, Dracunculus*
  B. *Ascaris, Trichinella, Ancylostoma*
  C. *Trichuris, Strongyloides, Enterobius*
  D. *Ancylostoma, Strongyloides, Necator*

CASE STUDY 8-2 UNDER THE MICROSCOPE

Paz, a 32-year-old woman originally from the Philippines, emigrated to the United States 2 years ago. She has since married and, at the time of admission, was pregnant with her first child. Economic restraints prevented the woman from seeking prenatal care. At the onset of labor, Paz was rushed to the local emergency room. During her labor, Paz told the nurse that she felt nauseous and thought that she was going to be sick. Paz then proceeded to cough up a large worm. The nurse placed the worm in a sterile urine cup and had it promptly sent to the laboratory for analysis. After the delivery of her child, a stool sample for parasite study was ordered, collected, and sent to the laboratory. The physician checked the baby and found him to be perfectly healthy.

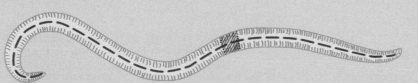 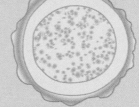

Once the worm (as seen in the figure) arrived in the laboratory, the clinical laboratorian on duty observed it under a dissecting microscope and noted that the worm was pregnant. The worm measured 30 cm in length and had the shape and thickness of a lead pencil. The worm was creamy white and possessed fine circular striations around the cuticle.

On receipt, the stool sample was promptly processed for parasite examination. Oval forms (as seen in the figure), which measured 60 by 40 μm, were observed in both the saline and iodine wet preparations. A trichrome stain was later performed and revealed the same organisms.

Questions and Issues for Consideration
1. State the scientific name and morphologic forms of the parasite you suspect to be present in this case. (Objectives 8-10C and 8-11A)
2. What is the common name associated with the parasite present? (Objective 8-11A)
3. Construct a life cycle for the parasite present in this case. (Objective 8-11C)
4. Which treatment option(s) and prevention and control strategies could be put into place to stop this parasite from replicating? (Objective 8-11D)

COMPARISON DRAWINGS
Intestinal Nematode Eggs

FIGURE 8-2A. *Enterobius vermicularis* egg

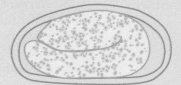

Size range: 48-60 μm long by 20-35 μm wide

FIGURE 8-4A. *Trichuris trichiura* egg

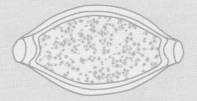

Average length: 50-55 μm
Average width: 25 μm

FIGURE 8-6A. *Ascaris lumbricoides* egg, unfertilized

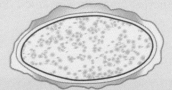

Size range: 85-95 μm by 38-45 μm

FIGURE 8-7A. *Ascaris lumbricoides* egg, fertilized

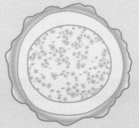

Size range: 40-75 μm by 30-50 μm

FIGURE 8-8. *Ascaris lumbricoides* egg, decorticated

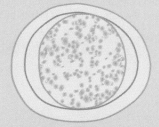

Size range: 40-75 μm by 30-50 μm

FIGURE 8-11A. Hookworm egg

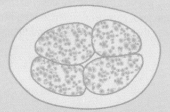

Necator size range: 60-75 μm by 35-40 μm
Ancylostoma size range: 55-60 μm by 35-40 μm

FIGURE 8-18. *Strongyloides stercoralis* egg

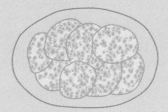

Average size: 48 μm by 35 μm

COMPARISON DRAWINGS
Nematode Larvae

FIGURE 8-12A. Hookworm rhabditiform larva

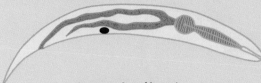

Average size of immature,
newly hatched rhabditiform larvae: 270 μm by 15 μm
Size range at 5 days old: 540-700 μm long

FIGURE 8-13. Hookworm filariform larva

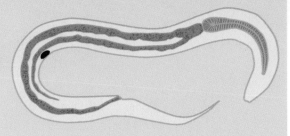

FIGURE 8-19A. *Strongyloides stercoralis* rhabditiform larva

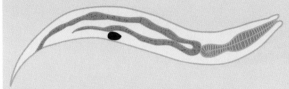

Average size: 220 μm by 15 μm

FIGURE 8-20. *Strongyloides stercoralis* filariform larva

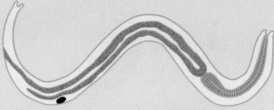

Average length: 690 μm

FIGURE 8-21A. *Trichinella spiralis* encysted larva

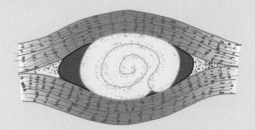

Size range—juvenile: 75-120 μm by 4-7 μm
Fully developed: up to 1 mm long

COMPARISON DRAWINGS
Nematode Adults

FIGURE 8-3. *Enterobius vermicularis,* adult female

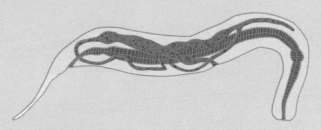

Size range: 7-14 mm long by up to 0.5 mm wide

FIGURE 8-5. *Trichuris trichiura,* adult male

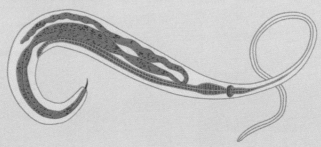

Size range: 2.5-5 cm long

FIGURE 8-9. *Ascaris lumbricoides,* adult male

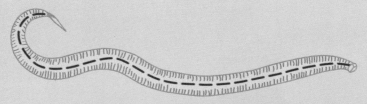

Average size: length is seldom up to 30 cm

FIGURE 8-10A. *Ascaris lumbricoides,* adult female

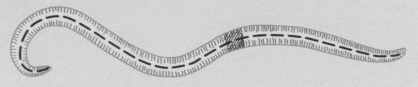

Average size: 22-35 cm long

COMPARISON DRAWINGS
Nematode Adults—cont'd

FIGURE 8-14. *Necator americanus,* buccal capsule

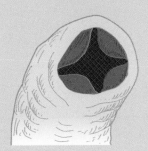

FIGURE 8-15. *Necator americanus,* adult male

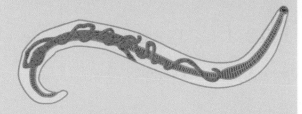

Size range: 9-12 mm long by 0.25-0.5 mm wide

FIGURE 8-16. *Ancylostoma duodenale,* buccal capsule

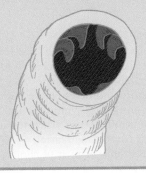

FIGURE 8-17. *Ancylostoma duodenale,* adult female

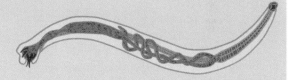

Size range: 5-10 mm long by 0.2-0.4 mm wide

The Filariae

Teresa A. Taff and Elizabeth Zeibig

WHAT'S AHEAD

Focusing In
Morphology and Life Cycle
  Notes
Laboratory Diagnosis
Pathogenesis and Clinical
  Symptoms

Filariae Classification
  Wuchereria bancrofti
  Brugia malayi
  Loa loa
  Onchocerca volvulus

Other Filarial Organisms
  Mansonella ozzardi
  Mansonella perstans
Looking Back

LEARNING OBJECTIVES

On completion of this chapter and review of its diagrams, tables, and corresponding photomicrographs, the successful learner will be able to:

9-1. Define the following key terms:
  Calabar swelling
  Diurnal
  Elephantiasis
  Filaria (*pl.*, filariae)
  Filarial
  Microfilaria (*pl.*, microfilariae)
  Nematode (*pl.*, nematodes)
  Nocturnal
  Occult
  Periodicity
  Sheath
  Subperiodic
  Vector (*pl.*, vectors)

9-2. State the geographic distribution of the filariae.

9-3. State the common name associated with each of the filariae.

9-4. Given a list of parasites, select those belonging to the filariae.

9-5. Briefly describe the life cycle of each of the filaria.

9-6. List the vectors responsible for filarial transmission.

9-7. Identify and describe the populations prone to contracting symptoms and clinically significant disease processes associated with each pathogenic filarial.

9-8. Select the specimen of choice, collection and processing protocol, and laboratory diagnostic technique(s) for the recovery of each of the filarial parasites.

9-9. Identify and describe each of the following as they relate to the filariae:
  A. Disease or condition, prognosis
  B. Treatment options
  C. Prevention and control measures

9-10. Explain the significance of collection time as it relates to successful filarial organism recovery.

9-11. Given a description, photomicrograph and/or diagram of a filarial parasite:
  A. Correctly label the designated characteristic structure(s).
  B. State the purpose of designated characteristic structure(s).
  C. Identify the organism by scientific name, common name, and morphologic form.

D. State the common name for associated conditions or diseases, if applicable.

9-12. Analyze case studies that include pertinent patient information and laboratory data and do the following:

A. Identify each responsible filarial organism by scientific name, common name, and morphologic form.

B. Identify the associated diseases and conditions associated with the responsible parasite.

C. Construct a life cycle associated with each filarial parasite present that includes corresponding epidemiology, route of transmission, infective stage, and diagnostic stage.

D. Propose each of the following related to stopping and preventing nematode infections:
1. Treatment options
2. Prevention and control plan

E. Recognize sources of error, including but not limited to those involved in specimen collection, processing, and testing and propose solutions to remedy them.

F. Interpret laboratory data, determine specific follow-up tests to be done, and predict the results of those identified tests.

9-13. Identify, compare, and contrast the similarities and differences among the parasites discussed in this and other chapters in this text.

9-14. Describe standard and alternative laboratory diagnostic approaches as appropriate for the recovery of filarial parasites in clinical specimens.

9-15. Given prepared laboratory specimens and with the assistance of this manual, the learner will be able to do the following:

A. Differentiate filarial organisms from artifacts.

B. Correctly name each filaria parasite based on its key characteristic structure(s).

CASE STUDY 9-1   UNDER THE MICROSCOPE

Lois is a distraught 44-year-old female visiting her primary care physician at 9:00 a.m. She describes looking in the mirror that morning and seeing a worm crawl across her eye and then disappear. On her updated patient history, she notes she had visited the African rainforest the previous year. The physician orders a stool for ova and parasite examination, as well as a complete blood count and differential. The blood is drawn at 11:30 a.m. on the same day as the office visit at a draw site near Lois' home. The stool parasite examination proves to be negative. The automated blood count shows increased eosinophils and a Giemsa stained blood film is prepared. An evening shift medical laboratory scientist obeserves a worm-like form on the blood smear that is 275 μm in length. There is a stained sheath and nuclei extend to the tip of the tail.

Questions to Consider
1. What is the scientific name of the organism observed? (Objective 9-12A)
2. What is the significance of her travel history? (Objective 9-2)
3. Determine if the blood sample was drawn appropriately. (Objective 9-10)
4. Propose treatment options for this individual. (Objective 9-12D)

FOCUSING IN

This chapter describes a group of nematodes, known as the **filariae** or **filarial nematodes**, in which the adult worms live in tissue or the lymphatic system and are thus rarely seen. The adult filariae produce larvae called **microfilariae** that are usually detected in the blood. These microfilariae may exhibit periodicity (a concept detailed later in the laboratory diagnosis section). Vectors of filarial nematodes include biting insects such as mosquitoes. Distribution of these organisms includes Asia, Africa, South and Central Americas and the Carribean.

MORPHOLOGY AND LIFE CYCLE NOTES

There are two known morphologic forms of the filariae, adult worms and larvae known as microfilariae. The adults usually appear creamy white and assume a threadlike appearance. Adult males may measure from 20 to 500 mm in length, which is often half that of typical adult females. The microfilariae are slender and may range in size from just under 150 μm to 350 μm in length. The distribution of nuclei within the tip of the tail, as well as the presence or absence of a delicate transparent covering known as a **sheath**, are the two key characteristics helpful in speciating the microfilariae forms of these organisms.

The basic life cycle is the same for all members of the filariae. Only one to four infective larvae, injected by an infected arthropod at the feeding site, are required to initiate human infection. Once inside the body, the larvae migrate to the tissues, where they complete their development, a process that may take up to 1 year. The resulting adult worms may reside in the lymphatics, subcutaneous tissue or internal body cavities. Fertilized adult female worms lay live microfilariae, which take up residence in the blood or dermis. The microfilariae exit the body via a blood meal by the appropriate arthropod vector. The arthropod serves as the intermediate host for the parasite. Larvae development into the infective stage takes place in the insect host. Once the infective stage is reached, the parasite is ready to be transferred into an uninfected human, thus initiating a new cycle.

The location of the adult worms and microfilariae in the body and specific arthropod vector all vary by individual species. The specifics of these differences are addressed on an individual basis.

Quick Quiz! 9-1

Speciation of the microfilariae can be done by recognition of the distribution of nuclei in the tip of the tail and the presence or absence of a delicate transparent covering known as the: (Objective 9-1)
A. Flilariform
B. Cuticle
C. Sheath
D. Nucleus

LABORATORY DIAGNOSIS

Some species of filarial parasites exhibit **periodicity,** a phenomenon whereby the parasites are present in the bloodstream during a specific time period; this feature is helpful in selecting the appropriate time for specimen collection. There is evidence to suggest that this periodicity, which may be **nocturnal** (occurring at night), **diurnal** (occurring during the day), or **subperiodic** (timing of occurrences not clear-cut) is connected to the corresponding vector's feeding schedule. The periodicity for each of the filarial parasites is described on an individual basis.

The primary method of filarial diagnosis is microscopic examination of the microfilariae in a Giemsa-stained smear of blood or a tissue scraping of an infected nodule. Whole blood samples may also be collected. Processing of these samples consists of lysing the cells followed by concentrating and examining the sample for microfilariae using the Knott technique. Although a number of serologic tests have been developed and are available, there is some concern as to their specificity, and thus they are not universally considered as viable diagnostic techniques. Representative laboratory diagnostic methodologies are found in Chapter 2 as well as in each individual parasite discussion, as appropriate.

Quick Quiz! 9-2

What type of periodicity is exhibited if microfilariae appear in the blood of an individual at 2:00 p.m. each day? (Objective 9-1)
A. Nocturnal
B. Diurnal
C. Subperiodic
D. Biannual

PATHOGENESIS AND CLINICAL SYMPTOMS

The clinical symptoms experienced by persons infected with filarial organisms vary, depending on the species. Such symptoms range from involvement of the lymphatics, with subsequent granulomatous lesions, eosinophilia, fever, chills,

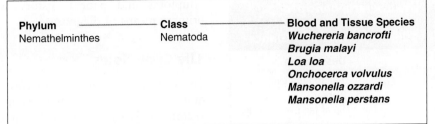

Phylum	Class	Blood and Tissue Species
Nemathelminthes	Nematoda	*Wuchereria bancrofti*
		Brugia malayi
		Loa loa
		Onchocerca volvulus
		Mansonella ozzardi
		Mansonella perstans

FIGURE 9-1 Parasite classification: The filariae.

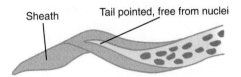
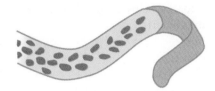

Sheath

Tail pointed, free from nuclei

Size range: 240-300 µm long

FIGURE 9-2 *Wuchereria bancrofti* microfilaria.

and enlargement of skin and subcutaneous tissue known as **elephantiasis,** to **Calabar swellings** (transient swelling of subcutaneous tissues), eye involvement, and even blindness.

 Quick Quiz! 9-3

Which of the following is similar for all microfilariae discussed? (Objective 9-13)
A. Presence of a sheath
B. Ability to exhibit periodicity
C. Location of the adult worms
D. The basic life cycle

FILARIAE CLASSIFICATION

The filariae belong to the same phylum and class as the nematodes introduced in Chapter 8, Nemathelminthes and Nematoda, respectively. All six of the organisms discussed in this chapter are blood and tissue species, listed in Figure 9-1.

Wuchereria bancrofti
(wooch-ur-eer′ee-uh/ban-krof′tye)

Common name: Bancroft's filaria.

Common associated disease and condition names: Bancroft's filariasis or elephantiasis.

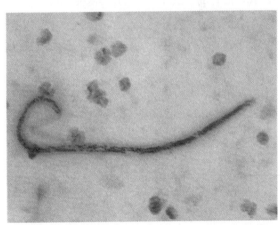

FIGURE 9-3 *Wuchereria bancrofti* microfilaria. Note the presence of a sheath and absence of nuclei in the tip of the tail (Giemsa stain, ×400). *(Courtesy of WARD'S Natural Science Establishment, Rochester, NY.)*

Morphology

Microfilariae. The average microfilaria measures 240 to 300 µm in length (Figs. 9-2 and 9-3; Table 9-1). A thin and delicate sheath surrounds the organism. Numerous nuclei are contained in the body. The cephalic or anterior end is blunt and round. The posterior or tail end culminates in a point that is free of nuclei. This is a key

TABLE 9-1	*Wuchereria bancrofti* Microfilaria: Typical Characteristics at a Glance
Parameter	**Description**
Size range	240-300 µm long
Sheath	Present
Arrangement of nuclei in tail	Tip of tail free of nuclei

characteristic that helps distinguish it from other sheathed microfilariae.

Adults

The adult *Wuchereria bancrofti* worms are white and assume a threadlike appearance. The females are typically larger than the males, measuring 40 to 100 mm and 20 to 40 mm, respectively.

Laboratory Diagnosis

The examination of fresh Giemsa-stained blood for *W. bancrofti* microfilariae serves as the laboratory diagnostic method of choice. A more sensitive method for microfilariae recovery involves filtering heparinized blood through a special filter, known as a nuclepore filter, and then staining and examining the filter contents. The Knott technique may also be used. Light infections may be diagnosed by immersing 1 mL of blood in 10 mL of a 2% solution of formalin, which lyses the red cells. Microscopic examination of the stained sediment is then performed. In all these methods, the optimal sample is collected at night because this organism generally exhibits nocturnal periodicity. Peak hours for specimen collection are between 9:00 p.m. and 4:00 a.m. which correlates with the appearance of its vector, the mosquito. However, subperiodic organisms are sometimes detected throughout the day. They are more prevalent in the late afternoon. Serologic tests, including antigen and antibody detection and PCR assays, have been developed. The sensitivity and specificity of these tests vary widely. With all these techniques available, it is interesting to note that in endemic areas, clinical symptoms and patient history serve as the primary means of diagnosis.

Life Cycle Notes

The *Culex, Aedes,* and *Anopheles* spp. of mosquitoes serve as the intermediate hosts and vectors of *W. bancrofti*. In the human host, the adult worms take up residence in the lymphatics, where they lay their microfilariae. These microfilariae live in the blood and lymphatics.

Epidemiology

W. bancrofti may be found in the subtropical and tropical areas of the world. These include central Africa, the Nile Delta, India, Pakistan, Thailand, the Arabian sea coast, the Philippines, Japan, Korea, and China in the Eastern Hemisphere and in Haiti, the Dominican Republic, Costa Rica, and coastal Brazil in the Western Hemisphere. Mosquito breeding occurs in contaminated water in these areas. It is interesting to note that indigenous inhabitants of the endemic areas are at a greater risk of contracting *W. bancrofti* than are non-indigenous individuals living in these areas.

Clinical Symptoms

Asymptomatic. Adult patients, who as children were most likely exposed to *W. bancrofti*, may become infected and experience no symptoms. Microfilariae are usually recovered in blood samples from these patients. Eosinophilia may also be noted in these samples. Physical examination reveals only enlarged lymph nodes, particularly in the inguinal region, the groin area. Infections of this type are self-limiting because the adult worms eventually die and there are no signs of microfilariae being present. A patient may undergo the entire process and not even know it.
Symptomatic Bancroftian Filariasis. A wide variety of symptoms may be experienced by patients infected with *W. bancrofti*. In general, they develop a fever, chills, and eosinophilia. The invasion of the parasite may result in the forma-

tion of granulomatous lesions, lymphangitis, and lymphadenopathy. Bacterial infections with *Streptococcus* may also occur. Elephantiasis or swelling of the lower extremities especially the legs develop due to obstruction of the lymphatics. The genitals and breasts may also be involved. On the death of the adult worms, calcification or the formation of abscesses may occur.

Treatment

Medications that have known effectiveness against *W. bancrofti* include diethylcarbamazine (DEC) and ivermectin (Stromectol) when used in combination with albendazole. DEC and ivermectin kill microfilariae. Increased doses are necessary to kill adults. Surgical removal of excess tissue may be appropriate for the scrotum but is only rarely successful when performed on the extremities. The use of special boots, known as Unna's paste boots, as well as elastic bandages and simple elevation, have proven successful in reducing the size of an infected enlarged limb.

Prevention and Control

Prevention and control measures for *W. bancrofti* include using personal protection when entering known endemic areas, destroying breeding areas of the mosquitoes, using insecticides when appropriate, and educating the inhabitants of endemic areas. Avoiding mosquito infested areas is ideal. Mosquito netting and insect repellants are more practical and useful in endemic areas.

Notes of Interest and New Trends

The origin of *W. bancrofti* is thought to date back as far as the second millennium BC. This parasite appears to have been spread via people around the world exploring and relocating over the years. For example, early explorers of the 17th and 18th centuries learned about bancroftian filariasias when they visited Polynesia.

Circa 1930, an epidemic caused by *W. bancrofti* died out in Charleston, South Carolina. It is suspected that the infection was brought to the

United States by African slaves who were sent to Charleston.

Quick Quiz! 9-4

Diagnosis of infection with *Wuchereria bancrofti* is best accomplished by: (Objective 9-8)
A. Examination of stained peripheral blood taken during the night
B. Examination of stained tissue biopsy taken during the night
C. Use of serologic testing with blood taken during the day
D. Examination of stained lymph fluid taken during the day

Quick Quiz! 9-5

Which of the following, in combination with albendazole, has proven to be an important drug for the treatment of Bancroft's filariasis? (Objective 9-9C)
A. Doxycycline
B. Ivermectin
C. Metronidazole
D. None of the above

Brugia malayi
(broog'ee-uh/may-lay-eye)

Common name: Malayan filaria.

Common associated disease and condition names: Malayan filariasis or elephantiasis.

Morphology

Microfilariae. The typical *Brugia malayi* microfilaria ranges in length from 200 to 280 μm (Figs. 9-4 and 9-5; Table 9-2). This organism, like *W. bancrofti*, possesses a sheath, rounded anterior end, and numerous nuclei. The characteristic that distinguishes it from the other sheathed organisms is the presence of two distinct nuclei in the tip of the somewhat pointed tail. These two nuclei are distinct and separated from the other nuclei present in the body of the organism, as shown in Figure 9-4.

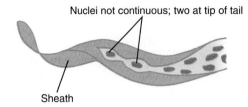

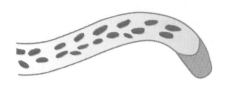

Nuclei not continuous; two at tip of tail

Sheath

Size range: 200-280 μm long

FIGURE 9-4 *Brugia malayi* microfilaria.

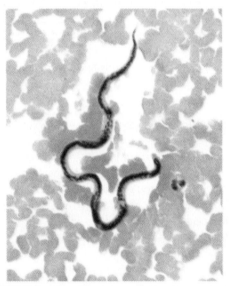

FIGURE 9-5 *Brugia malayi* microfilaria. Note the sheath and characteristic nuclei in the tip of the tail (Giemsa stain, ×400).

■ **Adults.** The adult worms of *B. malayi* resemble those of *W. bancrofti* in that members of both species are white in color and threadlike in appearance. The typical adult female worm measures 53 mm in length, whereas the adult male measures 24 mm in length.

Laboratory Diagnosis

Although a limited number of documented *B. malayi* microfilariae have been recovered, examination of stained blood films serves as the best method for diagnosis. Because *B. malayi* generally exhibits nocturnal periodicity, specimens collected during the nighttime hours are most likely to yield large numbers of circulating microfilariae. Subperiodic organisms may appear and this possibility should be considered when determining specimen collection protocol. The Knott technique may also be used. Serologic methods have also been developed and are now available.

Life Cycle Notes

B. malayi may be transmitted by the mosquito genera *Aedes*, *Anopheles* or *Mansonia* depending on the location and animal reservoirs present. The *Anopheles* mosquito can also transmit *W. bancrofti* so co-infection can theoretically be possible. All other aspects of the life cycle of *B. malayi* are similar to that of *W. bancrofti*.

Epidemiology

Areas of the world in which the mosquitoes breed are the primary locations in which *B. malayi* may be found. These include the

TABLE 9-2	*Brugia malayi* Microfilaria: Typical Characteristics at a Glance	
Parameter	**Description**
Size range	200-280 μm long
Sheath	Present
Arrangement of nuclei in tail	Presence of two distinct nuclei in the tip of the tail; the organism tissue tends to bulge around each of the two nuclei

Philippines, Indonesia, Sri Lanka, New Guinea, Vietnam, Thailand, and specific regions of Japan, Korea, and China. Although humans are considered to be the primary definite host, *B. malayi* is also known to infect felines and monkeys.

Clinical Symptoms

Infections with *B. malayi* are often asymptomatic even with the presence of microfilariae in the blood. Fevers may take months to years to develop after the inital infection. Additional symptoms include the formation of granulomatous lesions following microfilarial invasion into the lymphatics, chills, lymphadenopathy, lymphangitis, and eosinophilia. Eventually the result is elephantiasis of the legs. Elephantiasis of the genitals is possible but less common.

Treatment

Treatment for *B. malayi* is similar to that for *W. bancrofti*, with the most useful medication being diethylcarbamazine (DEC). Inflammatory reactions are more common after treatment and can be severe. Therefore, anti-inflammatory drugs may be necessary.

Prevention and Control

The prevention and control measures for *B. malayi* are identical to those for *W. bancrofti*.

Notes of Interest and New Trends

In addition to *B. malayi*, Malayan filariasis may also be caused by another species of *Brugia*, *Brugia timori*, first isolated in 1964 on the island of Timor. Readily distinguishable from *B. malayi*, the microfilariae of *B. timori* measure approximately 310 μm. The organism has a sheath, which is difficult to observe using Giemsa stain and distinct nuclei in the tip of the tail. The body tissue of this organism does not bulge around the two nuclei like that of *B. malayi*.

A condition called tropical eosinophilia or **occult** (meaning hidden or not apparent) filariasis is known to occur in persons who reside in the areas of the world in which both *B. malayi* and *W. bancrofti* are endemic. These patients experience a number of pulmonary and asthmatic symptoms. On thorough examination of infected patients, no microfilariae are found in their blood. It is suspected that a filarial parasite is present and is responsible for this condition but remains hidden deep in the body such as in the lungs. The signs and symptoms may be due to the body's inflammatory response. Successful resolution of symptoms with DEC therapy confirms the diagnosis of filarial infection but failure to respond to DEC suggests another cause for the symptoms.

Quick Quiz! 9-6

Which of the following can be used in the differentiation and identification of *Brugia malayi*? (Objective 9-13)
A. Absence of a sheath
B. Absence of nuclei in the tail
C. Presence of a sheath that is very difficult to observe on Giemsa stain
D. Presence of two terminal nuclei in the tail

Quick Quiz! 9-7

Select the ideal time period to collect blood samples for examination for the presence of the microfilariae of *Brugia malayi*. (Objective 9-8)
A. 10:00 p.m. to 4:00 a.m.
B. 10:00 a.m. to 4:00 p.m.
C. 4:00 p.m. to 8:00 p.m.
D. Any time of the day or night

Loa loa
(lo'uh/lo'uh)

Common name: Eye worm (African).

   Common associated disease and condition names: Loiasis.

Morphology

Microfilariae. The sheathed *Loa loa* microfilaria usually measures 248 to 300 μm in length

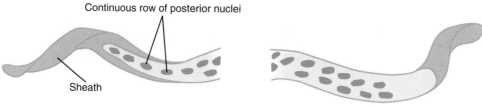

Size range: 248-300 μm long

FIGURE 9-6 *Loa loa* microfilaria.

TABLE 9-3	*Loa loa* Microfilaria: Typical Characteristics at a Glance
Parameter	**Description**
Size range	248-300 μm long
Sheath	Present
Arrangement of nuclei in tail	Distinct continuous row of nuclei; extend to tip of tail

(Fig. 9-6; Table 9-3). Nuclei fill the organism and are continuous to the tip of the pointed tail. This characteristic helps distinguish it from the other sheathed microfilariae.

◼ **Adults.** The adult *L. loa* worms are typically white in color and exhibit a cylindrical threadlike appearance. The adult females are large, relatively speaking, measuring 38 to 72 mm in length. The adult males are significantly smaller, measuring 28 to 35 mm in length.

Laboratory Diagnosis

The specimen of choice for the recovery of *L. loa* microfilariae is Giemsa-stained blood. The Knott technique may also be used. These samples yield the best recovery rate when collected during the midday hours, between 10:15 AM and 2:15 PM, because this organism displays diurnal periodicity. The migrating adult worms may be extracted from a variety of body locations, including the eye. Residence in an endemic area and the presence of eosinophilia and Calabar or transient subcutaneous swellings also aid in diagnosis. As with the other microfilariae discussed, serologic testing is also available.

Life Cycle Notes

Human infection of *L. loa* is initiated by the bite of an infected *Chrysops* fly. Adult worms take up residence and multiply throughout the subcutaneous tissues. The microfilariae are present in the blood but not until years after the initial infection making the diagnosis more difficult.

Epidemiology

As with all the filarial organisms, the endemic regions of infections correlate with the areas where the vector flourishes. In the case of *L. loa*, the *Chrysops* fly inhabits Africa especially the rainforest belt region. It is estimated that infection rates may be over 70% in the areas in which a large vector population exists. A less than 10% infection rate occurs in regions in which minimal numbers of vectors reside.

Clinical Symptoms

◼ **Loiasis.** After the initial bite, individuals infected with *L. loa* may experience pruritus or itchiness and localized pain. Development of Calabar swellings at the site of initial discomfort usually follows. This localized subcutaneous edema may occur anywhere on the body and is thought to result from the migration and death of the microfilariae. It is interesting to note that the presence of circulating adult worms in the subcutaneous tissues usually causes no discomfort. The adult worms may only be noticeable when seen migrating under the conjunctiva of the eye or crossing under the skin of the bridge of the nose.

No sheath (found in tissue only)

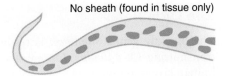

Size range: 148-355 μm long

FIGURE 9-7 *Onchocerca volvulus* microfilaria.

Treatment

Surgical removal of adult *L. loa* worms is the treatment of choice. Extracting these worms when they are attempting to cross the eye or the bridge of the nose is the ideal time to remove them. Unfortunately, it is impossible to select the appropriate time to perform such a procedure in advance.

The medication of choice for the treatment of *L. loa* is diethylcarbamazine (DEC). Although this antiparasitic drug is known to be effective, it should be used with caution. Its use to treat heavily infected patients may result in serious side effects, including encephalitis.

Prevention and Control

Personal protection measures are essential to stop the spread of *L. loa* infection. In addition, destroying the vector breeding areas, although probably not economically or logistically feasible, would also help in halting the spread of infection. The use of prophylactic DEC, particularly for non-natives visiting endemic areas, has also proven effective.

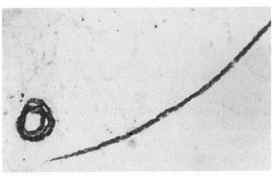

FIGURE 9-8 *Onchocerca volvulus* microfilaria. Note the absence of a sheath (Giemsa stain, ×400). *(Courtesy of WARD'S Natural Science Establishment, Rochester, NY.)*

 Quick Quiz! 9-9

What type of periodicity does *Loa loa* exhibit? (Objective 9-8)
A. Nocturnal
B. Subperiodic
C. Diurnal
D. None

Onchocerca volvulus
(onk'o-sur'kuh/vol'vew-lus)

Common name: Blinding filaria.

Common associated disease and condition names: River blindness, onchocerciasis.

Morphology

 Microfilariae. *Onchocerca volvulus* ranges in length from 150 to 355 μm (Figs. 9-7 and 9-8; Table 9-4). The one primary characteristic that distinguishes this organism from the other

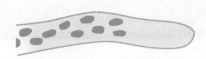 *Quick Quiz! 9-8*

A small threadlike worm is observed under the conjunctiva of the eye. What organism and form is most likely? (Objective 9-8)
A. *Wuchereria bancrofti* adult
B. *Brugia malayi* microfilaria
C. *Onchocera volvulus* larva
D. *Loa loa* adult

TABLE 9-4	*Onchocerca volvulus* Microfilaria: Typical Characteristics at a Glance	
Parameter		**Description**
Size range		150-355 µm long
Sheath		Absent
Arrangement of the nuclei in tail		Do not extend to tip of tail

microfilariae is that it does not possess a sheath. The body contains numerous nuclei that extend from the rounded anterior end, almost to but not including the tip of the somewhat pointed tail. Another distinction that helps in its identification is the location of the microfilariae. Those of *O. volvulus* are found in the subcutaneous tissue and not blood specimens.

Adults. The adult *O. volvulus* worms are thin and wirelike in appearance. They typically coil up in knots inside infected skin nodules. The adult females may measure up to 500 mm in length, whereas the adult males are 25 to 50 mm long.

Laboratory Diagnosis

Multiple Giemsa-stained slides of tissue biopsies, known as skin snips, collected from suspected infected areas are the specimens of choice for the recovery of *O. volvulus* microfilariae. The skin snips should be obtained with as little blood as possible. The reason is to avoid contamination of the sample with other species of microfilariae that may be present in the blood. Adult worms may be recovered from infected nodules. Organisms residing in the eye are best seen by ophthalmologic examination using a slit lamp. As with *L. loa*, patient history, particularly travel and residence, as well as the presence of eosinophilia and ocular discomfort, may be helpful in the diagnosis of *O. volvulus*. Serologic methods are also available. PCR can successfully detect low level infections.

Life Cycle Notes

The blackfly genus *Simulium* is responsible for transmitting *O. volvulus*. On entrance into the human host and following maturation, the resulting adult worms encapsulate in subcutaneous fibrous tumors. It is here that the adults become coiled and microfilariae emerge. The microfilariae may migrate throughout infected nodules, subcutaneous tissues, and skin and into the eye. The microfilariae are rarely seen in the peripheral blood making this a poor specimen for diagnosis.

Epidemiology

O. volvulus is distributed primarily in equatorial Africa and Central America. Specific endemic areas include East Africa, Zaire, Angola, parts of Mexico, Colombia, Brazil, and portions of Venezuela. All these areas harbor the vector, the *Simulium* blackfly. This insect breeds in running water, particularly along streams and rivers. Persons entering these areas are at risk for becoming infected via a vector bite. There are known animal reservoirs.

Clinical Symptoms

Onchocerciasis: River Blindness. Infection with *O. volvulus* usually results in a chronic and nonfatal condition. Patients typically experience localized symptoms caused by the development of infected nodules. Some patients may also suffer severe allergic reactions to the presence of the microfilariae. Scratching leads to secondary bacterial infections. When the eye becomes involved, lesions, due to the body's reaction to the microfilariae, may lead to blindness. Blindness has proven to be a significant complication for many infected adults. The specific symptoms associated with *O. volvulus* infection, particularly changes in overall skin appearance, such as loss of elasticity, and location of nodules on the body, vary based on whether the patient contracted the parasite in the Eastern or Western Hemisphere.

Treatment

The drug of choice for the treatment of *O. volvulus* microfilariae is ivermectin. There is no known medication on the market that effectively destroys both the adult worms and microfilariae without some toxic effects or complications. Therapy may be necessary for very long periods of time due to the long life of the adult worms. They can live for 15 years or more. When appropriate, surgical removal of the adult worms from an infected nodule may be performed to reduce the number of microfilariae present in the subcutaneous tissue.

Prevention and Control

Exercising personal protection when entering endemic areas is crucial to halting the spread of *O. volvulus*. In addition, controlling the vector breeding grounds with the use of insecticides, as well as areas in which the adult insects reside, is also essential to eradicate the parasite but has been proven to be very difficult.

Quick Quiz! 9-10

How do the microfilariae of *Onchocerca volvulus* differ from those of other filarial? (Objective 9-13)

A. The presence of a sheath.
B. Nuclei are present continuous to the end of the tail
C. They exhibit diurnal periodicity
D. They are found in the skin rather than blood

Quick Quiz! 9-11

Skin snips are the specimen of choice for diagnosis of infection with: (Objective 9-8)

A. *Loa loa*
B. *Onchocerca volvulus*
C. *Brugia malayi*
D. *Wuchereria bancrofti*

OTHER FILARIAL ORGANISMS

Other microfilarial parasites do exist. Although primarily nonpathogenic, there are times when treatment is indicated. Despite their varying pathogenicity, these organism produce microfilariae that must differentiated from others known to be pathogenic. Two filarial parasites (*Mansonella ozzardi* and *Mansonella perstans*) that fit into this category are described in the sections that follow.

Mansonella ozzardi
(man"so-nel'ah/o-zar'de)

Common name: New World filaria.

   Common associated disease and condition names: None (considered as a nonpathogen).

Morphology

Microfilariae. As with the other microfilariae, the average *Mansonella ozzardi* microfilaria has a rounded, blunt anterior end and measures approximately 220 μm (Fig. 9-9; Table 9-5). The posterior end is short and not as tapered as that of *Onchocerca*. The organism contains numerous nuclei that do not extend to the tip of the long, narrow and tapered tail. There is no sheath present. It is similar in appearance to that of *O. volvulus* but is found in blood rather than skin snips. The microfilariae do not exhibit any periodicity in the blood.

Adults. The typical adult female *M. ozzardi* may range in length from 65 to 80 mm, with an

TABLE 9-5	*Mansonella ozzardi* Microfilaria: Typical Characteristics at a Glance
Parameter	**Description**
Size range	220 μm in length
Sheath	Absent
Arrangement of nuclei in tail	Numerous; do not extend to tip of tail

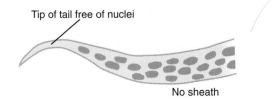
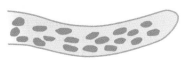

Tip of tail free of nuclei

No sheath

Approximate length: 88 μm

FIGURE 9-9 *Mansonella ozzardi* microfilaria.

average of 70 mm. The posterior section of the adult male worm, measuring approximately 32 mm in length, has been recovered and documented from humans. The location of the adults in humans is currently unknown.

Laboratory Diagnosis

M. ozzardi microfilariae may be recovered in peripheral blood. The organism is nonperiodic because there is no known optimum time for collecting the blood sample. Giemsa-stained microscopic examination is necessary to identify the characteristic microfilariae.

Life Cycle Notes

M. ozzardi is transferred by the injection of infective larvae to the human definitive host. This transmission is carried out by the *Culicoides* sucking midge or, depending on the geographical location, the *Simulium* blackfly. The microfilariae are found in the blood as well as in the capillaries and intravascular spaces of the skin. The emerging adults may take up residence in the body cavities, visceral fat, and mesenteries but is still undocumented.

Epidemiology

Found exclusively in the Western Hemisphere, *M. ozzardi* is known to exist in North America and Central and South Americas, as well as in parts of the West Indies and Caribbean. Specific countries known to harbor this organism include Bolivia, Colombia, Peru, Haiti, the Dominican Republic, and Puerto Rico. The parasite may be transmitted by *Culicoides* midges or *Simulium* blackflies, depending on the geographic location.

Clinical Symptoms

Although asymptomatic infections are common, symptoms such as urticaria, lymphadenitis, skin itching, and arthralgias may occur. As with several of the other microfilariae, eosinophilia is common. The adult worms cause minimal damage to the areas they inhabit.

Treatment

Asymptomatic infections are not typically treated. Individuals who require treatment usually receive ivermectin. Diethylcarbamazine (DEC) has proven to be ineffective against *M. ozzardi*.

Prevention and Control

Controlling the sucking midge and *Simulium* populations is crucial to halting *M. ozzardi*. Unfortunately, there are no known control programs in place at this time. Both vectors are so small that they are not deterred by nets or screening equipment.

Quick Quiz! 9-12

How are the microfilariae of *Mansonella ozzardi* differentiated from those of *Ochocerca volvulus*? (Objective 9-13)

A. Location of the microfilariae

B. Absence of a sheath

C. Lack of terminal nuclei in the tail

D. Presence of a sheath

Mansonella perstans
(man"so-nel'ah/per'stans)

Common name: Perstans filaria.

Common associated disease and condition names: None (considered as a nonpathogen).

Morphology

Microfilariae. The average *Mansonella perstans* microfilaria measures about 200 μm in length (Fig. 9-10; Table 9-6). The organism does not have a sheath and the body is filled with nuclei that extend all the way to the tip of the tail. The anterior or tail end is rounded and blunt.

TABLE 9-6	*Mansonella perstans* Microfilaria: Typical Characteristics at a Glance	
Parameter	**Description**
Size range	about 200 μm in length
Sheath	Absent
Arrangement of nuclei in tail	Numerous; extend to tip of tail

Adults. The typical adult female worm measures 82 mm in length, whereas the adult male measures a little over half that, 43 mm in length. They reside in peritoneal and pleural cavities as well as the mesentery.

Laboratory Diagnosis

Blood is the specimen of choice for the recovery of *M. perstans*. The sample may be collected at any time because there is no known peak time for the circulating microfilariae to be present, that is, the organism is non-periodic.

Life Cycle Notes

The life cycle of *M. perstans* is similar to that of *M. ozzardi*. The only known vector is the *Culicoides* sucking midge. In this life cycle, the insects usually settle in areas in and around the eye. As in the life cycle of *M. ozzardi*, humans are the primary definitive hosts in the life cycle of *M. perstans*. The incubation period of this organism once inside the host is unknown.

Epidemiology

Infection rates are high in areas endemic to the *Culicoides* sucking midge. These include parts of Africa, selected areas in the Caribbean Islands, Panama, and northern South America. Primates are thought to harbor *M. perstans* or a closely related species as reservoir hosts.

Clinical Symptoms

Because adult *M. perstans* worms usually appear singly, damage to affected tissue is minimal. As

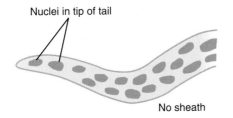
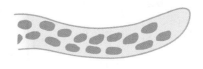

Nuclei in tip of tail

No sheath

Average length: 93 μm

FIGURE 9-10 *Mansonella perstans* microfilaria.

a result, symptoms, such as a minor allergic reactions, or no symptoms at all, are experienced by the infected individual. These individuals may exhibit moderate eosinophilia. The presence of Calabar swellings, similar to those of *Loa loa* headache, edema, and lymphatic discomfort are also associated with this infection. There is evidence to suggest that this organism may be responsible for joint and bone pain, as well as enlargement and associated pain in the liver.

Treatment

Asymptomatic infections are often not treated. However, it has been suggested that treatment in some cases may be of benefit. The treatment of choice, when deemed necessary, is diethylcarbamazine (DEC). It may require multiple treatments. An effective alternative is mebendazole. Ivermectin has not been proven effective.

Prevention and Control

The use of insecticides targeted against the vector, as well as other measures of controlling the vector population, is crucial to the prevention of *M. perstans* infection. Personal protection is also necessary to prevent the insect bites.

Quick Quiz! 9-14

If a physician suspects an individual has the potential for infection with *Mansonella perstans*, what specimen type would you suggest for recovery of the organism? (Objective 9-8)
A. Skin snips
B. Lymphatic fluid
C. Blood
D. Infected nodules

Quick Quiz! 9-15

What type of periodicity does *Mansonella perstans* exhibit? (Objective 9-8)
A. Nocturnal
B. Diurnal
C. Subperiodic
D. None

LOOKING BACK

When examining specimens for microfilariae or adult filarial worms, it is important to keep several points in mind. First, noting the specimen source is helpful in determining which organisms and morphologic forms may be found. Because the appearance of almost all adult filarial worms is similar, careful examination of microfilariae for the presence of a sheath and for arrangement of nuclei in the tail are necessary to ensure proper identification. Organism size may be helpful in some cases when screening adult worms as well as microfilariae. However, because of overlapping of sizes among the species, an identification based solely on size is not recommended.

Microfilariae are the typical forms recovered in blood and tissue specimens submitted for diagnosis of infection with the filarial nematodes. This morphologic form is the focus of the comparison drawings in this chapter.

TEST YOUR KNOWLEDGE!

9-1. You live by a fast moving river in Eastern Africa. Which of the following filarial nematodes poses the greatest risk of infection for you? (Objective 9-5)
A. *Brugia malayi*
B. *Onchocerca volvulus*
C. *Wuchereria bancrofti*
D. *Loa loa*

9-2. Which of the following filarial nematodes is known as the blinding filaria? (Objective 9-3)
A. *Brugia malayi*
B. *Onchocera volvulus*
C. *Loa loa*
D. *Mansonella ozzardi*

9-3. The microfilariae of *Brugia malayi* are recognized by the: (Objective 9-11)
A. presence of a sheath and two distinct terminal nuclei in the tail
B. presence of a sheath and absence of nuclei in the tail
C. absence of a sheath and nuclei continuous to the tip of the tail

D. absence of a sheath and absence of nuclei in the tail

9-4. Which of the filarial nematodes uses the mosquito as its vector?(Objective 9-5)
   A. *Loa loa*
   B. *Onchocera volvulus*
   C. *Wuchereria bancrofti*
   D. *Mansonella ozzardi*

9-5. Swelling of the lower extremities due to obstruction of the lymphatic system by adult filarial nematodes is known as: (Objective 9-1)
   A. Periodicity
   B. Lymphangitis
   C. Eosinophilia
   D. Elephantiasis

9-6. All of the following microfilariae lack a sheath *except*: (Objective 9-13)
   A. *Mansonella ozzardi*
   B. *Mansonella perstans*
   C. *Onchocera volvulus*
   D. *Brugia malayi*

9-7. 9-7. Diagnosis of infection with *Wuchereria bancrofti* can be accomplished by all of the following methods *except*: (Objective 9-8)
   A. Serologic testing
   B. Tissue biopsies
   C. Knott technique
   D. Thick and thin peripheral blood smears

9-8. Which of the following filarial nematodes is transmitted by the *Chrysops* fly? (Objective 9-6)
   A. *Onchocerca volvulus*
   B. *Mansonella ozzardi*
   C. *Loa loa*
   D. *Brugia malayi*

9-9. Which of the following filarial nematode infections is diagnosed by using skin snips rather than a peripheral blood smear? (Objective 9-8)
   A. *Onchocerca volvulus*
   B. *Loa loa*
   C. *Mansonella perstans*
   D. *Wuchereria bancrofti*

9-10. If an individual was planning to visit Africa, which of the following filarial nematodes would *not* be a concern for potential infection? (Objective 9-2)
   A. *Loa loa*
   B. *Wuchereria bancrofti*
   C. *Brugia malayi*
   D. *Mansonella ozzardi*

CASE STUDY 9-2   UNDER THE MICROSCOPE

Sir Robert, a 42-year-old male, returned to his home in England after an adventure along the Nile Delta. On arrival at his estate, Sir Robert began to experience chills and a fever. The fever remained high for about 2 days and then subsided but spiked again after 5 days. He also noticed an abscess on his right leg, which had become swollen, inflamed, and hot. After a few days, his leg began to enlarge. At this point, Sir Thomas promptly set-up an appointment and went to the office of his physician at 4:00 p.m. the next day to seek medical treatment. On determining the patient's recent travel history and performing a physical examination, the physician ordered blood and stool samples for parasite study. In addition, the physician surgically opened the abscess and obtained a sample of the contents for parasitic examination.

Laboratory examination of the abscess and stool specimens revealed no parasites. However, the Giemsa-stained slide of the blood contained suspicious organisms, each measuring approximately 260 μm in length. The diagram below depicts these structures.

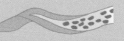 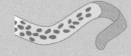

Questions to Consider
1. Identify the scientific name and morphologic form of the organism observed in the stained blood smear. (Objective 9-12A)
2. Determine if the appropriate timing of the blood collection was utilized for this individual. (Objective 9-8)
3. What is the vector for transmission of the organism? (Objective 9-12C)
4. What disease is Sir Robert exhibiting? (Objective 9-12B)
5. Determine a prevention and control plan that Sir Robert should have used while on his adventure. (Objective 9-12D)

COMPARISON DRAWINGS
The Filariae

FIGURE 9-2. *Wuchereria bancrofti* microfilaria

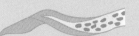 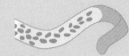

Size range: 240-300 μm long

FIGURE 9-4. *Brugia malayi* microfilaria

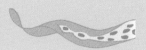 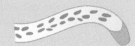

Size range: 200-280 μm long

FIGURE 9-6. *Loa loa* microfilaria

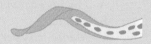 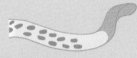

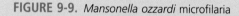

Size range: 248-300 μm long

FIGURE 9-7. *Onchocerca volvulus* microfilaria

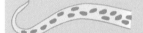 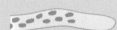

Size range: 148-355 μm long

FIGURE 9-9. *Mansonella ozzardi* microfilaria

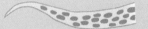 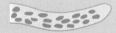

Approximate length: 88 μm

FIGURE 9-10. *Mansonella perstans* microfilaria

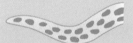 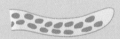

Average length: 93 μm

The Cestodes

John Seabolt and Elizabeth Zeibig

WHAT'S AHEAD

Focusing In
Morphology and Life Cycle
  Notes
Laboratory Diagnosis
Pathogenesis and Clinical
  Symptoms

Cestode Classification
  Taenia saginata
  Taenia solium
  Hymenolepis diminuta
  Hymenolepis nana
  Dipylidium caninum

Diphyllobothrium latum
Echinococcus granulosus
Looking Back

LEARNING OBJECTIVES

On completion of this chapter and review of its diagrams, tables, and corresponding photomicrographs, the successful learner will be able to:

10-1. Define the following key terms:
  Anaphylactic shock
  Brood capsule (*pl.*, brood capsules)
  Cestoda
  Cestode (*pl.*, cestodes)
  Coracidium
  Cysticercoid larval stage
  Cysticercosis
  Cysticercus larva
  Daughter cyst (*pl.*, daughter cysts)
  Embryophore
  Gravid
  Hermaphroditic
  Hexacanth embryo
  Hooklets
  Hydatid cyst
  Hydatid sand
  Oncosphere
  Operculum
  Platyhelminthes
  Pleurocercoid
  Procercoid
  Proglottid (*pl.*, proglottids)

  Rostellum
  Scolex (*pl.*, scolices)
  Sparganosis
  Sparganum
  Strobila
  Suckers
  Tegument
  Viscera
  Zoonosis
  Zoonotic
10-2. State the geographic distribution of the cestodes.
10-3. State the common name associated with each of the cestodes.
10-4. Given a list of parasites, select those belonging to the class Cestoda.
10-5. Briefly describe the life cycle of each cestode.
10-6. Identify and describe the symptoms and clinically significant disease processes associated with each of the pathogenic cestodes.
10-7. Identify and describe each of the following as they relate to the cestodes:
  A. Treatment options
  B. Prevention and control measures

10-8. Select the specimen(s) of choice and diagnostic approach for the recovery of each of the cestodes.

10-9. Compare and contrast the cestodes in terms of the key features that the parasites have in common, as well as the features that distinguish them.

10-10. Given a description, photomicrograph, and/or diagram of a cestode, correctly:
A. Identify and/or label the designated characteristic structure(s)
B. State the purpose of the designated characteristic structure(s)
C. Identify the organism by scientific name, common name, and morphologic form.

10-11. Analyze case studies that include pertinent patient information and laboratory data and:
A. Identify each responsible cestode organism by scientific name, common name, and morphologic form.
B. Identify the associated diseases and conditions associated with the responsible parasite.
C. Construct a life cycle associated with each cestode parasite present that includes corresponding epidemiology, route of transmission, infective stage, and diagnostic stage.

D. Propose each of the following related to eliminating and preventing cestode infections:
1. Treatment options
2. A prevention and control plan
E. Recognize sources of error, including but not limited to those involved in specimen collection, processing, and testing and propose solutions to remedy them.
F. Interpret laboratory data, determine specific follow-up tests to be done, and predict the results of those identified tests.

10-12. Given prepared laboratory specimens, and with the assistance of this manual, the learner will be able to:
A. Differentiate cestode organisms and/or structures from artifacts.
B. Determine the cestode organisms from each other and from other appropriate categories of parasites.
C. Correctly identify each cestode parasite by scientific name, common name, and morphologic form based on its key characteristic structure(s).

CASE STUDY 10-1　**UNDER THE MICROSCOPE**

A 14-year-old, severely mentally disabled boy, who was institutionalized in a state facility, was evaluated for episodes of chronic diarrhea, anal pruritis, restless nights, and occasional vomiting. Significant laboratory findings were a 10% eosinophilia, an IgE level of 225 IU/mL, and microscopic examination of a stool concentrate that revealed two thin-shelled, oval-shaped eggs measuring 45 by 35 um in size and containing three pairs of hooklets and polar filaments.

Questions and Issues for Consideration
1. What is the most likely identification of the parasite in question? (Objective 10-11A)
2. Why is this organism unique among the intestinal cestodes? (Objective 10-9)
3. What is the preferred treatment for infection caused by this organism? (Objective 10-11D)

FOCUSING IN

This chapter consists of a discussion of the class of multicellular worms noted for their flat or ribbon-like appearance known as **Cestoda** (the **cestodes**). The characteristic appearance of the cestodes forms the basis for the common names associated with this group, flatworms or tapeworms.

MORPHOLOGY AND LIFE CYCLE NOTES

There are three morphologic forms that exist in the typical cestode life cycle—egg, one or more larval stages, and adult worm. With one exception, the egg consists of a **hexacanth embryo** (also known as an **oncosphere**) defined as the motile, first larval stage characterized by the presence of six small hooks (called **hooklets**), arranged in pairs, that are believed to pierce the intestinal wall of the infected host. In the intestinal tapeworm life cycle, human ingestion of an egg or larval stage results in an adult worm eventually emerging in the intestine. An intermediate host is required for the development of the larval form in certain life cycles. It is important to note that under no known circumstances is the larval form seen in human specimens. Adult tapeworms resemble a ribbon in appearance and range in length from several millimeters up to an impressive 15 to 20 m. These worms are very primitive in that they absorb nutrients and excrete waste products through their outer surface, called a **tegument.** Although this group of adult parasites possess a reproductive system, they lack sophisticated body parts and systems, such as a mouth, digestive tract, and internal means of excretion.

Three distinct features common to all adult tapeworms are the presence of a **scolex** (a defined anterior end), a neck region, and a series of **proglottids** (individual segments that in their mature form are equipped with both male and female reproductive organs), referred to as the **strobila.** The typical scolex contains four cup-shaped structures, known as **suckers,** that provide the worm with the ability to attach to the intestinal mucosa of the infected host. Some species have a fleshy extension of the scolex known as a **rostellum,** from which one or two rows of hooks might be present.

The internal structures that are visible vary with the age of the proglottid. Because all tapeworms are self-fertilizing (**hermaphroditic**), both male and female reproductive organs are present in the mature proglottid. Following self-fertilization, the resulting pregnant (**gravid**) proglottids each consist of a uterus filled with eggs. The gravid proglottids rupture when these eggs are released into the intestine. The resulting eggs are usually passed into the outside environment via the stool.

There are several other life cycle notes of importance. Because tapeworms are hermaphroditic, human ingestion of a single egg will usually initiate a new life cycle. Autoreinfection is known to occur in the life cycle of *Hymenolepis nana.* Most cestodes require at least one intermediate host for their life cycles to continue. Development of a cyst in tissue occurs in the intestinal-extraintestinal cestode species *Echinococcus granulosus.* Specifics of both organisms' morphology, as well as life cycle notes, are described individually.

Quick Quiz! 10-1

The cestode morphologic form characterized by a segmented appearance that houses male and female reproductive structures is referred to as a(an): (Objective 10-1)
A. Scolex
B. Proglottid
C. Egg
D. Cyst

LABORATORY DIAGNOSIS

The primary specimen necessary to recover and identify intestinal tapeworms is stool. These samples are generally examined for the presence of eggs and, occasionally, gravid proglottids, which may be partially degenerated. Rarely, a scolex may be recovered, particularly following treatment. A biopsy of tissue presumed to be infected with the atrial cestode *E. granulosus* may be examined for the presence of organisms. In addition, serologic tests are available for select organisms. Representative laboratory diagnosis methodologies are located in Chapter 2 as well as in each individual parasite discussion, as appropriate.

Quick Quiz! 10-2

Characteristics of the cestodes include all the following except: (Objective 10-9)
A. They are hermaphroditic.
B. They generally require intermediate host(s).
C. Their laboratory diagnosis consists of finding larvae in feces.
D. Their anatomic regions include the scolex, neck, and strobila.

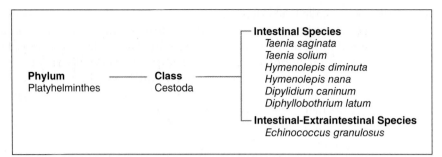

FIGURE 10-1 Parasite classification: The cestodes.

PATHOGENESIS AND CLINICAL SYMPTOMS

Many patients infected with intestinal cestodes remain asymptomatic. However, infected persons who experience symptoms often complain of vague, nondescript gastrointestinal discomfort, including diarrhea and abdominal pain. These patients may also develop nausea, dizziness, headache, and weight loss. Intestinal obstruction and vitamin B_{12}–induced macrocytic anemia may develop in persons infected with *Diphyllobothrium latum*. Liver and lung involvement are common in persons infected with *E. granulosus*. These patients may develop a persistent cough, localized pain, and eosinophilia. Under appropriate conditions, a serious allergic response may develop, known as **anaphylactic shock**, which produces large amounts of histamine and other chemical mediators and may be fatal.

> ### Quick Quiz! 10-3
>
> A persistent cough, localized pain, and liver and lung involvement are associated with an infection with which of the following cestodes? (Objective 10-6)
> A. *Diphyllobothrium latum*
> B. *Echinococcus granulosus*
> C. Both A and B
> D. Neither A nor B

CESTODE CLASSIFICATION

Members of the class Cestoda belong to the phylum that also contains the flukes (Chapter 11) known as **Platyhelminthes.** The species discussed in this chapter are listed in Figure 10-1 and may be divided into two categories, intestinal and intestinal-extraintestinal.

Taenia saginata
(tee'nee-uh/sadj-i-nay'tuh)

Common name: Beef tapeworm.

Common associated disease and condition names: Taeniasis, beef tapeworm infection.

Taenia solium
(tee'nee-uh/so-lee'um)

Common name: Pork tapeworm.

Common associated disease and condition names: Taeniasis, pork tapeworm infection.

There are two members of the *Taenia* species that are of clinical significance to humans, *Taenia solium* and *Taenia saginata*. With only a few notable exceptions (see later), the two organisms are similar in most respects. Thus, these two organisms will be discussed together.

Morphology

 Eggs. The eggs of *T. solium* and *T. saginata* are indistinguishable (Fig. 10-2; Table 10-1). Ranging in size from 28 to 40 μm by 18 to 30 μm, the average, somewhat roundish *Taenia* spp. egg measures 33 by 23 μm. The egg consists of a hexacanth embryo, including the standard

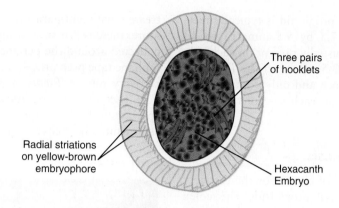

Three pairs
of hooklets

Radial striations
on yellow-brown
embryophore

Hexacanth
Embryo

Size range: 28-40 μm by 18-30 μm
Average length: 33 μm by 23 μm

A

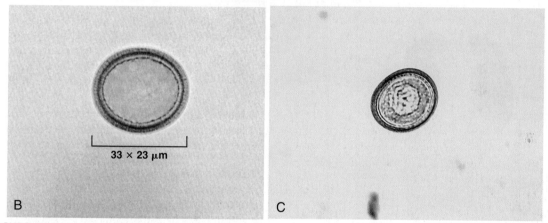

33 × 23 μm

B

C

FIGURE 10-2 **A,** *Taenia* spp. egg. **B,** *Taenia* spp. unembryonated egg, 400×. **C,** *Taenia* spp. embryonated egg, 400×. (**B, C** *courtesy of Carolina Biological Supply, Burlington, NC.*)

TABLE 10-1	*Taenia* Species Egg: Typical Characteristics at a Glance
Parameter	**Description**
Size range	28-40 μm by 18-30 μm
Hooklets	Three pairs; hexacanth embryo
Other features	Radial striations on yellow-brown embryophore

three pairs of hooklets. The embryo is surrounded by a yellow-brown shell present on select tapeworm eggs known as an **embryophore** on which distinct radial striations reside. These eggs may be nonembryonated (see Fig. 10-2*B*) or embryonated (see Fig. 10-2*C*).

Scolices. The typical *Taenia* spp. scolex measures from 1 to 2 mm in diameter and is equipped with four suckers (Figs. 10-3 and 10-4; Table 10-2). The primary difference between those of *T. saginata* and *T. solium* is that the latter contains a fleshy rostellum and double crown (row) of well-defined hooks (Fig. 10-4), whereas the former lacks these structures.

Proglottids. The average number of segments (proglottids) of typical *T. saginata* and *T. solium* adult worms is 1048 and 898, respectively (Table 10-2). There are two primary differences between the internal structures in the proglottids of the two *Taenia* organisms, appearance and number of uterine branches on each side of the uterus. A *T. saginata* proglottid is typically rect-angular, averaging 17.5 by 5.5 mm; 15 to 30 uterine branches are usually present on each side of the uterus (Fig. 10-5). In contrast, *T. solium* is square in appearance and only contains 7 to 15 uterine branches on each side of the uterus (Fig. 10-6).

Laboratory Diagnosis

Stool is the specimen of choice for the recovery of *Taenia* eggs and gravid proglottids. The scolex may be seen only after the patient has been treated with antiparasitic medication. Further-more, there is evidence to suggest that specimens collected around the perianal area using the cel-lophane tape prep procedure result in a very high recovery rate of *Taenia* eggs. It is important to note that the eggs of *Taenia* are identical. To speciate in the laboratory, a gravid proglottid or scolex must be recovered and examined.

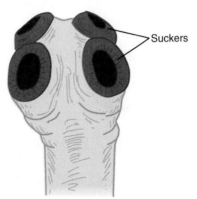

FIGURE 10-3 *Taenia saginata scolex.*

TABLE 10-2	*Taenia* spp. Adult: Typical Characteristics at a Glance	
Characteristic	***T. saginata***	***T. solium***
Scolex		
Number of suckers	Four	Four
Rostellum	Absent	Present
Hooks	Absent	Present; double crown
Gravid Proglottid		
Appearance, shape	Longer than wide; average, 17.5 by 5.5 μm	Somewhat square
Number of lateral branches on each side of uterus	15-30	7-15

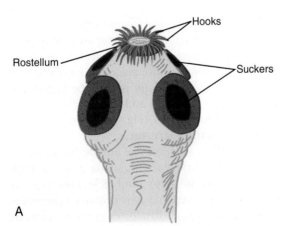

A

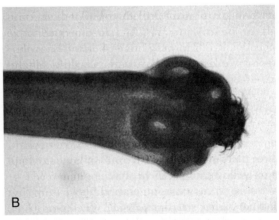

B

FIGURE 10-4 A, *Taenia solium* scolex. **B,** *Taenia solium* scolex, 40×. (*Courtesy of Carolina Biological Supply, Burlington, NC.*)

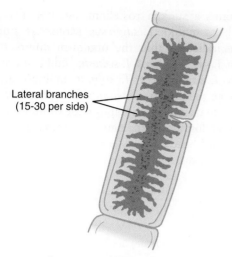

Lateral branches
(15-30 per side)

Average size: 17.5 by 5.5 mm

FIGURE 10-5 *Taenia saginata* proglottid.

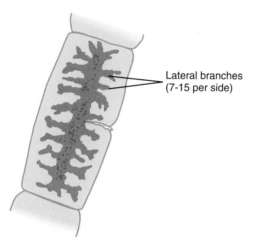

Lateral branches
(7-15 per side)

FIGURE 10-6 *Taenia solium* proglottid.

Life Cycle Notes

Infection with *Taenia* spp. occurs following the ingestion of raw or undercooked beef (*T. saginata*) or pork (*T. solium*) contaminated with a **cysticercus larva**, a type of larva that consists of a scolex surrounded by a bladder-like, thin-walled cyst that is filled with fluid. Scolex attachment to the intestinal mucosa occurs after the

larva emerges in the small intestine, in which maturation into an adult worm occurs. The resulting adult multiplies, producing numerous eggs, some of which may be passed into the feces. These eggs are then consumed by the proper animal species (cow or pig) in which the onco-sphere hatches. The oncosphere then migrates via the blood to the animal tissue and converts into the infective cysticercus larval stage. A new cycle is initiated on human ingestion of the infected animal meat.

Epidemiology

The distribution of *T. saginata* and *T. solium* directly correlates with areas of the world in which the inhabitants do not practice sanitary conditions and beef or pork is eaten on a routine basis. *T. saginata* is found primarily in these types of cosmopolitan areas, whereas *T. solium* is found worldwide. As noted, both organisms require an intermediate host, a cow or pig, depending on the species.

Clinical Symptoms

Asymptomatic. Most people who become infected with *Taenia* spp. typically remain asymptomatic.

Taeniasis: Beef or Pork Tapeworm Infection. Nondescript symptoms, such as diarrhea, abdominal pain, change in appetite, and slight weight loss, may be experienced by *Taenia*-infected patients. In addition, symptoms including dizziness, vomiting, and nausea may also develop. Laboratory tests often reveal the presence of a moderate eosinophilia. The prognosis is usually good.

Treatment

The most important and, in some cases, difficult aspect of treatment of *Taenia* infections is total eradication of the scolex. Fortunately, praziquantel has proven effective against the entire adult worm; however, it is not used when there is ocular or central nervous system

(CNS) involvement. Paramomycin and quinacrine hydrochloride (Atabrine) may also be used as alternative treatments.

Prevention and Control

There are three important prevention and control measures to alleviate *Taenia* spp.: exercising proper sanitation practices, thorough cooking of beef and pork prior to consumption, and promptly treating infected persons. Although each of these measures, on their own, will break the organism's life cycle if instituted, a combination of all three provides for an overall cleaner environment and healthier populations.

Notes of Interest and New Trends

Humans have been known to contract a human tissue infection associated with *T. solium* known as **cysticercosis**. This occurs when a human accidentally ingests the *T. solium* eggs that are passed in human feces. Food, water, and soil contamination are likely methods of transmitting the eggs from person to person. Once inside the body, the eggs lose their outer covering, allowing the developing oncosphere to invade the bloodstream and tissues, primarily the voluntary muscles. Although some patients remain asymptomatic, symptoms may vary by location of the infection. Manifestations of brain infections (neurocysticercosis) are common and may include headache, seizures, confusion, ataxia, and even death. Treatment is available, including surgical removal and medication. Immunologic tests are available for the diagnosis of cysticercosis, including indirect hemagglutination and the enzyme-linked immunosorbent assay (ELISA). Prevention measures are similar to those for the *Taenia* species, thorough cooking of pork and using proper sanitation practices.

Taenia saginata asiatica (Asian *Taenia*) or *Taenia asiatica* infections have been reported from various locations in Asia. Most reported cases have been acquired by eating raw pig liver, although consumption of cattle and goat has also been implicated. Morphologically, *T. asiatica*

contains a sunken rostellum and two rows of hooklets, unlike *T. saginata*. Molecular studies have indicated that the organism differs from both *T. saginatia and T. solium*. Unlike infections with *T. saginata* or *T. solium*, multiple adults may be present in *T. asiatica* infection. Infected individuals may be asymptomatic or may experience abdominal pain, nausea, weakness, weight loss, and headaches. The treatment of choice is praziquantel.

Quick Quiz! 10-4

Which of the following are key distinguishing factors in differentiating an infection between *T. saginata* and *T. solium*? (Objective 10-9)
A. Egg morphology and number of uterine branches in proglottid
B. Presence of hooklets on scolex and egg morphology
C. Presence of hooklets and number of uterine branches in proglottid
D. Egg morphology and presence of suckers on scolex

Quick Quiz! 10-5

The primary means of developing an intestinal infection with *Taenia* spp. is via which of the following? (Objective 10-5)
A. Skin penetration of larvae
B. Ingestion of raw or poorly cooked meat
C. Egg consumption
D. Drinking contaminated water

Quick Quiz! 10-6

Which is the preferred drug for treating intestinal infection by *Taenia* spp.? (Objective 10-7)
A. Praziquantel
B. Penicillin
C. Nicolasamide
D. Pentamidine

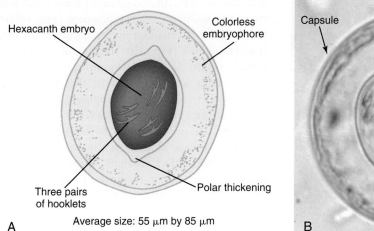

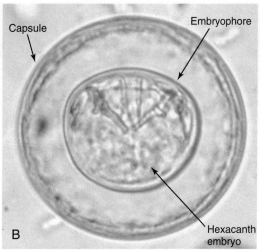

FIGURE 10-7 *A, Hymenolepis diminuta* egg. **B,** *Hymenolepis diminuta* egg. (***B*** *from Bowman DD: Georgis' parasitology for veterinarians, ed 9, St. Louis, 2009, Saunders.)*

TABLE 10-3	*Hymenolepis diminuta* Egg: Typical Characteristics at a Glance
Parameter	**Description**
Average size	55 by 85 μm
Hooklets	Three pairs; hexacanth embryo
Polar thickenings	Present
Polar filaments	Absent
Embryophore	Present; colorless

Hymenolepis diminuta
(high"men-ol'e-pis/dim-in-oo'tuh)

Common name: Rat tapeworm.

Common associated disease and condition names: Hymenolepiasis, rat tapeworm disease.

Morphology

▧ **Eggs.** The average *Hymenolepis diminuta* egg measures 55 by 85 μm. The hexacanth embryo contains three pairs of hooks (Fig. 10-7; Table 10-3). A shell surrounds the embryo that exhibits distinct polar thickenings and no polar filaments (see Fig. 10-10A, *H. nana* egg, for filaments). A colorless embryophore encloses the entire structure.

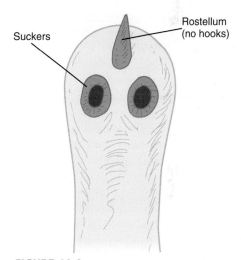

FIGURE 10-8 *Hymenolepis diminuta* scolex.

▧ **Scolices.** The *H. diminuta* scolex is equipped with four suckers. A small rostellum bearing no hooks protrudes from the anterior end of the scolex (Fig. 10-8; Table 10-4).

▧ **Proglottids.** Proglottids are typically rectangular, measuring just under 1 mm by over 2 mm (Table 10-4). Each mature segment contains one set of female and one set of male reproductive organs. The gravid proglottid (Fig. 10-9) consists

TABLE 10-4	*Hymenolepis diminuta* Adult: Typical Characteristics at a Glance
Parameter	**Description**
Scolex	
Number of suckers	Four
Rostellum	Present
Hooks	Absent
Gravid Proglottid	
Size	Twice as wide as long
Appearance	Saclike uterus filled with eggs

Sac-like uterus filled with eggs

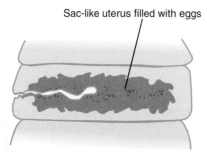

FIGURE 10-9 *Hymenolepis diminuta* proglottid.

of a saclike uterus filled with eggs that occupy most of the available space.

Laboratory Diagnosis

Laboratory diagnosis is based on the recovery of the characteristic eggs in stool specimens. It is interesting to note that the proglottids are typically not found in stool because they usually disintegrate in the human gut. Similarly, the scolex is rarely seen in these samples.

Life Cycle Notes

H. diminuta is primarily a parasite of rats. Contaminated droppings from infected rats are the source of parasite transmission into an intermediate host, such as the grain beetle or flea. Development of the **cysticercoid larva**, a larval stage consisting of a scolex surrounded by a bladder-like cyst that contains little or no fluid that emerges from select tapeworm eggs, occurs in this host. Consumption by a rat of infected insects, which typically reside in grains or cereal, results in the development of an adult worm. Eggs are produced in the infected rat and are excreted in its droppings, thus setting the stage for a new cycle. Human infection with *H. diminuta* is considered to be an accidental parasitic disease that normally infects animals but can also infect humans, known as a **zoonotic** occurrence, or **zoonosis**. In this case, the human takes the place of the rat in the parasite life cycle.

Epidemiology

The distribution of *H. diminuta* is worldwide. Areas in which foodstuffs such as grain or cereal are not protected from rats and insects are at risk of transmitting the parasite.

Clinical Symptoms

◢ **Asymptomatic.** Many patients infected with *H. diminuta* remain asymptomatic.
◢ **Hymenolepiasis: Rat Tapeworm Disease.** Persons infected with *H. diminuta* usually present with mild symptoms such as diarrhea, nausea, abdominal pains, and anorexia.

Treatment

The treatment of choice against *H. diminuta* is praziquantel. Niclosamide is an effective alternative therapy; however, it is not yet readily available in the United States.

Prevention and Control

There are three primary prevention and control measures against the spread of *H. diminuta*. First, administering effective rodent control measures is crucial to ensure the halt of the normal parasite life cycle, thus preventing rats from contaminating foodstuffs such as grains and cereals. Second, protection of these foods from both rat droppings and from intermediate host insects is critical to prevent consumption of contaminated food. Finally, thorough inspection of all potentially contaminated foodstuffs prior to human consumption is necessary to prevent transmission of the parasite to unsuspecting humans.

Quick Quiz! 10-7

Which of the following is characteristic of an *H. diminuta* egg? (Objective 10-10A)
A. Spherical, with radial striations
B. Ellipsoid, with terminal polar plugs
C. Oval, with thin shell and polar filaments
D. Oval, with polar thickenings and no filaments

Quick Quiz! 10-8

The infective stage of *H. diminuta* for humans is which of the following? (Objective 10-5)
A. Rhabditiform larva
B. Cysticeroid larva
C. Embryonated egg
D. Encysted form

Quick Quiz! 10-9

Prevention and control measures against *H. diminuta* include all except which of the following? (Objective 10-7B)
A. Vaccination program
B. Effective rodent control
C. Inspection of food prior to consumption
D. Protection of food from rodents

Hymenolepis nana
(high"men-ol'e-pis/nay'nuh)

Common name: Dwarf tapeworm.

Common associated disease and condition names: Hymenolepiasis, dwarf tapeworm disease.

Morphology

Eggs. The somewhat roundish to oval egg of *Hymenolepis nana* typically measures 45 by 38 μm in size (Fig. 10-10; Table 10-5). The centrally located hexacanth embryo is equipped with the standard three pairs of hooklets. A shell complete with polar thickenings protects the embryo. Numerous polar filaments originate from the polar thickenings, which, in addition to size, help distinguish it from the egg of

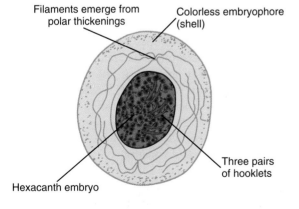

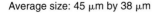

A   Average size: 45 μm by 38 μm

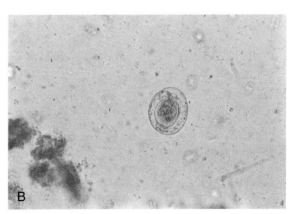

B

FIGURE 10-10 A, *Hymenolepis nana* egg. **B,** *Hymenolepis nana* egg, 400×. (**B** *from Mahon CR, Lehman DC, Manuselis G: Textbook of diagnostic microbiology, ed 4, St Louis, 2011, Saunders.*)

TABLE 10-5	*Hymenolepis nana* Egg: Typical Characteristics at a Glance
Parameter	**Description**
Average size	45 by 38 μm
Hooklets	Three pairs; hexacanth embryo
Polar thickenings	Present
Polar filaments	Present
Embryophore	Present; colorless

TABLE 10-6	*Hymenolepis nana* Adult: Typical Characteristics at a Glance
Parameter	**Description**
Scolex	
Number of suckers	Four
Rostellum	Present; short
Hooks	Present; one row
Gravid Proglottid	
Size	Twice as wide as long
Appearance	Saclike uterus filled with eggs

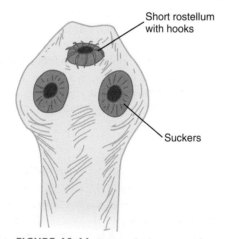

FIGURE 10-11 *Hymenolepis nana* scolex.

H. diminuta. A colorless embryophore serves as the outermost egg layer.

▓ **Scolices.** Like the other cestode scolices discussed thus far, the *H. nana* scolex contains four suckers (Fig. 10-11; Table 10-6). The presence of a short rostellum with one row of hooks helps distinguish it from that of *H. diminuta,* which has no hooks at all.

▓ **Proglottids.** The mature and gravid proglottids of *H. nana* resemble those of *H. diminuta* both in size and appearance (see Fig. 10-9 and Table 10-6). A brief description may be found in the *H. diminuta* proglottid morphology section.

Laboratory Diagnosis

Laboratory diagnosis of *H. nana* is accomplished by examining stool samples for the characteristic eggs.

Life Cycle Notes

Consumption of an infective egg initiates human *H. nana* infection. Development of the cysticercoid larva occurs in the intestine. On further maturation, the scolex emerges and attaches to the intestinal mucosa. The resulting adult worm resides in the intestine, in which it is capable of self-reproduction. Disintegration of gravid proglottids releases numerous eggs. At this point, a resulting egg may take one of two routes. The egg may be passed outside the body via the feces or initiate autoreinfection. An egg released into the outside environment is in the infective stage. No intermediate host is required to complete the cycle. Such an egg, when ingested by a new human host, initiates a new cycle. An egg that remains inside the human may hatch in the gastrointestinal tract and develop into an adult, never leaving the human host and thus initiating a new cycle.

As noted, *H. nana* does not require an intermediate host to complete its life cycle. However, this parasite may exist in a number of other animal transport hosts, such as fleas, beetles, rats, and house mice. It is interesting to note that the cysticercoid larval stage may develop in these hosts; when this occurs; such hosts are infective to both humans and rodents.

Epidemiology

H. nana is considered to be the most common tapeworm recovered in the United States, particularly in the southeastern part of the country.

In addition, tropical and subtropical climates worldwide are known to harbor this parasite. Persons residing in close quarters, such as in institutional settings, as well as children attending preschool or at day care centers, are at a particularly high risk of contracting *H. nana*. In addition to infective eggs generated by contaminated human feces, stool from contaminated rodents may also serve as a source of infection.

Clinical Symptoms

 Asymptomatic. Light infections with *H. nana* typically remain asymptomatic.

Hymenolepiasis: Dwarf Tapeworm Disease. Persons with heavy *H. nana* infections often develop gastrointestinal symptoms, such as abdominal pain, anorexia, diarrhea, dizziness, and headache.

Treatment

Praziquantel is considered to be the treatment of choice for infections with *H. nana*. Niclosamide is also known to be an effective alternative medication; however, it is not yet readily available in the United States.

Prevention and Control

Proper personal hygiene and sanitation practices are crucial to preventing the spread of *H. nana*. Controlling transport host populations and avoidance of contact with potentially infected rodent feces are also prevention and control measures aimed at halting the spread of the parasite.

Quick Quiz! 10-10

A primary differential feature between an *H. nana* egg and *H. diminuta* egg is which of the following? (Objective 10-9)
A. A flattened side for *H. diminuta* egg
B. A thick shell for *H. nana* egg
C. Polar filaments in *H. nana* egg
D. Radial striations in *H. diminuta* egg

Quick Quiz! 10-11

The characteristic of the life cycle of *H. nana* that differentiates it from the other cestodes is which of the following? (Objective 10-9)
A. Lack of an intermediate host.
B. Infective larval stage.
C. Need for external environment
D. Larval passage through the lungs

Quick Quiz! 10-12

Which of the following does not apply to *H. nana*? (Objectives 10-3, 10-6, 10-7A, 10-7B)
A. Dwarf tapeworm
B. Steatorrhea
C. Proper hygiene and sanitation procedures
D. Praziquantel therapy

Dipylidium caninum
(dip" ĭ-lid′e-um/kain-i′num)

Common names: Dog or cat tapeworm, pumpkin seed tapeworm.

Common associated disease and condition names: Dipylidiasis, dog or cat tapeworm disease.

Morphology

Egg Packets. The average *Dipylidium caninum* egg may range in diameter from 30 to 60 µm (Fig. 10-12; Table 10-7). It consists of the typical six-hooked oncosphere. Unlike the eggs of the other cestodes discussed thus far, which appear individually, those of *D. caninum* form membrane-enclosed packets; each packet may contain 5 to 30 eggs.

Scolices. The *D. caninum* scolex is equipped with four suckers and a club-shaped armed rostellum (Table 10-8). Rather than containing hooks, like some cestodes discussed earlier, *D. caninum* contains one to six or seven circlets of spines that reside on the rostellum.

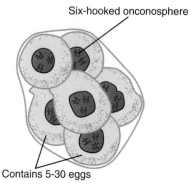

Six-hooked onconosphere

Contains 5-30 eggs

A   Size range of each egg: 30-60 μm in diameter

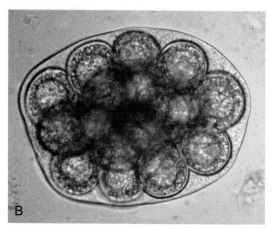

B

FIGURE 10-12 A, *Dipylidium caninum* egg packet. **B,** *Dipylidium caninum* egg packet. (**B** *from Bowman DD: Georgis' parasitology for veterinarians, ed 9, St. Louis, 2009, Saunders.*)

TABLE 10-7	*Dipylidium caninum* Egg Packet: Typical Characteristics at a Glance
Parameter	**Description**
Number of eggs in enclosed packet	5-30
Diameter range per egg	30-60 μm
Individual egg features	Six-hooked oncosphere

Proglottids. The mature and gravid proglottids of *D. caninum* resemble pumpkin seeds in shape (see Table 10-8). Each mature segment contains two sets of both male and female reproductive organs. Following self-fertilization, the resulting gravid proglottid is full of eggs enclosed in an embryonic membrane (Fig. 10-13).

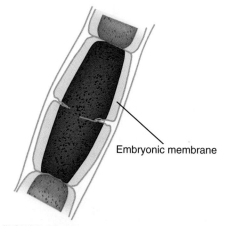

Embryonic membrane

FIGURE 10-13 *Dipylidium caninum* proglottid.

Laboratory Diagnosis

D. caninum diagnosis is based on the recovery of the characteristic egg packets or gravid proglottids in stool samples. The presence of a single egg in a stool sample may occur, but is extremely rare.

Life Cycle Notes

As the common name implies, *D. caninum* is primarily a parasite of dogs and cats. However, humans may become accidentally infected on

TABLE 10-8	*Dipylidium caninum* Adult: Typical Characteristics at a Glance
Parameter	**Description**
Scolex	
Number of suckers	Four
Rostellum	Present; club-shaped, with one to seven circlets of spines
Hooks	Absent
Gravid Proglottid	
Shape	Pumpkin seed
Appearance	Full of eggs in enclosed embryonic membrane

ingestion of an intermediate host's dog or cat fleas. These fleas may be transmitted by the lick of an infected dog or cat or by hand-to-mouth contamination. Ingestion of contaminated food has also been known to initiate infection. Intestinal infection occurs following human ingestion of the larval stage. The resulting adult worm self-fertilizes. Characteristic egg packets and gravid proglottids may be subsequently passed in the stool. To continue the cycle, the eggs must be ingested by a dog or cat flea, in which larval development occurs. The swallowing of an infected flea initiates a new cycle. It is important to note that humans take the place of the dog or cat in the life cycle when they become infected.

Epidemiology

The incidence of *D. caninum* infection is worldwide. Children appear to be the most at risk for infection transmission.

Clinical Symptoms

 Asymptomatic. Most infected persons experience no symptoms because of a light worm burden (infection).

 Dipylidiasis: Dog or Cat Tapeworm Disease. Patients with a heavy worm burden may develop appetite loss, diarrhea, abdominal discomfort, and indigestion. They may also experience anal pruritus caused by gravid proglottids migrating out of the anus.

Treatment

The treatment of choice for infections with *D. caninum* is praziquantel. Niclosamide (if available) and paromomycin have proven to be effective alternative treatments.

Prevention and Control

There are three primary prevention and control measures that if strictly instituted, would most likely eradicate human *D. caninum* infection. First, dogs and cats should be examined by a

veterinarian on a regular basis. Routine procedures should include deworming infected animals (the process of worm removal via medication) and periodic administration of prophylactic antihelminth medications. Second, dogs and cats should be treated and protected against flea infestation regularly. Finally, children should be taught not to let dogs or cats lick them in or near their mouths.

> **Quick Quiz! 10-13**
>
> A unique characteristic of *Dipylidium caninum* is which of the following? (Objective 10-10A)
> A. Lack of suckers on the scolex
> B. Formation of egg packets
> C. Proglottid resemblance to *Taenia solium*
> D. Alternation of female and male proglottids

> **Quick Quiz! 10-14**
>
> A 2-year-old girl and her pet dog were diagnosed with *D. caninum* infection. This infection was acquired by which of the following? (Objective 10-5)
> A. Ingestion of the parasite's egg
> B. Penetration of soil larva
> C. Ingestion of a flea
> D. Consumption of poorly cooked beef

> **Quick Quiz! 10-15**
>
> Prevention and control measures to prevent *D. caninum* infection include all except which of the following? (Objective 10-7B)
> A. Treat dog and cat pets to prevent fleas.
> B. Warn children against dog and cat licks.
> C. Deworm dog and cat pets, as needed.
> D. Neuter dog and cat pets.

Diphyllobothrium latum
(dye-fil"o-both-ree-um/lay'tum)

Common name: Broad fish tapeworm.

Common associated disease and condition names: Diphyllobothriasis, fish tapeworm infection, broad fish tapeworm infection.

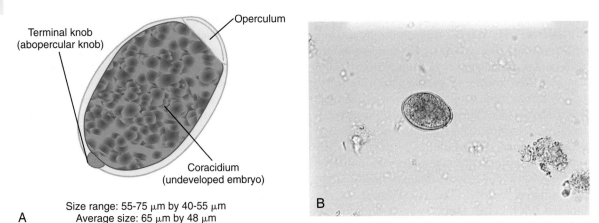

Terminal knob
(abopercular knob)

Operculum

Coracidium
(undeveloped embryo)

Size range: 55-75 μm by 40-55 μm
Average size: 65 μm by 48 μm

A

B

FIGURE 10-14 **A,** *Diphyllobothrium latum* egg. **B,** *Diphyllobothrium latum* egg, 400×. (**B** from Mahon CR, Lehman DC, Manuselis G: *Textbook of diagnostic microbiology, ed 4, St Louis, 2011, Saunders.*)

TABLE 10-9	*Diphyllobothrium latum* Egg: Typical Characteristics at a Glance	
Parameter	**Description**
Size range	55-75 μm long, 40-55 μm wide
Shape	Somewhat oblong
Embryo	Undeveloped, termed *coracidium*
Shell	Smooth; yellow-brown in color
Other features	Operculum on one end; terminal knob on opposite end

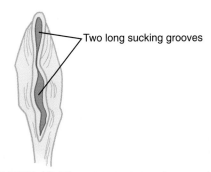

Two long sucking grooves

FIGURE 10-15 *Diphyllobothrium latum* scolex.

Morphology

Eggs. The eggs of *Diphyllobothrium latum* differ from the cestodes discussed thus far in that they are not comprised of the typical hexacanth embryo (Fig. 10-14; Table 10-9). Rather, the average *D. latum* egg consists of a ciliated larval stage known as a **coracidium**, surrounded by a smooth yellow to brown shell. The egg is somewhat oblong in shape. The typical size is from 55 to 75 μm by 40 to 55 μm, with an average of 65 by 48 μm. A lid structure, referred to as an **operculum**, consumes one end of the egg. A small but distinct terminal knob, also known as an abopercular knob, extends from the opposite end of the egg.

Scolices. The scolex of *D. latum* also varies from the four cuplike suckers present on the

other cestode species discussed thus far (Fig. 10-15; Table 10-10). The *D. latum* scolex is almond-shaped and contains two long, prominent, sucking grooves.

Proglottids. *D. latum* proglottids are wider than they are long (Fig. 10-16; Table 10-10). Gravid proglottids characteristically contain a centrally located uterine structure that frequently assumes a rosette formation.

Laboratory Diagnosis

Diagnosis of *D. latum* is accomplished by examining stool specimens for the presence of the characteristic eggs and/or, less frequently, the proglottids. On occasion, a scolex may also be

TABLE 10-10	*Diphyllobothrium Latum* Adult: Typical Characteristics at a Glance
Parameter	**Description**
Scolex	
Number of sucking grooves	Two
Shape of sucking groove	Almond
Gravid Proglottid	
Shape	Wider than long
Location and appearance of uterine structure	Central; rosette

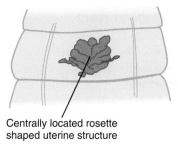

Centrally located rosette shaped uterine structure

FIGURE 10-16 *Diphyllobothrium latum* proglottid.

seen. Recovery of intact *D. latum* proglottids and scolices from untreated patients is rare. Stool samples from infected patients who have had drug treatment should be examined. To ensure that the treatment was successful, the expected findings consist of the passage of the scolex and absence of (new) proglottids.

Life Cycle Notes

The life cycle of *D. latum* is relatively complex in that it requires two intermediate hosts for its completion. Human *D. latum* infection is initiated when the **pleurocercoid**, defined as a precursor larval stage, is ingested when consuming contaminated freshwater fish that is raw or undercooked. In the small intestine, the scolex emerges from the pleurocercoid and attaches to the intestinal mucosa. The adult worm self-fertilizes and the undeveloped eggs are passed into the outside environment via the stool. If

these eggs were to come in contact with fresh water, the coracidium, or free-swimming larva, would hatch. This larva is ingested by the first intermediate host, the *Cyclops* species copepod.

The next stage in *D. latum* development, the larval stage known as the **procercoid**, occurs in the copepod. The infected copepod is ingested by the second intermediate host, a freshwater fish. Once inside the fish, the procercoid develops into a pleurocercoid larva in the muscle tissue. Human ingestion of the contaminated fish initiates a new cycle.

It is interesting to note that often the second intermediate host, a freshwater fish, is small in size. These fish have been known to become meals to larger fish before directly infecting humans. The larger fish harbor the parasite and serve as a transport host. Human consumption of these larger fish will result in the release of the pleurocercoid larva, which will develop and continue the life cycle.

Epidemiology

D. latum may be found in a variety of temperate regions worldwide. In the United States, Alaska and the Great Lakes region are known to harbor the parasite. Other noted endemic areas include parts of South America and Asia, Central Africa, the Baltic region, and Finland. It is in these areas that raw and/or freshwater fish are routinely consumed. In addition to humans, a number of fish-eating animals may also become infected with *D. latum* and serve as definitive hosts.

Clinical Symptoms

◾ **Asymptomatic.** It is estimated that most infected persons with adult *D. latum* worms exhibit no clinical symptoms.

◾ **Diphyllobothriasis: Fish Tapeworm Infection, Broad Fish Tapeworm Infection.** Persons infected with *D. latum* often experience symptoms consistent with digestive discomfort. Overall weakness, weight loss, and abdominal pain may also develop. When the adult *D. latum* worm takes up residence in and attaches itself to the proximal part of the jejunum, the patient is at risk for developing vitamin B_{12} deficiency. This condition mimics that of pernicious anemia.

Inhabitants of select areas, such as Finland, appear to be at higher risk for contracting this parasite-induced condition. Some of them also appear to be inherently predisposed to contracting pernicious anemia. This is important because it suggests that otherwise healthy patients infected with *D. latum* appear not to exhibit excessive symptoms, as might be expected considering the predisposition and mimicry of symptoms noted earlier.

Treatment

The drugs of choice for the treatment of *D. latum* infections are praziquantel and niclosamide, if available.

Prevention and Control

There are three primary prevention and control measures that may be initiated to halt the spread of *D. latum*. These include proper human fecal disposal, avoidance of eating raw or undercooked fish, and thorough cooking of all fish before consumption.

Notes of Interest and New Trends

Humans have been known to suffer from **sparganosis**. This condition results from ingesting the procercoid larvae of *D. latum* as well as that of other related *Diphyllobothrium* species. There are two primary routes whereby humans can contract this form of the parasite, water contaminated with infected copepods and medicines contaminated with infected animal by-products. The formation of a **sparganum** (infected subcutaneous tissue often described as white, wrinkled, and ribbon-shaped) typically results. It is interesting to note that in the life cycle of certain species, humans serve as the intermediate host for the parasite. In that of other species, the life cycle ceases once it is consumed by a human. Surgical removal of the sparganum is the

treatment of choice. Praziquantel has also proven effective against the sparganum.

Quick Quiz! 10-16

The egg of *D. latum* is unique among the cestodes in that it contains which of the following? (Objective 10-10A)
A. An operculum and terminal knob
B. Radial striations and oncosphere
C. An operculum and lateral spine
D. A ciliated rhabditiform larva

Quick Quiz! 10-17

Which of the following associations is correct for *D. latum*? (Objective 10-5)
A. Snail-coracidium
B. Copepod-procercoid
C. Fish-cysticercus
D. Beetle-pleurocercoid

Quick Quiz! 10-18

The primary pathology associated with a *D. latum* infection is which of the following? (Objective 10-6)
A. Eosinophilic pneumonitis
B. Vitamin D deficiency
C. Vitamin B_{12} deficiency
D. Fat malabsorption

Echinococcus granulosus
(eh-kigh"no-kock'us/gran-yoo-lo'sus)

Common names: Dog tapeworm, hydatid tapeworm.

Common associated disease and condition names: Echinococcosis, hyatid cyst, hyatid disease, hyatidosis.

Morphology

▨ **Eggs.** The eggs of *Echinococcus granulosus* are identical to, and thus indistinguishable from, those of *Taenia* spp. (see Fig. 10-2). Fortunately, the diagnostic stage of *E. granulosus* is that of the larval stage described later.

▌ **Hydatid Cysts.** The **hydatid cyst** larval stage of *E. granulosus*, found in human tissue, consists of several structures (Table 10-11). These structures overlap somewhat in their definitions, resulting in a confusion of the terms and making a clear and concise description of them a challenge. The following description should be clear.

The entire structure is termed a *hydatid cyst.* Within the cyst, miniaturizations of the entire hydatid cyst may occur; these are referred to as

TABLE 10-11	*Ecbhinococcus granulosus* Hydatid Cyst: Typical Characteristics at a Glance
Parameter	**Description**
Protective coverings	Cyst wall; multiple laminated germinal tissue layers
Basic cyst makeup	Fluid-filled bladder
Structures that arise from inner germinal layer	Daughter cysts Brood capsules
Other possible structures present	Hydatid sand

daughter cysts. Both types of cysts are surrounded by a protective cyst wall and laminated layers of germinal tissue. In addition, **brood capsules**, which lack a protective cyst wall, form from the inner germinal layer. Developing scolices are found within these structures. Each scolex, once fully developed, has the capability of developing into an adult worm when present in the definitive host. A **hydatid sand**, defined as components found in the fluid of older *E. granulosus* cysts that typically include daughter cysts, free scolices, hooklets, and miscellaneous nondescript material may evolve, as shown in Figure 10-17.

Some hydatid cysts fail to produce all or some of these structures. In this case, some hydatid cysts may start out by developing such structures but, because of the onset of secondary bacterial infections, may result in sterility or death of the cyst, with subsequent calcification.

▌ **Adults.** The average adult *E. granulosus* is small, relatively speaking, measuring only 4.5 mm in length. The worm consists of a scolex, small neck, and three proglottids, one at each developmental stage—immature, mature, and gravid. The scolex contains four suckers and has approximately 36 hooks. This form is not typically seen in humans but is commonly found in canines, which serve as definitive hosts.

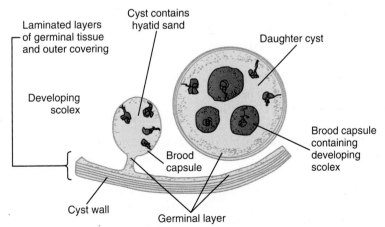

FIGURE 10-17 *Echinococcus granulosus* hydatid cyst.

Laboratory Diagnosis

E. granulosus may be diagnosed in several ways. Hydatid cyst fluid may be examined on biopsy samples for the presence of scolices, daughter cysts, brood capsules, or hydatid sand. Care must be used when choosing this method of diagnosis because infected patients may suffer from anaphylaxis if fluid escapes from the hydatid cyst during specimen collection. Serologic tests such as ELISA, indirect hemagglutination, and the Western blot test are available. Detection of the hydatid cyst may be accomplished using radiography, computed tomography (CT), or ultrasound scan techniques.

Life Cycle Notes

Humans serve as accidental intermediate hosts for *E. granulosus*. The typical intermediate host is sheep, although other herbivores may also serve in this role. Human infection begins following the ingestion of *Echinococcus* eggs obtained by contact with contaminated dog feces. Larvae from the eggs penetrate the intestine and migrate via the bloodstream to a number of tissue sites, particularly the lung and liver. A hydatid cyst develops in the infected tissue. Humans are considered to be dead-end hosts because the *Echinococcus* life cycle ceases in human tissue.

When the sheep serves as the intermediate host, the life cycle may be completed. The hydatid cyst forms in the **viscera** (soft parts and internal organs of major cavities in the body) of the sheep. The definitive host, the dog or wild canine, contracts the parasite by consuming infected sheep viscera. On ingestion of the cyst, each scolex develops into an adult worm. The adult worms reside in the definitive host's intestine. Eggs are produced and passed into the environment via the feces, in which they are capable of initiating a new cycle.

Epidemiology

E. granulosus is primarily found in areas in which sheep or other herbivores are raised and are in close contact with dogs or wild canines. Other criteria for areas at risk include those in which close contact between canines and humans occurs. These areas include Great Britain, parts of South America, Australia, parts of Africa, Asia, and China, and select portions of the Middle East. There have been several cases reported in the United States, particularly in Alaska, as well as in the West and Southwest.

Clinical Symptoms

Echinococcosis: Hydatid Cyst, Hydatid Disease, Hydatidosis. The extent to which infected patients may experience discomfort varies, depending on the size and location of the hydatid cyst. In general, patients experience little if any symptoms for approximately one year or more following ingestion of the *Echinococcus* eggs. As the cyst continues to enlarge, necrosis of the infected tissues, accompanied by a buildup of pressure on these tissues, usually results. Death may also occur. Rupture of a cyst may occur naturally or during the process of obtaining a biopsy for microscopic examination. Patients may suffer from anaphylactic shock, eosinophilia, and allergic reactions, or even death. The cyst fluid that emerges from the rupturing cyst, under the right conditions, can spread to other sites and form new cysts.

Patients suffering from *E. granulosus* lung infection may develop chest pain, coughing, and shortness of breath. Liver involvement may result in obstructive jaundice. Symptoms related to cyst development in other body organs are site-specific. Further discussion of these symptoms is beyond the scope of this chapter.

Treatment

Surgical removal of the hydatid cyst, when located in a suitable area for surgery, has historically been considered as the treatment of choice for *Echinococcus*. However, the advent of antiparasitic medications has offered an alternative to surgery, if appropriate. The medications mebendazole, albendazole, and praziquantel have particularly been useful in situations in which the hydatid cyst was inoperable.

Prevention and Control

To break the *E. granulosus* life cycle and subsequently halt the spread of human disease, the implementation of several measures is essential. These include implementing appropriate personal hygiene practices to prevent ingestion of the eggs, discontinuing the practice of feeding canines potentially contaminated viscera, promptly treating canines and humans who become infected, and instituting a thorough education program for those in high-risk areas for transmission of the parasite.

Notes of Interest and New Trends

Echinococcus multilocularis is an accidental cause of hydatid disease in humans living in the Subarctic, as well as central Europe and India. Foxes are the primary definitive hosts; rodents, such as mice and voles, are the usual intermediate hosts. Disease manifestion in humans is similar to that of *E. granulosus*.

Quick Quiz! 10-19

Which of the following procedures would not be appropriate for diagnosing an infection with *Echinococcus granulosus*? (Objective 10-8)
A. Serologic procedure, such as ELISA
B. O&P examination of stool specimen
C. CT scan of suspect organ
D. Biopsy of cyst

Quick Quiz! 10-20

In humans, *Echinococcus granulosus* infection results in which of the following? (Objective 10-5)
A. Eggs similar to those of *H. nana*
B. A nutritional deficiency
C. A hydatid cyst
D. Filariform larva

Quick Quiz! 10-21

Which of the following is not a usual site for *Echinococcus granulosus* infection in humans? (Objective 10-8)
A. Brain
B. Liver
C. Lung
D. Genitalia

LOOKING BACK

Careful examination of the cestode eggs, scolices, and proglottids is essential for speciation of the organism. Comparison drawings, such as those provided at the end of this chapter, can be a useful resource and may aid in the determination of the cestodes.

With the exception of *D. latum*, all the remaining intestinal tapeworm eggs consist of a hexacanth embryo with six hooklets. The presence of structures such as radial striations, polar thickenings, and filaments are helpful in species identification. The presence of egg packets suggests the presence of *D. caninum*. *D. latum* is unique in that it consists of a coracidium, operculum, and terminal knob.

Similarly, with the exception of *D. latum*, all the remaining intestinal tapeworm scolices have four cuplike suckers. The presence of a rostellum and row(s) of hooks aid in identifying the species. Two long almond-shaped suckers comprise the scolex of *D. latum*, making this organism easy to distinguish from the others.

The proglottids of the intestinal tapeworms, particularly those that are gravid, vary in several respects. These include shape, number of uterine branches, if present, and location of the uterine structure, where appropriate.

The *E. granulosus* hydatid cyst, the only intestinal tissue tapeworm species, may be identified by the presence of all or some of the following: a fluid-filled bladder surrounded by a cyst wall and multiple layers of laminated germinal tissue from which daughter cysts and/or brood capsules may develop. Older cysts may evolve into and be seen as hydatid sands.

TEST YOUR KNOWLEDGE!

10-1. Match each of the key terms (column A) with the corresponding definition (column B). (Objective 10-1)

Column A	Column B
___ **A.** Hermaphroditic	**1.** Smaller cyst within a hydatid cyst
___ **B.** Scolex	**2.** Series of proglottids
___ **C.** Zoonotic	**3.** Contains both male and female organs
___ **D.** Oncosphere	**4.** Develops from a procercoid larva
___ **E.** Cysticerus	**5.** Segment of a tapeworm
___ **F.** Brood capsule	**6.** Free-swimming larva of *D. latum*
___ **G.** Strobila	**7.** Acquired from animals
___ **H.** Proglottid	**8.** Hexacanth embryo
___ **I.** Coracidium	**9.** Head of a tapeworm
___ **J.** Sparaganosis	**10.** Larval form of *Taenia* spp.

10-2. State the common name of each of the following cestodes. (Objective 10-3)
   A. *Taenia saginata*
   B. *Dipylidium caninum*
   C. *Hymenolepis nana*
   D. *Diphyllobothrium latum*
   E. *Taenia solium*
   F. *Echinococcus granulosus*
   G. *Hymenolepis diminuta*

10-3. In what parts of the world is *Diphyllobothrium latum* endemic? (Objective 10-2)

10-4. Specify the infective stage name for each of the cestodes listed in question 10-2. (Objective 10-5)

10-5. What is the pathology most commonly associated with each of the following? (Objective 10-6)
   A. *Diphyllobothrium latum*
   B. *Echinococcus granulosus*

10-6. What is the specimen of choice for the laboratory diagnosis of each cestode listed in question 10-2? (Objective 10-8)

10-7. Describe the appearance of the scolex of the cestodes listed in question 10-2. (Objective 10-9).

10-8. Differentiate the proglottids of *Taenia saginata* and *Taenia solium*. (Objective 10-9).

10-9. A 30-year-old recent immigrant from Mexico, living in Colorado, presented to the Hispanic Health Clinic after experiencing a seizure at his worksite His history revealed numerous headaches for several weeks. The basic neurologic examination was normal; however, fearing a malignancy, the physician ordered a CT scan. Calcified lesions were noted. A biopsy revealed a parasitic infection. What organism is suspected? (Objective 10-11A)

10-10. A 55-year-old man and his family had returned to the United States after a visit to his native Finland. While there, he enjoyed fishing and cooking the fish over an open fire. After his return, he visited his physician with complaints of diarrhea, abdominal pain, and some cramping. Bacterial culture of a stool specimen was negative for enteric pathogens. However, the microscopic O&P examination revealed several large, oval, operculated eggs. With this brief history, which tapeworm is suspected? (Objective 10-11A)

CASE STUDY 10-2   UNDER THE MICROSCOPE

Renota, a 51-year-old Slavic woman, lived in Romania with her family on a pig farm. She routinely slaughtered pigs and cooked pork for family meals. She had a wide variety of recipes that called for pork. A few days after preparing one of her famous pork dishes, Renota experienced diarrhea, abdominal pain, and chronic indigestion. She went to her family physician and explained her symptoms to him. The physician, who knew the family well and was familiar with the family business, immediately suspected a bacterial or parasitic infection. A stool sample for routine bacterial culture and O&P study was collected from Renota and submitted to the local diagnostic laboratory.

Routine processing procedures were conducted on the stool sample. Gross examination of the stool revealed a portion of the infecting worm (Fig. A). An egg, measuring 36 by 25 um (Fig. B), was seen on the permanent O&P slide. No intestinal bacterial pathogens were isolated.

Questions and Issues for Consideration
1. What is the morphologic form of Figure A? (Objective 10-11A)
2. Label the designated structures in Figures A and B. (Objective 10-10A)
3. Which genus of organism do you suspect? Which species? (Objective 10-11A)
4. What is the common name for this parasite? (Objective 10-11A)
5. Which of the figures shown here, A or B, is most helpful for speciating this parasite? Why? (Objective 10-9)
6. Note the differential characteristics of this species compared with those of its closest relative species. (Objective 10-9)

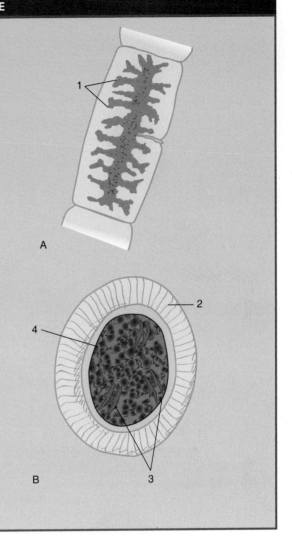

COMPARISON DRAWINGS
Cestode Eggs

FIGURE 10-2A. *Taenia* spp. egg

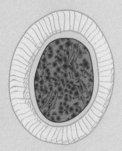

Size range: 28-40 μm by 18-30 μm
Average length: 33 μm by 23 μm

FIGURE 10-10A. *Hymenolepis nana* egg

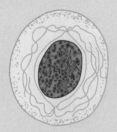

Average size: 45 μm by 38 μm

FIGURE 10-14A. *Diphyllobothrium latum* egg

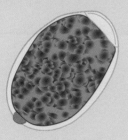

Size range: 55-75 μm by 40-55 μm
Average size: 65 μm by 48 μm

FIGURE 10-7A. *Hymenolepis diminuta* egg

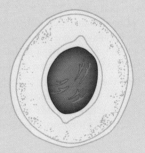

Average size: 55 μm by 85 μm

FIGURE 10-12A. *Dipylidium caninum* egg packet

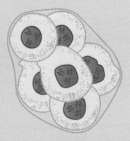

Size range of each egg: 30-60 μm in diameter

COMPARISON DRAWINGS
Cestode Scolices, Proglottids, and Hydatid Cyst

FIGURE 10-5. *Taenia saginata proglottid*

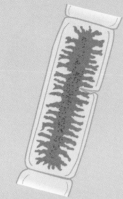

Average size: 17.5 by 5.5 mm

FIGURE 10-6. *Taenia solium proglottid*

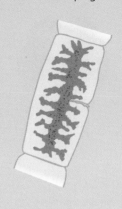

FIGURE 10-9. *Hymenolepis diminuta proglottid*

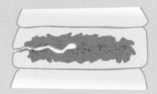

FIGURE 10-13. *Dipylidium caninum proglottid*

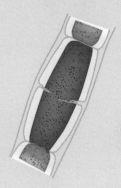

FIGURE 10-16. *Diphyllobothrium latum proglottid*

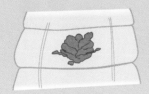

Continued

COMPARISON DRAWINGS
Cestode Scolices, Proglottids, and Hydatid Cyst—cont'd

FIGURE 10-3. *Taenia saginata scolex*

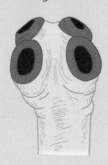

FIGURE 10-4A. *Taenia solium scolex*

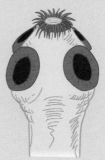

FIGURE 10-8. *Hymenolepis diminuta scolex*

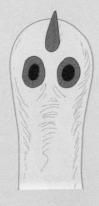

FIGURE 10-11. *Hymenolepis nana scolex*

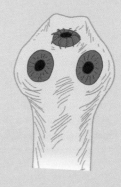

FIGURE 10-15. *Diphyllobothrium latum scolex*

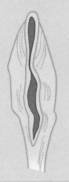

FIGURE 10-17. *Echinococcus granulosus hydatid cyst*

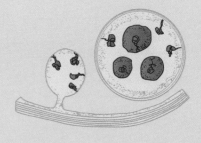

The Trematodes

Lynda Britton and Elizabeth Zeibig

WHAT'S AHEAD

Focusing In
Morphology and Life Cycle
  Notes
Laboratory Diagnosis
Pathogenesis and Clinical
  Symptoms

Trematode Classification
  Fasciolopsis buski
  Fasciola hepatica
  Clonorchis sinensis
  Heterophyes heterophyes
  Metagonimus yokogawai
  Paragonimus westermani

Schistosoma Species
  Schistosoma mansoni
  Schistosoma japonicum
  Schistosoma haematobium
Looking Back

LEARNING OBJECTIVES

On completion of this chapter and review of its figures, tables, and corresponding photomicrographs, the successful learner will be able to:

11-1. Define the following key terms:
  Cercaria (*pl.*, cercariae)
  Dioecious
  Digenea
  Distomiasis
  Katayama fever
  Metacercaria (*pl.*, metacercariae)
  Miracidium
  Operculum
  Redia operculum (*pl.*, rediae)
  Schistosomule
  Sporocyst (*pl.*, sporocysts)
  Swimmer's itch
  Trematoda
  Trematode (*pl.*, trematodes)

11-2. State the geographic distribution of the trematodes.

11-3. State the common name associated with the trematodes.

11-4. Given a list of parasites, select those organisms belonging to the class Digenea.

11-5. Briefly summarize the life cycle of each of the trematodes.

11-6. Identify and describe the symptoms and clinically significant disease processes associated with each pathogenic trematode.

11-7. Identify and describe each of the following as they relate to the trematodes:
  A. Treatment options
  B. Prevention and control measures

11-8. Select the specimen of choice, collection and processing protocol, and laboratory diagnostic techniques for the recovery of each of the nematodes.

11-9. Compare and contrast the trematodes in terms of the key features that the parasites have in common, as well as features that distinguish them.

11-10. Given a description, photomicrograph, and/or diagram of a trematode, correctly:
  A. Identify and/or label the designated characteristic structure(s).
  B. State the purpose of the designated characteristic structure(s).
  C. Identify the organism by scientific name, common name, and morphologic form.

11-11. Analyze case studies that include pertinent patient information and laboratory data and:
   A. Identify each responsible trematode organism by scientific name, common name, and morphologic form, with justification.
   B. Identify the associated diseases and conditions associated with the responsible parasite.
   C. Construct a life cycle associated with each trematode parasite present that includes corresponding epidemiology, route of transmission, infective stage, and diagnostic stage.
   D. Propose each of the following related to stopping and preventing trematode infections:
      1. Treatment options
      2. Prevention and control plan

   E. Recognize sources of error, including but not limited to those involved in specimen collection, processing, and testing and propose solutions to remedy them.
   F. Interpret laboratory data, determine specific follow-up tests to be performed, and predict the results of those identified tests.
11-12. Given prepared laboratory specimens, and with the assistance of this manual, the learner will be able to:
   A. Differentiate trematode organisms from artifacts.
   B. Differentiate the trematode organisms from each other and from other appropriate categories of parasites.
   C. Correctly identify each trematode parasite by scientific, common name, and morphologic form based on its key characteristic structure(s).

CASE STUDY 11-1 | UNDER THE MICROSCOPE

Mr. Park, a 62-year-old Korean man, was seen for fatigue, fever, and abdominal pain. On questioning the patient, it was learned that Mr. Park is a commercial fisherman. His liver function test results were abnormal, showing elevated aspartate aminotransferase (350 IU/liter), alanine amino-transferase (352 IU/liter), alkaline phosphatase (204 IU/liter), and conjugated bilirubin (3.9 mg per deciliter) levels; total bilirubin was 6.4 mg/dL. His white blood cell (WBC) count was 13,000/mm³ and eosinophilia value was 26%. A computed tomography (CT) scan of the abdomen showed dilation of the common bile duct. A tube was inserted into the common bile duct and numerous leaf-shaped worms

were aspirated. The patient was given praziquantel and had a quick and uneventful recovery.

Questions and Issues for Consideration
1. What parasite(s) do you suspect? Why? (Objective 11-11A)
2. Briefly describe the life cycle of the parasite(s). (Objective 11-11C)
3. What is the name of the disease/condition associated with this parasite? (Objective 11-11B)
4. Propose a plan that Mr. Park could follow to prevent future encounters with this parasite. (Objective 11-11D)

FOCUSING IN

This chapter covers the class of helminth parasites belonging to the class known as **Trematoda** or **Digenea**. Commonly known as the flukes, these parasites vary in egg, larva, and adult morphology and reproduction processes. The **trematodes** (another name for the parasites that belong to Trematoda) can be divided into two groups, the hermaphroditic (self-fertilizing) flukes that infect organs and are foodborne, and the blood flukes or schistosomes that are **dioecious** (parasites that reproduce via separate sexes) and infect

by direct penetration. Common to all trematodes is their complex life cycles, which almost always include mollusks (snails) as an intermediate host.

MORPHOLOGY AND LIFE CYCLE NOTES

The trematodes pass through three morphologic forms during their life cycle—eggs, multiple larval stages, and adult worms. The eggs, which are the primary morphologic form recovered in human specimens, vary in appearance. Some contain a lidlike structure that under the appropriate conditions flips open to release its contents for further development, called an **operculum**, such as in *Fasciolopsis* and *Fasciola*. Other members of the trematodes may be distinguished by the presence and location of spines, as seen in the *Schistosoma* spp. The various larval stages typically occur outside the human host and are rarely if ever encountered. The rarely seen adult flukes are thin and nonsegmented, resembling leaves in shape and thickness. They typically range in length from 1 to 5 cm. Each adult fluke is equipped with two muscular, cup-shaped suckers, one oral and the other located ventrally, a simple digestive system, and a genital tract. Like the typical cestode, the average trematode uses its body surface as a means for absorbing and releasing essential nutrients and waste products.

Based on the organism's life cycle, the trematodes may be placed into two categories, those that reside in the intestine, bile duct, or lung (organ-dwelling) and those that reside in the blood vessels around the intestine and bladder (blood-dwelling). A brief general description of each type of life cycle follows. Only the specifics related to each parasite are discussed on an individual basis.

The organ-dwelling flukes include all trematodes except those belonging to the genus *Schistosoma*. Human infection of such organ-dwelling flukes occurs following the ingestion of water plants (e.g., water chestnuts), fish, crab, or crayfish contaminated with the encysted form of the parasite known as **metacercaria**.

On entrance into the intestinal tract, the encysted metacercaria excysts and migrates to the intestine, bile duct, or lung. Development into the adult stage occurs here. Following self-fertilization (all organ-dwelling flukes are hermaphroditic), the resulting eggs exit the host via the feces or sputum. On contact with fresh water, the **miracidium** (contents of the egg) emerges from each egg. Specific species of snails serve as the first intermediate host. The miracidium penetrates into the snail, where the development of a larval form consisting of a saclike structure (**sporocyst**) occurs. Numerous **rediae** (a larval

stage that forms in the sporocyst) result and ultimately produce many **cercariae** (final-stage larvae). The cercariae emerge from the snail and encyst on water plants or enter a fish, crab, or crayfish, which serves as the second intermediate host. Human consumption of these contaminated items initiates a new cycle.

The blood-dwelling flukes consist of the *Schistosoma* spp. Human infection of these flukes occurs following the penetration of cercariae into the skin. This typically happens when an unsuspecting human swims or wades in contaminated water. Following penetration, the resulting **schistosomule** (the morphologic form that emerges from cercariae following human penetration) takes up residence in the blood vessels around the liver, intestinal tract, or urinary bladder, where maturation into adulthood occurs. Because sexes are separate, the presence of both an adult male and an adult female is necessary for copulation to take place. Completion of this mating process results in numerous eggs. Passage of the eggs may take place in the urine or stool, depending on the species. The development of the miracidium, **sporocyst** (daughter sporocysts are produced in place of rediae in this cycle), and cercariae occur in the same manner as those of the organ-dwelling flukes. The cercariae emerge from the snail. An additional host is not required in this cycle. The cercariae, on penetrating the skin of a new human host, initiate a new cycle.

Quick Quiz! 11-1

The first intermediate host for all the trematodes is which of the following? (Objective 11-5)

A. Fish
B. Snail
C. Shrimp
D. Water plant

LABORATORY DIAGNOSIS

The specimen of choice for the recovery of trematode organisms is species-dependent. Samples

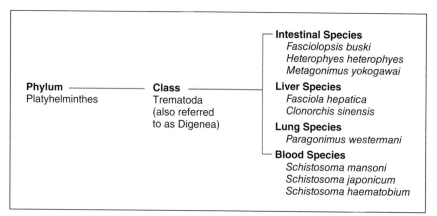

FIGURE 11-1 Parasite classification: The trematodes.

include feces, duodenal drainage, rectal biopsy, sputum, and urine. Eggs are the primary morphologic form seen in these specimens. Under appropriate conditions, adult worms may be recovered. Serologic tests, such as the enzyme-linked immunofluorescence assay (ELISA), are also available for the diagnosis of the blood flukes (*Schistosoma* spp.). Representative laboratory diagnostic methodologies are presented in Chapter 2 as well as in each individual parasite discussion, as appropriate.

Quick Quiz! 11-2

Adult trematodes are readily recoverable in clinical samples. (Objective 11-5)
A. True
B. False

PATHOGENESIS AND CLINICAL SYMPTOMS

The pathogenesis and clinical symptoms experienced by patients infected with flukes vary by species. Such symptoms typically correlate with the infected area of the body, such as the intestinal tract or lung. Symptoms associated with trematode infections include eosinophilia, allergic and toxic reactions, tissue damage, jaundice, and diarrhea.

Quick Quiz! 11-3

Individuals suffering from trematode infections experience a variety of species-dependent symptoms. (Objective 11-6)
A. True
B. False

TREMATODE CLASSIFICATION

Like the cestodes, the trematodes belong to the phylum Platyhelminthes. For classification purposes, the flukes may be divided into four categories (Fig. 11-1) based on the areas of the body that primarily harbor the parasites: intestinal, liver, lung, and blood.

Up until this point, an attempt has been made to discuss the organisms individually in order based on their classification category—that is, a description of extraintestinal parasites follows that of the intestinal organisms. However, the trematodes are introduced in a slightly different order. Because of the similarity of egg morphology that overlaps the various classification categories, discussion of the organ-dwelling flukes is organized in a way that best highlights such similarities. Primarily because of morphologic similarities, appropriate organ-dwelling parasites are presented as units. Similarly, the blood flukes, which are similar in other respects, are also described as a unit.

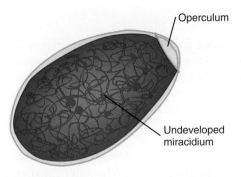

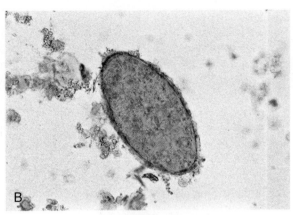

FIGURE 11-2 **A,** *Fasciolopsis buski* egg. **B,** *Fasciolopsis buski, Fasciola hepatica* egg. (**B** *from Mahon CR, Lehman DC, Manuselis G: Textbook of diagnostic microbiology, ed 4, St Louis, 2011, Saunders.*)

Fasciolopsis buski
(fa-see'o-lop'sis/bus'kee)

Common name: Large intestinal fluke.
    Common associated disease and condition names: Fasciolopsiasis.

Fasciola hepatica
(fa-see'o-luh/he-pat'i-kuh)

Common name: Sheep liver fluke.
    Common associated disease and condition names: Fascioliasis, sheep liver rot.

Morphology

▰ **Eggs.** Even though a size range has been established for the eggs of *Fasciolopsis buski* as well as for *Fasciola hepatica*, there is significant overlapping of the numbers (Fig. 11-2; Table 11-1). The typical *F. buski* egg measures 128 to 140 μm by 78 to 85 μm, whereas that of *F. hepatica* measures 128 to 150 μm by 60 to 90 μm. The eggs are identical in all other respects. They consist of an oblong undeveloped miracidium equipped with a distinct operculum. The eggs of the two species are considered to be indistinguishable.

▰ **Adults.** The somewhat oblong, fleshy adult *F. buski* (Fig. 11-3) averages 5 by 1.5 cm in size.

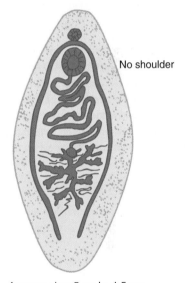

Average size: 5 cm by 1.5 cm

FIGURE 11-3 *Fasciolopsis buski* adult.

TABLE 11-1	*Fasciolopsis buski* and *Fasciola hepatica* Egg: Typical Characteristics at a Glance
Parameter	**Description**
Size range	*F. buski*, 128-140 μm by 78-85 μm; *F. hepatica*, 128-150 μm by 60-90 μm
Shape	Somewhat oblong
Egg contents	Undeveloped miracidium
Other features	Presence of a distinct operculum

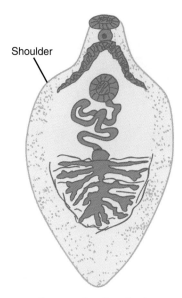

Shoulder

Average size: 3 cm by 1 cm

FIGURE 11-4 *Fasciola hepatica* adult.

The adult *F. hepatica* (Fig. 11-4) is comparable in size to *F. buski*, measuring approximately 3 by 1 cm. Unlike *F. buski, F. hepatica* is equipped with so-called shoulders (see Fig. 11-4).

Laboratory Diagnosis

The specimen choice for recovery of the eggs of *F. buski* and *F. hepatica* is stool. Because the eggs are indistinguishable, information regarding patient symptoms and travel history is necessary to diagnose the causative species. Speciation may also be accomplished by recovery of the adult *Fasciolopsis* worm. Other methodologies available for the detection of *Fasciola* include the Enterotest, ELISA, and gel diffusion.

Life Cycle Notes

The primary difference in the life cycles of *F. buski* and *F. hepatica* is where the adult worms reside in the human host. *F. buski* adults live in the small intestine—thus, the common name intestinal fluke. The adults of *F. hepatica* take up residence in the bile ducts—hence, the common name liver fluke.

Epidemiology

Although the transmission of infection to humans is the same, through ingestion of raw infected water plants, the geographic distribution of these two parasites, *F. buski* and *F. hepatica*, varies. *F. buski* is limited to areas of the Far East, including parts of China, Thailand, Taiwan, and Vietnam, as well as regions in India and Indonesia. Several animals, including rabbits, pigs, and dogs, may serve as reservoir hosts. The water chestnut, lotus, and water caltrop are common food sources.

F. hepatica is found worldwide, particularly in areas in which sheep and cattle are raised. The natural host for the completion of the *F. hepatica* life cycle is the sheep. Humans serve as accidental hosts.

Clinical Symptoms

▶ **Fasciolopsiasis.** Patients suffering from *F. buski* infection usually develop abdominal discomfort because of irritation at the site of worm attachment in the small intestine. This is often accompanied by inflammation and bleeding of the affected area, jaundice, diarrhea, gastric discomfort, and edema. These symptoms often mimic those of a person suffering from a duodenal ulcer. Patients may also suffer from malabsorption syndrome, similar to that seen in patients with giardiasis. Intestinal obstruction, and even death, although rare, may result.

▶ **Fascioliasis: Sheep Liver Rot.** Persons infected with *F. hepatica* experience symptoms caused by the presence and attachment of the adult worm to the biliary tract. These include headache, fever, and chills, and pains in the liver area of the body (because of tissue damage), some of which may extend to the shoulders and back. Eosinophilia, jaundice, liver tenderness, anemia, diarrhea, and digestive discomfort are sometimes seen. Biliary obstruction may also result.

Treatment

Infections with *F. buski* may be treated with praziquantel. Patients suffering from *F. hepatica* infection have been successfully treated with dichlorophenol (bithionol). Triclabendazole is more effective but is not available in the United States.

Prevention and Control

Prevention of future potential infections with *F. buski* and *F. hepatica* may be accomplished by exercising proper human fecal disposal and sanitation practices, particularly in areas in which animal reservoir hosts reside, controlling the snail population, and avoiding the human consumption of raw water plants or contaminated water.

Quick Quiz! 11-4

Fasciolopsis buski infects which organ in humans? (Objective 11-5)
A. Bile ducts
B. Liver
C. Colon
D. Small intestine

Quick Quiz! 11-5

The determination of *Fasciolopsis* versus *Fasciola* can only be accomplished in the laboratory by the recovery of which of the following? (Objective 11-5)
A. Eggs
B. Larvae
C. Adults
D. Sporocysts

Quick Quiz! 11-6

The eggs of *Fasciolopsis* and *Fasciola* possess a caplike structure from which their contents are released under the appropriate conditions; this is called a (an): (Objective 11-1)
A. Operculum
B. Shoulder
C. Coracidium
D. Digenea

TABLE 11-2	*Clonorchis sinensis* Egg: Typical Characteristics at a Glance
Parameter	**Description**
Average size	30 by 15 μm
Egg contents	Developed miracidium
Operculum	Present
Other features	Presence of distinct shoulders and presence of small knob opposite operculum

Clonorchis sinensis
(klo-nor'kis/si-nen'sis)

Common name: Chinese liver fluke.

Common associated disease and condition names: Clonorchiasis.

Morphology

Eggs. The typical *Clonorchis sinensis* egg measures 30 by 15 μm (Fig. 11-5; Table 11-2). The developed miracidium takes up the interior of the egg. The egg is equipped with a distinct operculum opposite a small knob. A thick rim is strategically located around the operculum and is referred to as shoulders.

Adults. The average adult *C. sinensis* measures 2 by 0.5 cm (Fig. 11-6). Each end of the adult worm is narrower than the midportion of the body.

Laboratory Diagnosis

Diagnosis of *C. sinensis* is accomplished by recovery of the characteristic eggs from stool specimens or duodenal aspirates. The Enterotest (see Chapter 2) may also be performed. The rarely encountered adult worms are only seen when removed during a surgery or autopsy procedure.

Life Cycle Notes

Human *C. sinensis* infection occurs following the ingestion of undercooked fish contaminated with

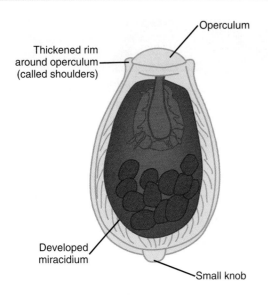

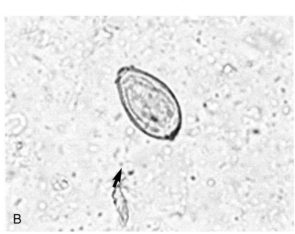

A   Average size: 30 μm by 15 μm

FIGURE 11-5 A, *Clonorchis sinensis* egg. **B,** *Clonorchis sinensis* egg. **(B** *from Mahon CR, Lehman DC, Manuselis G: Textbook of diagnostic microbiology, ed 4, St Louis, 2011, Saunders.)*

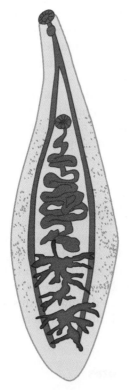

Average size: 2 cm by 0.5 cm

FIGURE 11-6 *Clonorchis sinensis* adult.

encysted metacercariae. Maturation of the immature flukes takes place in the liver. The adult worms take up residence in the bile duct.

Epidemiology

C. sinensis is endemic in areas of the Far East, including China, especially the northeast portions, Taiwan, Korea, Vietnam, and Japan. Reservoir hosts include fish-eating mammals, dogs, and cats. More than 35 million people are infected, and the numbers have tripled to 15 million in China alone in the last decade. Much of this increase may be the result of aquaculture.

Clinical Symptoms

▨ **Asymptomatic.** Light infections typically occur without any obvious symptoms.
▨ **Clonorchiasis.** Persons infected with a heavy worm burden often experience symptoms that include fever, abdominal pain, eosinophilia, diarrhea, anorexia, epigastric discomfort, and occasional jaundice. Enlargement and tenderness of the liver and leukocytosis may also occur. Liver

dysfunction may result in persons severely infected over a long period of time.

Treatment

The treatment for *C. sinensis* infection is praziquantel or albendazole.

Prevention and Control

Prevention and control measures for halting the spread of *C. sinensis* include practicing proper sanitation procedures, especially in regard to fecal disposal by the human and reservoir host (dogs and cats) and avoiding the ingestion of raw, undercooked, or freshly pickled freshwater fish and shrimp.

Quick Quiz! 11-7

The number of *Clonorchis* cases has tripled in which country because of aquaculture? (Objective 11-2)
A. Japan
B. Vietnam
C. China
D. Korea

Quick Quiz! 11-8

What procedures must be done to recover the adult form of *Clonorchis sinensis*? (Objective 11-8)
A. Direct examination of stool and after autopsy
B. Direct and concentration examinations of stool
C. Following surgery and after autopsy
D. Following surgery and duodenal aspiration

Quick Quiz! 11-9

Which of the following is a recommended prevention and control strategy designed to halt the spread of *Clonorchis*? (Objective 11-7B)
A. Consuming raw, pickled, freshwater fish
B. Protecting food from flies
C. Avoidance of swimming in fresh water
D. Proper human and reservoir host fecal disposal

Heterophyes heterophyes
(het-ur-off'ee-eez/het″ur-off'ee-eez)

Common name: Heterophid fluke.
   Common associated disease and condition names: Heterophyiasis.

Metagonimus yokogawai
(met'uh-gon'imus/yo-ko-gah-wah'eye)

Common name: Heterophid fluke.
   Common associated disease and condition names: Metagonimiasis.

Morphology

■ **Eggs.** The eggs of *Heterophyes heterophyes* and *Metagonimus yokogawai* are basically indistinguishable and may be easily confused with those of *C. sinensis* (Table 11-3; see Fig. 11-5). These eggs measure approximately the same as *C. sinensis*, 30 by 15 μm. There are only two somewhat discrete differences among the eggs of *H. heterophyes* and *M. yokogawai* versus those of *C. sinensis*. First, although the *Heterophyes* and *Metagonimus* eggs have shoulders, they are less distinct than those of *Clonorchis*. Second, the eggs of *Heterophyes* and *Metagonimus* may lack the small terminal knob found on those of *Clonorchis*.

TABLE 11-3	*Heterophyes heterophyes* and *Metagonimus yokogawai* Egg: Typical Characteristics at a Glance*
Parameter	**Description**
Average size	30 by 15 μm
Egg contents	Developing miracidium
Operculum	Present
Shoulders	Present but discrete
Small knob	May be absent
Shell thickness	*Heterophyes*, thick; *Metagonimus*, thin

*These eggs may be confused easily with those of *Clonorchis sinensis*.

The eggs of both species consist of a developing miracidium, similar to those of *Clonorchis*. In addition, they both exhibit an operculum like that of *Clonorchis*. However, it is important to note that *Heterophyes* eggs typically have a much thicker shell than those of *Metagonimus*. This is generally not considered enough of a difference to distinguish between the two species.

 Adults. The adult *Heterophyes* worm is small, measuring just over 1.0 by 0.5 mm in size. The pyriform organism is grayish in color and is protected by an outer layer of fine spines that are scaly in appearance. The adult *Metagonimus* is similar in size, measuring approximately 1.5 by 0.5 mm. The worm is also pyriform in shape, with tapering at the anterior end and rounding at the posterior end. A tiny layer of scaly spines covers the organism, which is heavily distributed over the anterior end.

Laboratory Diagnosis

Identification of *Heterophyes* and *Metagonimus* is based on the recovery of the eggs in stool samples. Careful microscopic examination is essential to ensure proper species identification. This is difficult to achieve because the eggs of *Heterophyes*, *Metagonimus*, and *Clonorchis* are so similar.

Life Cycle Notes

Human infection of *Heterophyes* and *Metagonimus* occurs after the ingestion of contaminated undercooked fish. The adult worms of both species reside in the small intestine.

Epidemiology

H. heterophyes is found in parts of Africa, the Near East, and the Far East. These areas include Taiwan, the Philippines, Korea, Japan, Israel, and Egypt, especially the lower Nile valley. *Heterophyes* is found in a variety of wild and domestic animals, particularly fish-eating mammals.

Metagonimus has been reported in areas of Japan, Siberia, China, the Philippines, Spain, Greece, and the Balkans. A number of animals are known to harbor the parasite, including dogs, cats, hogs, and fish-eating birds such as pelicans.

Clinical Symptoms

 Asymptomatic. Light infections typically remain asymptomatic.

Heterophyiasis/Metagonimiasis. Heavy infections of *H. heterophyes* and *M. yokogawai* produce similar symptoms. In addition to abdominal pain and discomfort, patients often experience a chronic mucous diarrhea and eosinophilia. The eggs of both organisms have the ability to escape into the lymphatics or venules via intestinal wall penetration and to migrate to other areas of the body, such as the heart or brain. Granulomas in these areas often result.

Treatment

The treatment of choice for *Heterophyes* and *Metagonimus* infection is praziquantel.

Prevention and Control

The easiest and most logistically possible measure to prevent and control *Heterophyes* and *Metagonimus* is the avoidance of consuming undercooked fish. In addition, practicing proper fecal disposal is also essential for halting the spread of disease. Because of the numerous animal hosts that may harbor both parasites, control of these populations, as well as that of the snails, is physically and economically impossible.

> ### Quick Quiz! 11-10
>
> The key feature that distinguishes *Heterophyes* from *Clonorchis* is which of the following? (Objective 11-9)
> A. Size
> B. Shape
> C. Appearance of shoulders
> D. Location of operculum

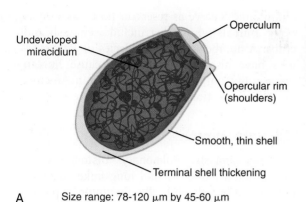

Operculum

Undeveloped
miracidium

Opercular rim
(shoulders)

Smooth, thin shell

Terminal shell thickening

A Size range: 78-120 μm by 45-60 μm

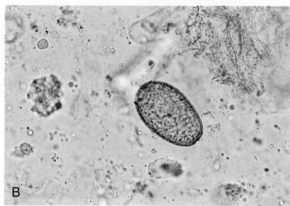

B

FIGURE 11-7 **A,** *Paragonimus westermani* egg. **B,** *Paragonimus westermani* egg. (**B** from Mahon CR, Lehman DC, Manuselis G: *Textbook of diagnostic microbiology, ed 4,* St Louis, 2011, Saunders.)

Quick Quiz! 11-11

The treatment of choice for *Heterophyes* and *Metagonimus* is which of the following? (Objective 11-7A)
A. Niclosamide
B. Praziquantel
C. Pyrantel pamoate
D. Metronidazole

Quick Quiz! 11-12

The specimen of choice for the recovery of *Heterophyes* and *Metagonimus* is which of the following? (Objective 11-8)
A. Stool
B. Duodenal contents
C. Urine
D. Sputum

Paragonimus westermani
(par″i-gon-′i-mus/wes-tur-man′eye)

Common name: Oriental lung fluke.

Common associated disease and condition names: Paragonimiasis, pulmonary distomiasis.

Morphology

 Eggs. The average egg of *Paragonimus westermani* ranges in size from 78 to 120 μm by 45

TABLE 11-4	*Paragonimus westermani* Egg: Typical Characteristics at a Glance
Parameter	**Description**
Size range	78-120 μm long; 45-60 μm wide
Shape	Somewhat oval
Egg contents	Undeveloped miracidium surrounded by a thin, smooth shell
Other features	Prominent operculum with shoulders; obvious terminal shell thickening opposite operculum

to 60 μm (Fig. 11-7; Table 11-4). The somewhat oval egg consists of an undeveloped miracidium protected by a thin smooth shell. An opercular rim (shoulders) surrounds the prominent operculum. An obvious terminal shell thickening is located on the end opposite the operculum. *Diphylobothrium latum* eggs have similar morphology to *P. westermani* but lack opercular shoulders and are more rounded in shape. *D. latum* eggs also have an abopercular knob lacking in *P. westermania.* Size is also helpful in distinguishing the two eggs in stool specimens.

 Adults. The typical somewhat oval, red- to brown-colored adult *P. westermani* measures 1 by 0.7 cm (Fig. 11-8). The cuticle of *P. westermani* possesses spines, similar to the other adult trematodes.

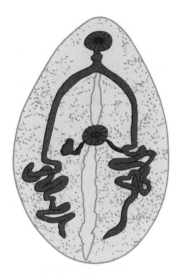

Average size: 1 cm by 0.7 cm

FIGURE 11-8 *Paragonimus westermani* adult.

Laboratory Diagnosis

Diagnosis of *P. westermani* is accomplished by the recovery of eggs in sputum specimens. These eggs are commonly found in bloody samples. Occasionally, the eggs may be seen in stool samples when sputum is swallowed. Serologic tests have also been developed.

Life Cycle Notes

P. westermani is transmitted in undercooked crayfish or crabs. On ingestion of such freshwater products, the immature flukes (often occurring in pairs) are released into the body, where they migrate through the intestinal wall, through the peritoneal cavity, into the diaphragm, and finally into lung tissue, where encystation occurs. Migration of immature flukes to other areas of the body, such as the brain or liver, has been known to take place.

Epidemiology

Infections caused by *P. westermani* occur in several areas of the world, including portions of Asia and Africa, India, and South America. Pigs and monkeys serve as reservoir hosts, as well as other animals whose diet includes crayfish and crabs. A number of related species of *Paragonimus* have also been known to cause human disease, not only in Central and South America but also in portions of the United States.

Clinical Symptoms

■ **Paragonimiasis: Pulmonary Distomiasis.** As the common name oriental lung fluke suggests, patients infected with *Paragonimus* typically experience symptoms associated with pulmonary discomfort—cough, fever, chest pain, and increased production of blood-tinged sputum. Individuals infected with this parasite (the corresponding condition is known at paragonimiasis and as pulmonary **distomiasis**) may also experience chronic bronchitis, eosinophilia, and the production of fibrous tissue. These symptoms often mimic those seen in persons infected with tuberculosis.

Patients who develop infections in areas other than the lung experience symptoms corresponding to the affected organ or tissue. One area is the brain, as described in the next section.

■ **Cerebral Paragonimiasis.** Migration of immature *P. westermani* organisms to the brain may result in the development of a serious neurologic condition. Patients experience seizures, visual difficulties, and decreased precision of motor skills.

Treatment

Praziquantel is the medication of choice for the treatment of *Paragonimus*. An acceptable alternative drug is bithionol.

Prevention and Control

As for other trematodes discussed in this chapter, the primary prevention and control measures for the eradication of *Paragonimus* include avoiding human ingestion of undercooked crayfish and crabs and exercising proper disposal of human waste products.

Quick Quiz! 11-13

In addition to its typical location, *Paragonimus* eggs are also known to cause serious complications when recovered in which of the following? (Objective 11-8)
A. Bile
B. Cerebrospinal fluid
C. Brain tissue
D. Feces

Quick Quiz! 11-14

A key feature that distinguishes *Paragonimus* from the other trematode eggs is which of the following? (Objective 11-9)
A. Prominent operculum
B. Obvious terminal shell thickening
C. Discrete shoulders
D. Three pairs of hooklets

Quick Quiz! 11-15

The typical transmission route of *Paragonimus* to humans consists of which of the following? (Objective 11-5)
A. Consumption of contaminated crayfish or crabs
B. Swimming in contaminated water
C. Hand-to-mouth contamination
D. Walking barefoot on contaminated sandy soil

SCHISTOSOMA SPECIES

Schistosoma mansoni
(shis'to-so'muh/man-so'nigh)

Common name: Manson's blood fluke.

Schistosoma japonicum
(shis'to-so'muh/ja-pon'i-kum)

Common name: Blood fluke.

Schistosoma haematobium
(shis'to-so'muh/hee-muh'-toe'bee-um)

Common name: Bladder fluke.

Common *Schistosoma* spp. disease and condition names: Schistosomiasis, bilharziasis, swamp fever, Katayama fever.

There are many species of schistosomes but only five infect humans. *Schistosoma intercalatum* is found in small pockets of Africa and *Schistosoma mekongi* is found in Southeast Asia. Neither will be discussed further because they are of lesser importance. Although the differences among the *Schistosoma* are numerous, the three species of human significance have many similarities. To avoid repeating much of the same information, these organisms are discussed as a unit in this section.

Schistosomiasis has recently been recognized as a major parasite cause of morbidity and occasional mortality, especially in sub-Saharan Africa. Along with HIV and malaria, disability from schistosomiasis caused by anemia, chronic pain, diarrhea, exercise intolerance, and undernutrition makes it a major problem in many parts of Africa and other areas of the world.

Morphology

Eggs. The average *Schistosoma* egg is comprised of a developed miracidium (Table 11-5). The presence of lateral or terminal spines, as well as the organism's shape and size, aid in species identification.

Schistosoma mansoni (Fig. 11-9) is relatively large, measuring 112 to 182 μm by 40 to 75 μm. The organism is somewhat oblong and possesses a prominent large lateral spine.

The somewhat roundish *Schistosoma japonicum* (Fig. 11-10) is the smallest of the *Schistosoma* spp., measuring 50 to 85 μm by 38 to 60 μm. The egg is characterized by the presence of a small lateral spine, which is often difficult to detect on microscopic examination.

Schistosoma haematobium (Fig. 11-11) resembles *S. mansoni* in size and shape. The somewhat oblong egg measures 110 to 170 μm by 38 to

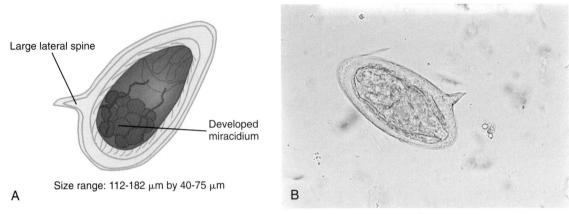

A

Large lateral spine

Developed miracidium

Size range: 112-182 μm by 40-75 μm

B

FIGURE 11-9 A, *Schistosoma mansoni* egg. **B,** *Schistosoma mansoni* egg. (**B** *from Mahon CR, Lehman DC, Manuselis G: Textbook of diagnostic microbiology, ed 4, St Louis, 2011, Saunders.*)

TABLE 11-5	*Schistosoma* Species Eggs: Typical Characteristics at a Glance		
	S. mansoni	**S. japonicum**	**S. haematobium**
Size Range	112-182 μm by 40-75 μm	50-85 μm by 38-60 μm	110-170 μm by 38-70 μm
Shape	Oblong	Somewhat roundish	Somewhat oblong
Egg Contents	Developed miracidium	Developed miracidium	Developed miracidium
Appearance and Location of Spine	Large; lateral	Small; lateral*	Large; terminal

*Difficult to see.

70 μm. The presence of a large, prominent, terminal spine distinguishes the egg from that of other *Schistosoma* spp.

▶ **Adults.** As noted, the adults of *Schistosoma* are the only trematodes discussed in this chapter that have separate sexes. Unlike the other adult trematodes discussed thus far, the schistosomes are rounder in appearance. Although the typical female measures 2 cm in length and the male measures 1.5 cm, the male surrounds the female almost completely, facilitating copulation (Fig. 11-12).

Laboratory Diagnosis

Laboratory diagnosis of *S. mansoni* and *S. japonicum* is accomplished by recovery of the eggs in stool or rectal biopsy specimens. The specimen of choice for the recovery of *S. haematobium* eggs is a concentrated urine specimen. In addition, a number of immunodiagnostic techniques, including ELISA, are also available.

Life Cycle Notes

Human infection with *Schistosoma* occurs in fresh water following the penetration of fork-tailed cercariae into the skin. The resulting schistosomule migrates into the bloodstream, where maturation into adulthood is completed. The location of the adult flukes varies by species. *S. mansoni* and *S. japonicum* reside in the veins that surround the intestinal tract, as well as in the blood passages of the liver. *S. haematobium* resides in the veins surrounding the bladder. Females lay thousands of eggs daily, which make their way from the bloodstream through the tissue into the colon (*S. mansoni* and *S. japonicum*) or the urine (*S. haematobium*). The eggs produce enzymes that help them travel through the tissue to be excreted. Once an egg reaches fresh water, the miracidium is released from the egg and must locate a snail, where it develops into the cercariae.

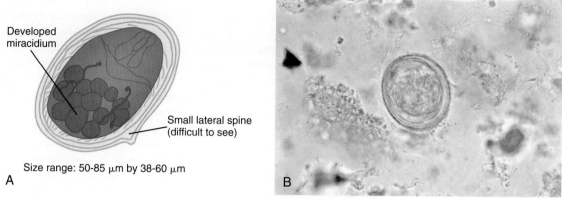

FIGURE 11-10 **A,** *Schistosoma japonicum* egg. **B,** *Schistosoma japonicum* egg. (**B** *from Mahon CR, Lehman DC, Manuselis G: Textbook of diagnostic microbiology, ed 4, St Louis, 2011, Saunders.*)

Developed miracidium

Small lateral spine (difficult to see)

Size range: 50-85 μm by 38-60 μm

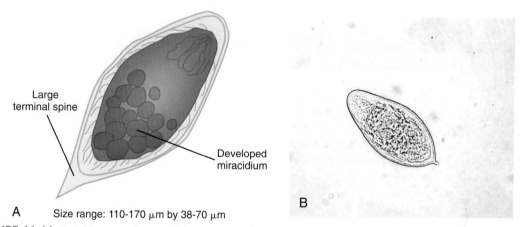

Large terminal spine

Developed miracidium

Size range: 110-170 μm by 38-70 μm

FIGURE 11-11 **A,** *Schistosoma haematobium* egg. **B,** *Schistosoma haematobium* egg. (**B** *from Mahon CR, Lehman DC, Manuselis G: Textbook of diagnostic microbiology, ed 4, St Louis, 2011, Saunders.*)

Epidemiology

There are a number of reservoir hosts capable of carrying *Schistosoma* spp. These include monkeys, cattle and other livestock, rodents, and domesticated animals such as dogs and cats. The specific geographic distribution of each of the three *Schistosoma* spp. vary by species.

It is believed that *S. mansoni* originated in the Old World because it is prevalent primarily in parts of Africa. Transport of the organism to the New World most likely occurred via the slave trade. Known endemic areas include Puerto Rico, the West Indies, and portions of Central and South America.

The geographic distribution of *S. japonicum* is limited to the Far East. Areas known to harbor the parasite include parts of China, Indonesia, and the Philippines. There is evidence to suggest that although portions of Japan were once known endemic areas, it may no longer be considered as such.

S. haematobium has been known to occur primarily in the Old World. Almost all of Africa and portions of the Middle East, including Iran, Iraq, and Saudi Arabia are considered endemic regions.

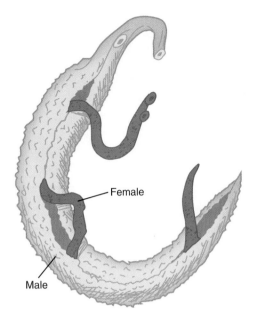

Average length: females — 2 cm, males — 1.5 cm

FIGURE 11-12 Schistosomes in copula.

Clinical Symptoms

▶ **Asymptomatic.** It is believed that most chronic *Schistosoma* infections contracted in known endemic areas remain asymptomatic. It is interesting to note that a brown hematin pigment, similar to the pigment seen in persons infected with malaria, is present in the macrophages and neutrophils (microphages is not used very often) of these patients.

▶ **Schistosomiasis, Bilharziasis, Swamp Fever.** The first symptom experienced by most symptomatic persons infected with *Schistosoma* is inflammation at the cercaria penetration site. Symptoms of acute infection include abdominal pain, fever, chills, weight loss, cough, bloody diarrhea, and eosinophilia. Painful urination and hematuria may also occur in persons infected with *S. haematobium*. The development of necrosis, lesions, and granulomas is common and occurs in the area(s) infected with the parasite. Obstruction of the bowel or ureters, as well as secondary bacterial infections and involvement of the central nervous system and other tissues, may also result.

Katayama fever is a systemic hypersensitivity reaction to the schistosomulae migrating through tissue. Rapid onset of fever, nausea, myalgia, malaise, fatigue, cough, diarrhea, and eosinophilia occur 1 to 2 months after exposure. Although rare in chronically exposed persons, it is common in people new to endemic areas, such as tourists and travelers.

A number of associated conditions have been identified in patients with *Schistosoma*. For example, those infected with *S. japonicum* or *S. haematobium* are also at risk of suffering from nephrotic syndrome. Similarly, there appears to be a connection between *S. haematobium* infection and bladder cancer. In addition, *S. mansoni* and *S. japonicum* may be associated with repeated *Salmonella* infections.

Treatment

Praziquantel is the drug of choice for the treatment of schistosomal infections. Oxamniquine is only used for *S. mansoni*. The antimalarial artemisinins, artemether and artesunate, have proven effective for schistosomal infections but, in areas endemic for malaria, concern for resistance by *Plasmodium* may limit their usefulness. Surgery may be necessary for patients in whom obstruction has occurred.

Prevention and Control

Older methods of preventing schistosomiasis included proper human waste disposal and control of the snail population, primarily their breeding areas, prompt diagnosis and treatment of infected persons, the avoidance of human contact with potentially contaminated water, and educational programs for the inhabitants of known endemic areas. Current focus is on anthelminthic chemotherapy with praziquantel because of its low cost, few side effects, and rapid results. The World Health Organization (WHO) has recommended the following measures: mass treatment of everyone in a community in which there is a high prevalence and/or high risk of schistosomiasis (7 of 15 or more children test positive), treatment of all children in moderately prevalent areas (2 of 15 children test positive), and only treating diagnosed cases in low-prevalence areas. National control programs for schistosomiasis are frequently being linked to control of other parasitic diseases in endemic areas, especially in sub-Saharan Africa.

Notes of Interest and New Trends

Human *Schistosoma* infections are predicted to increase and spread in endemic areas because of the establishment of water control projects on a massive scale. Unfortunately, additional snail breeding areas have been generated. Schistosomiasis is now considered the second most serious parasitic infection, only after malaria, in terms of mortality and morbidity.

A condition referred to as **swimmer's itch** has been known to occur in persons who accidentally become infected with the cercariae of select *Schistosoma* spp., other than those discussed in this chapter, which would otherwise infect certain animals (mammals and birds). Human infection is initiated following the penetration of the fork-tailed cercariae into the skin. Severe allergic reactions and secondary bacterial infections may occur. The life cycle of these parasites is not completed. Topical medications targeted at relieving the allergic response and swelling are available. Prevention and control measures include controlling the snail population and preventing the cercariae from penetrating the skin by vigorously rubbing the body with a towel after exposure to potentially infected water.

Quick Quiz! 11-16

The adults of this species of *Schistosoma* dwell in the veins surrounding the urinary bladder: (Objective 11-5)
A. *S. haematobium*
B. *S. mansoni*
C. *S. japonicum*
D. All of the above

Quick Quiz! 11-17

The specimen of choice for the recovery of *Schistosoma japonicum* is which of the following? (Objective 11-8)
A. Tissue biopsy
B. Urine
C. Sputum
D. Stool

Quick Quiz! 11-18

A systemic hypersensitivity reaction caused by the presence of *Schistosoma* is called which of the following? (Objective 1-1)
A. Bilharziasis
B. Katayama fever
C. Swamp fever
D. Schistosomiasis

LOOKING BACK

Laboratory diagnosis of the flukes depends primarily on the careful microscopic examination of stool, biliary drainage, duodenal drainage, sputum, or urine samples for the presence of eggs. In addition to noting the specific specimen type, because select organisms are found in certain samples, the organism's size, shape, and features (e.g., operculum, shoulders, and presence and location of a spine) aid in identification. It is important to stress that the eggs of certain flukes, such as *Fasciolopsis* and *Fasciola*, are indistinguishable and require further investigation for speciation. Patient travel history, as well as clinical signs and symptoms and the possible recovery of the adult *Fasciolopsis* organisms, aid in this determination. The presence of shoulders helps distinguish *Fasciola* from *Fasciolopsis*.

Overall recovery of the adult flukes is considered to be a rare occurrence. Nonetheless, it is important to have some idea of their appearance. With the exception of the schistosomes, the flukes are basically flattened, leaf-shaped organisms. Unlike the organ-dwelling trematodes, the schistosomes appear much more rounded and elongated. Comparison drawings of the trematode eggs and adults are provided at the end of this chapter as a reference guide for study and as an aid in identifying organisms in patient specimens.

TEST YOUR KNOWLEDGE!

11-1. Trematodes that mature in the lung and produce eggs that appear in the sputum are most probably which of the following? (Objective 11-5)
A. *Fasciolopsis buski*
B. *Schistosoma japonicum*
C. *Paragonimus westermani*
D. *Clonorchis sinensis*

11-2. Consumption of the infective larval stage encysted on aquatic plants that have not been cooked results in infection with: (Objective 11-5)
A. *Clonorchis sinensis*
B. *Fasciola hepatica*
C. *Heterophyes heterophyes*
D. *Paragonimus westermani*

11-3. The largest fluke infecting humans measuring as much as 5 cm in length is which of the following? (Objective 11-9)
A. *Fasciolopsis buski*
B. *Fasciola hepatica*
C. *Paragonimus westermani*
D. *Clonorchis sinensis*

11-4. A schistosoma egg with a terminal spine would be most likely found in which of the following? (Objective 11-9)
A. Feces
B. Bile
C. Sputum
D. Urine

11-5. The infective form of *Schistosoma mansoni* is which of the following? (Objective 11-5)
A. Cercaria swimming in water
B. Metacercaria on or in fish
C. Metacercaria encysted on water chestnuts or vegetables
D. Cercaria on water chestnuts, bamboo shoots, or vegetables

11-6. In the life cycle of hermaphroditic flukes, the infective stage for the snail is which of the following? (Objective 11-5)
A. Cercaria
B. Miracidium
C. Metacercaria
D. Redia

11-7. The adult form of the sheep liver fluke produces large, ovoid, unembryonated eggs with a yellowish-brown shell and an inconspicuous operculum. These eggs are morphologically most similar to which of the following? Objective 10-9)
A. *Fasciola hepatica*
B. *Fasciolopsis buski*
C. *Clonorchis sinensis*
D. *Paragonimus westermani*

11-8. The incidence of small, yellowish, oval, operculated eggs with a short, comma-like extension of the shell opposite the operculum increased markedly in stools examined in the United States with the influx of refugees from Vietnam and nearby countries. Although not transmitted in the United States, human infection in endemic areas is acquired by which of the following? (Objective 11-5)
A. Consumption of infected water vegetation
B. Direct larval penetration of human skin
C. Eating infected crabs or crayfish
D. Ingestion of infected fresh water fish

11-9. A child visited his grandparents in rural Egypt for a summer. While there, he played in irrigation ditches and developed salmonellosis. Blood cultures were positive for *Salmonella* and a stool examination revealed eggs of a parasite common to that part of the world. The egg would appear as which of the following? (Objective 11-10A)
A. Large (80 × 140 μm), with an operculum
B. Oval (40 × 48 μm), with a mammillated coat

C. Small (12 × 30 µm), with an operculum

D. Large (60 × 150 µm), with a large lateral spine

11-10. Match the host for metacercariae with the parasite. Answers can be used more than once. (Objective 11-5)

Column A	Column B
A. Fish	**1.** *Fasciolopsis buski*
B. Water plants	**2.** *Fasciola hepatica*
C. Crawfish	**3.** *Clonorchis sinensis*
	4. *Paragonimus westermani*
	5. *Metagonimus yokogawai*
	6. *Heterophyes heterophyes*

CASE STUDY 11-2 | **UNDER THE MICROSCOPE**

Anthony, a 30-year-old Italian man, worked as an archeologist in the Nile Valley. Anthony and his team recently made an important historical discovery, the Providence Stone. This stone allows a person's mind and soul on his or her death to be transferred into another person's body. To celebrate this find, the team went out to a local pub for champagne and escargot (snails). The team members became somewhat rowdy and insisted on ending the evening with a dip in the Nile.

Approximately 1 month later, Anthony experienced increased urination with spots of blood. He was also frequently tired and complained of a slight fever. Anthony explained his symptoms to a local physician and was asked if he had eaten or done anything unusual lately. Embarrassed, Anthony admitted only to an early morning swim in the Nile. On examination, the physician ordered a complete blood count (CBC), Chem 6 (a battery of chemistry tests for Na^+, K^+, Cl^-, CO_2, glucose, and BUN-blood urea nitrogen), and urinalysis (UA).

The samples were sent to a laboratory. The CBC revealed eosinophilia. The Chem 6 results were normal. The UA showed a trace of blood. Microscopic examination of the concentrated urine showed a yellowish-brown ovoid organism that measured approximately 115 by 50 µm.

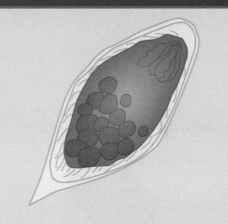

Questions and Issues for Consideration

1. What parasite, including its morphologic form, is suspected? (Objective 11-11A)
2. Name the disease caused by this parasite. (Objective 11-11B)
3. What is the first intermediate host associated with the life cycle of this parasite? (Objective 11-11C)
4. What is the mode of transmission for this parasite? (Objective 11-11C)

COMPARISON DRAWINGS
Trematode Eggs

FIGURE 11-2A. *Fasciolopsis buski, Fasciola hepatica* egg

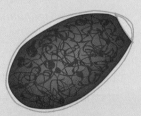

Fasciolopsis size range: 128-140 μm by 78-85 μm
Fasciola size range: 128-150 μm by 60-90 μm

FIGURE 11-5A. *Clonorchis sinensis* egg

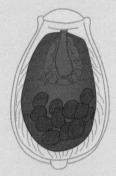

Average size: 30 μm by 15 μm

FIGURE 11-7A. *Paragonimus westermani* egg

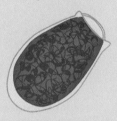

Size range: 78-120 μm by 45-60 μm

FIGURE 11-9A. *Schistosoma mansoni* egg

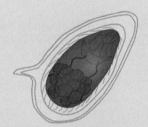

Size range: 112-182 μm by 40-75 μm

FIGURE 11-10A. *Schistosoma japonicum* egg

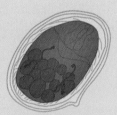

Size range: 50-85 μm by 38-60 μm

FIGURE 11-11A. *Schistosoma haematobium* egg

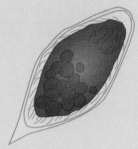

Size range: 110-170 μm by 38-70 μm

COMPARISON DRAWINGS
Trematode Adults

FIGURE 11-3. *Fasciolopsis buski* adult

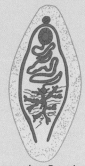

Average size: 5 cm by 1.5 cm

FIGURE 11-4. *Fasciola hepatica* adult

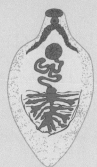

Average size: 3 cm by 1 cm

FIGURE 11-6. *Clonorchis sinensis* adult

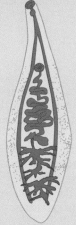

Average size: 2 cm by 0.5 cm

FIGURE 11-8. *Paragonimus westermani* adult

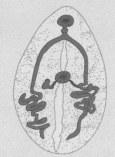

Average size: 1 cm by 0.7 cm

FIGURE 11-12. Schistosomes in copula

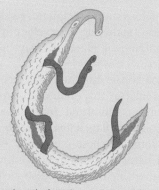

Average length: females — 2 cm, males — 1.5 cm

Artifacts and Confusers

Charity Accurso and Elizabeth Zeibig

WHAT'S AHEAD

Focusing In
White Blood Cells
Pollen Grains
Vegetable Cells
Vegetable Spirals
Charcot-Leyden Crystals

Yeast
Plant Hair
Plant Material
Epithelial Cells
Fungal Elements
Starch Cells

Clumped or Fused Platelets
Stain Precipitate
Red Cell Abnormalities
Looking Back

LEARNING OBJECTIVES

On completion of this chapter and review of its figures and corresponding photomicrographs, the successful learner will be able to:

12-1. Differentiate the artifacts and confusers discussed from parasites based on their key characteristics.

12-2. State the derivation and significance of Charcot-Leyden crystals, when present.

12-3. Given a diagram of an artifact or confuser, correctly name it as one, and not as a parasite.

12-4. Given prepared laboratory specimens, and with the assistance of this manual, the learner will be able to:
Differentiate the artifact and confusers discussed from parasites.

FOCUSING IN

There are a number of structures that closely resemble parasites but in reality are not. These structures, termed **artifacts** and **confusers**, are found primarily in stool and blood samples. Such stool artifacts and confusers may be the result of disease processes, medications, and/or dietary habits, such as those seen in Figure 12-1. The presence of free-living organisms in stool caused by specimen contact with water, sewage, or soil may often cause confusion. Artifacts and confusers, such as stain precipitate, red blood cell abnormalities, including Howell-Jolly bodies, and the clumping of platelets, may be seen on blood smears.

In addition to the common artifacts and confusers mentioned in this chapter, others may be seen in samples submitted for parasite study. Free-living amebae, flagellates, ciliates, and nematodes are some of these confusers. Accidental ingestion of parasite forms in which humans are not part of their life cycle may also yield confusers. Fourteen of the most common artifacts and

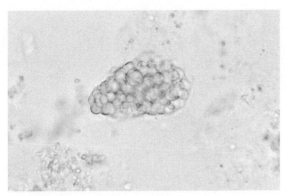

FIGURE 12-1 Cluster of fat globule artifacts. *(Courtesy of Carolina Biological Supply Company.)*

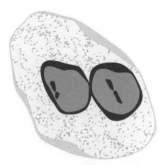

Average size: 15 μm
FIGURE 12-2 White blood cell.

confusers are briefly discussed in the following sections.

WHITE BLOOD CELLS

Polymorphonuclear white blood cells (WBCs), which typically have an average size of 15 μm, are often mistaken for amebic cysts, especially those of *Entamoeba histolytica,* whose average size range is 12 to 18 μm (Fig. 12-2).

WBCs are usually present in patients suffering from ulcerative colitis, bacterial dysentery, or intestinal amebiasis. Along with falling into the amebic cyst size range, these WBCs have a two- to four-lobed nucleus, similar in appearance to the *E. histolytica* nucleus. Even though these WBC lobes may appear as separate nuclei, they are connected by thin chromatin bands. Protozoan nuclear inclusions, such as karyosomes and peripheral chromatin, are absent in WBCs.

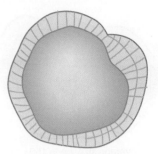

Size range: 12-20 μm
FIGURE 12-3 Pollen grain.

Careful microscopic focusing is necessary because these bands are often difficult to detect.

Mononuclear WBCs, also known as macrophages or monocytes, may range in size from 28 to 62 μm (less on permanently stained preparations) and closely resemble the *E. histolytica* trophozoite, which measures 8 to 65 μm. Both structures may ingest red blood cells (RBCs) and debris, but only the macrophages ingest polymorphonuclear WBCs. The macrophage has one irregularly shaped nucleus that is often absent on examination. Although the macrophage size range overlaps that of *E. histolytica,* the macrophage may be significantly smaller (5 to 10 μm). Red-staining round bodies may be seen in the macrophages.

POLLEN GRAINS

Thick-walled pollen grains resemble the eggs of *Taenia* spp. but are smaller, measuring 12 to 20 μm (Fig. 12-3). Pollen grains may appear round or symmetrically lobed. Unlike *Taenia,* there are no notable interior structures.

Quick Quiz! 12-1

Which of the following findings can help differentiate WBCs from amebic cysts? (Objective 11-1)
A. Size
B. Number of nuclei
C. Absence of protozoan nuclear inclusions
D. None of the above

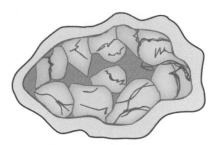

Average size: up to 150 μm

FIGURE 12-4 Vegetable cell.

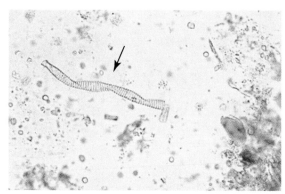

FIGURE 12-6 Vegetable spiral, Iron hematoxylin stain, 1000X. Arrow indicates a vegetable spiral artifact. *(Courtesy of Carolina Biological Supply Company.)*

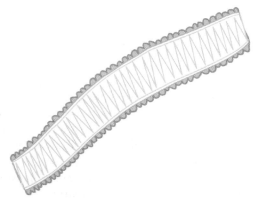

FIGURE 12-5 Vegetable spiral.

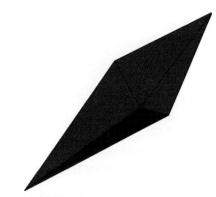

FIGURE 12-7 Charcot-Leyden crystal.

VEGETABLE CELLS

Vegetable cells may easily be confused with helminth eggs (Fig. 12-4). These cells are typically large and roundish oval to irregularly round in shape and may measure up to 150 μm in size. Thick cell walls are usually present. The interior portion of vegetable cells is unorganized and often appears to consist primarily of large vacuoles.

VEGETABLE SPIRALS

Vegetable spirals often resemble helminth larvae in their shape and size (Figs. 12-5 and 12-6). Unlike helminth larvae, however, vegetable spirals do not have a head or tail region. Vegetable spirals are readily distinguished from parasitic forms by their ladder-like appearance. The ladder consists of a series of rungs that are spaced closely together.

Quick Quiz! 12-2

Which of the following characteristics can help differentiate vegetable spirals from helminth larvae? (Objective 11-1)
A. Presence of head or tail region
B. Ladder-like appearance
C. Characteristic worm shape
D. Length of spiral

CHARCOT-LEYDEN CRYSTALS

Of all of the confusers and artifacts discussed in this chapter, Charcot-Leyden crystals have the most clinical significance (Fig. 12-7). They are typically found in stool or sputum specimens and are reported when seen. The presence of these diamond-shaped crystals, which develop from eosinophil breakdown products, indicates that an immune response of unknown origin has taken place. Because such an immune response may be caused by the presence of parasites, it is important to examine specimens that contain Charcot-Leyden crystals closely.

YEAST

The round to oval yeast cells measure 4 to 8 μm in size and may be confused with protozoan cysts, especially those of *Entamoeba hartmanni* (5 to 12 μm), *Entamoeba nana* (4 to 12 μm), and *Entamoeba hominis* (3 to 10 μm; Fig. 12-8). Furthermore, there is a considerable resemblance of a yeast cell to the oocyst of *Cryptosporidium* (4 to 6 μm). As with the other artifacts and confusers, yeast cells typically show no definite internal structures. Occasionally, however, small granules resembling karyosomes may be seen. Yeast may be easily distinguished from parasites when seen in their budding stage.

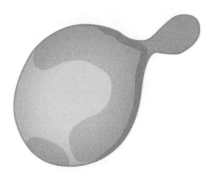

Size range: 4-8 μm
FIGURE 12-8 Budding yeast.

Quick Quiz! 12-3

What is the clinical significance of the presence of Charcot-Leyden crystals in a stool or sputum specimen? (Objective 12-2)
A. Indicative of an immune response of unknown origin
B. Indicative of a parasitic infection
C. Indicative of a bacterial infection
D. Not a significant finding

PLANT HAIR

Plant hair may resemble helminth larvae in size and shape (Fig. 12-9). In addition, plant hair may appear to have a nondescript internal structure. Upon further examination, plant hair does not have diagnostic structures, such as a buccal cavity, esophagus, intestine, or genital primordium. There is no head or tail region.

PLANT MATERIAL

Plant material may range in diameter from 12 to 150 μm and resemble helminth eggs, particularly an unfertilized *Ascaris lumbricoides* (38 to 45 μm), in size and shape (Fig. 12-10). This artifact is typically round to oval in shape and may or may not have a definite cell wall. Plant material is often rough in appearance and may have hairs (pseudocilia) extending from its periphery. The interior of the cell looks like a cluster of odd-shaped vacuoles.

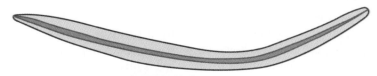

FIGURE 12-9 Plant hair.

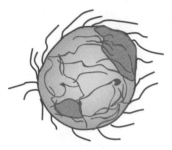

Size range: 12-150 μm in diameter

FIGURE 12-10 Plant material.

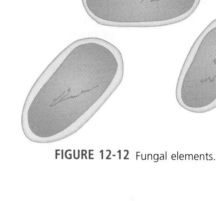

FIGURE 12-12 Fungal elements.

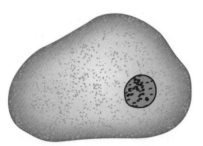

FIGURE 12-11 Epithelial cell.

FUNGAL ELEMENTS

Fungal elements may be similar to the size and shape of protozoan cysts (Fig. 12-12). The lack of interior structures easily distinguishes these artifacts from parasitic forms.

Quick Quiz! 12-4

Plant material differs from a helminth eggs in that plant material may have peripheral pseudocilia. (Objective 12-1)
A. True
B. False

Quick Quiz! 12-5

Which parasite may be confused with epithelial cells because of their similar size and shape? (Objective 12-1)
A. Helminth eggs
B. *Plasmodium* spp.
C. Amebic trophozoites
D. *Dientamoeba fragilis*

EPITHELIAL CELLS

Epithelial cells often show a striking resemblance to amebic trophozoites in size and shape (Fig. 12-11). In addition, epithelial cells have a single nucleus and often show a distinct cell wall, just like those of the amebic trophozoites. Epithelial cells lack the typical amebic trophozoite interior structures. For example, the cytoplasm of epithelial cells is usually smooth and contains no inclusions. The large epithelial cell nucleus, however, may consist of a large chromatin mass that resembles a nucleus.

STARCH CELLS

Round to irregular round-shaped starch cells (Fig. 12-13), also referred to as starch granules, measure less than 10 μm and may appear at first glance to be protozoan cysts, particularly those of *E. hartmanni* and *E. nana* (both measure 5 to 12 μm). These cells are readily differentiated from parasitic forms because they lack internal structures. A nondescript mass located inside the cell is often present and may resemble a nucleus. Further investigation of this structure reveals

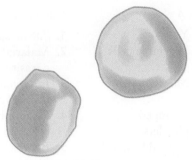

FIGURE 12-13 Starch cells.

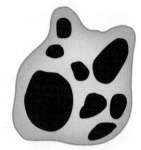

FIGURE 12-14 Clumped/fused platelets.

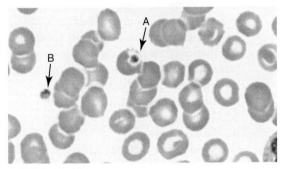

FIGURE 12-15 Giemsa stain, 1000×. Platelet artifacts. (A) intracellular (inside a red blood cell) and (B) outside a red blood cell (extracellular). *(Courtesy of WARD'S Natural Science Establishment, Inc.)*

that no karyosome or peripheral chromatin is present. In addition, starch cells may be differentiated from parasites because of their dark blue-black appearance when stained with iodine.

CLUMPED OR FUSED PLATELETS

Clumped or fused platelets often appear on Giemsa-stained blood film smears and may be mistaken for malarial parasites, especially the young trophozoite form (Figs. 12-14 and 12-15).

FIGURE 12-16 Stain precipitate.

Unlike a malarial parasite, which typically appears as a blue cytoplasm with a red chromatin, clumped or fused platelets appear in various shades of purple. In addition, malarial parasites possess a more definite outline than clumped or fused platelets.

> **Quick Quiz! 12-6**
>
> The major feature that distinguishes starch cells from protozoan cysts is which of the following? (Objective 12-1)
> A. Presence of bacteria in the cytoplasm
> B. Unusually large size
> C. Shape
> D. Lack of defined internal structures

STAIN PRECIPITATE

Giemsa-stain precipitate may be visible on blood smears and may be mistaken for malarial parasites (Fig. 12-16 and 12-17). Stain precipitate is usually bluer in color than malarial parasites and varies in size and shape.

RED CELL ABNORMALITIES

Red blood cell abnormalities, such as Howell-Jolly bodies or Cabot's rings, may be present on Giemsa-stained blood smears. These abnormalities may be easily distinguished from malarial parasites by their different staining characteristics.

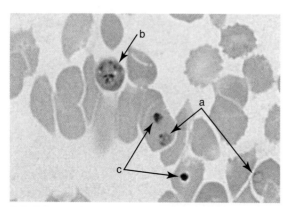

FIGURE 12-17 Giemsa stain, 1000x. Plasmodium faciparum ring form (a) and schizont (b) and stain precipitate (c).

   Quick Quiz! 12-7

Which of these characteristics distinguish(es) stain precipitate from malarial parasites? (Objective 12-1)
A. Color
B. Size
C. Shape
D. More than one: _____ (specify)

LOOKING BACK

Artifacts and confusers are defined as microscopic forms that resemble parasites but are not parasites. Therefore, it is important to screen all specimens carefully and take all features of suspicious microscopic forms seen into consideration before deciding on their final identity. One artifact in particular, Charcot-Leyden crystals, is of importance and should be reported when seen because they are indicative of an immune response that may or may not be caused by a parasitic infection. Especially careful screening should be completed before deciding that these specimens have no parasites present.

The most common artifacts are visually summarized and distinguished from true parasites at the end of this chapter in the three comparison drawings—protozoan look-alikes, malarial look-alikes, and helminth look-alikes.

TEST YOUR KNOWLEDGE!

12-1. Match the following artifacts or confusers (column A) with the appropriate parasite (column B). (Objective 12-1)

Column A

____ **A.** Yeast
____ **B.** Vegetable cells
____ **C.** Macrophages
____ **D.** Clumped platelets
____ **E.** Vegetable spirals
____ **F.** White blood cells
____ **G.** Pollen grains

Column B

1. *Taenia* spp. eggs
2. Malarial parasites
3. *Entamoeba histolytica* cysts
4. Helminth larvae
5. *Entamoeba histolytica* trophozoites
6. Helminth eggs
7. *Entamoeba hartmanni* cysts

12-2. When examining a sputum specimen, you notice the presence of diamond shaped crystals. What are these crystals called? Which clinical condition should be suspected when these crystals are observed? (Objective 11-2)

12-3. When examining a specimen for parasites, it appears that there are helminth larvae present. However, it is difficult to discern whether they are helminth larvae or a confuser, such as plant hair. Which of the following findings substantiates that it is plant hair? (Objective 12-1)
A. Presence of head or tail region
B. Buccal cavity
C. Nondescript internal structure
D. Intestine

12-4. When examining a specimen, you think that you have identified amebic trophozoites; however, the structures also look similar to epithelial cells. Describe how to differentiate the possible parasites from epithelial cells. (Objective 12-1)

12-5. Which of the following confusers may cause difficulties when identifying *E. hartmanni* or *E. nana*? (Objective 12-1)
A. Epithelial cells
B. Plant material
C. Vegetable cells
D. Starch cells

12-6. List the artifacts or confusers that may be confused with malarial parasites. (Objective 12-1)

COMPARISON DRAWINGS
Protozoan Look-Alikes

Parasites	**Look-Alikes**

Parasites

FIGURE 3-5A. Entamoeba histolytica cyst

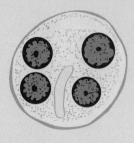

Size range: 8-22 μm
Average size: 12-18 μm

FIGURE 3-8. Entamoeba hartmanni cyst

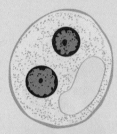

Size range: 5-12 μm
Average size: 7-9 μm

FIGURE 3-15. Endolimax nana cyst

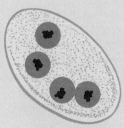

Size range: 4-12 μm
Average size: 7-10 μm

Look-Alikes

FIGURE 12-2. White blood cells

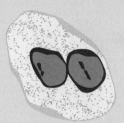

Average size: 15 μm

FIGURE 12-8. Budding yeast

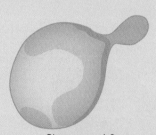

Size range: 4-8 μm

FIGURE 12-13. Starch cells

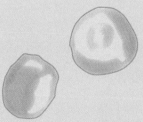

Average size: less than 10 μm

Continued

COMPARISON DRAWINGS
Protozoan Look-Alikes—cont'd

Parasites

FIGURE 3-2A. Entamoeba histolytica trophozoite

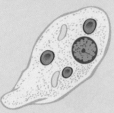

Size range: 8-65 μm
Average size: 12-25 μm

Look-Alikes

FIGURE 12-11. Epithelial cell

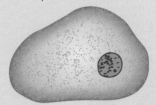

COMPARISON DRAWINGS
Malarial Look-Alikes

Parasites

FIGURE 6-4D. *Plasmodium ovale* (mature schizont)

Mature schizont

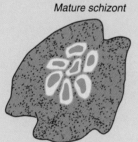

FIGURE 6-2A, B. *Plasmodium vivax* (ring for m and developing trophozoite)

Ring form
(early trophozoite)

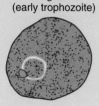

Developing trophozoite

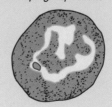

Look-Alikes

FIGURE 12-14. Clumped or fused platelets

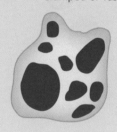

FIGURE 12-16. Stain precipitate

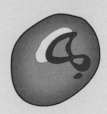

COMPARISON DRAWINGS
Helminth Look-Alikes

Parasites	**Look-Alikes**

Parasites

FIGURE 10-2A. *Taenia* spp. egg.

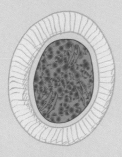

Size range: 28-40 μm by 18-30 μm
Average length: 33 μm by 23 μm

FIGURES 8-6A, 8-7A, and 8-8. Ascaris lumbricoides eggs

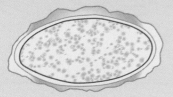

Size range: 85-95 μm by 38-45 μm

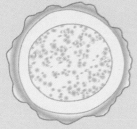

Size range: 40-75 μm by 30-50 μm

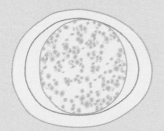

Size range: 40-75 μm by 30-50 μm

Look-Alikes

FIGURE 12-3. Pollen grain

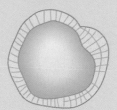

Size range: 12-20 μm

FIGURE 12-4. Vegetable cells

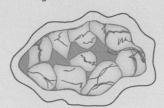

Average size: up to 150 μm

FIGURE 12-10. Plant material

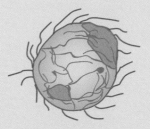

Size range: 12-150 μm in diameter

Continued

COMPARISON DRAWINGS
Helminth Look-Alikes—cont'd

Parasites	Look-Alikes

Parasites

FIGURE 8-13. Hookworm filariform larva

Look-Alikes

FIGURE 12-5. Vegetable spiral

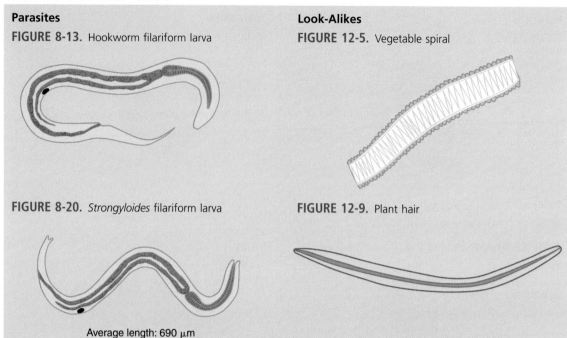

FIGURE 8-20. *Strongyloides* filariform larva

FIGURE 12-9. Plant hair

Average length: 690 μm

The Arthropods

Janice Conway-Klaassen and Elizabeth Zeibig

WHAT'S AHEAD

Focusing In
Morphology and Life Cycle
  Notes
Laboratory Diagnosis
Arthropod-Human
  Relationships
Pathogenesis and Clinical
  Symptoms

Treatment
Prevention and Control
Arthropod Classification
  Ticks
  Mites
  Spiders
  Scorpions
  Fleas

Flies
Lice
Mosquitoes
Bugs
Looking Back

LEARNING OBJECTIVES

*On completion of this chapter and review
of its figures, tables, and corresponding
photomicrographs, the successful learner will be
able to:*

13-1. Define the following key terms:
  Capitulum
  Chitinized exoskeleton
  Ectoparasite (*pl.*, ectoparasites)
  Excrement
  Genal ctenidia
  Hemocele
  Infestation
  Larva (*pl.*, larvae)
  Metamorphosis
  Myiasis (*pl.*, myiases)
  Nymph (*pl.*, nymphs)
  Pediculosis
  Pronotal ctenidia
  Pupa (*pl.*, pupae)
  Pupal
  Scutum
  Vertical transmission
13-2. State the three distinguishing
  characteristics common to all arthropods.

13-3. Classify the arthropods discussed in this
  chapter by phylum and class.
13-4. Describe the primary laboratory diagnosis
  technique used to identify the arthropods.
13-5. Describe the distinguishing characteristics
  of each arthropod discussed.
13-6. Briefly describe each arthropod life cycle
  and which portions affect humans.
13-7. State the general geographic distribution
  of each arthropod discussed.
13-8. Match the parasite(s) and other
  microorganisms studied with their
  corresponding arthropod vector.
13-9. Briefly identify the populations at risk for
  complications from and the clinical
  symptoms and associated diseases and
  conditions relevant to the presence of each
  arthropod studied.
13-10. Identify and describe treatment,
  prevention, and control measures for each
  arthropod discussed.
13-11. Provide the common and scientific names
  for the arthropods discussed in this
  chapter.

13-12. Given a case study, including pertinent patient information and laboratory data, correctly name the arthropod responsible.
13-13. Given prepared laboratory specimens, and with the assistance of this manual, the student will be able to identify and differentiate the arthropods discussed in this chapter based on their key characteristics.

CASE STUDY 13-1   UNDER THE MICROSCOPE

Ed and Sue went for a romantic walk in a heavily wooded area. After completing their excursion, Sue looked down at her watch to check the time and noticed a small black object partially buried under her skin on her right forearm. The area had already become red and irritated. Ed drove her home immediately, where he attempted to remove the unwelcomed guest with a pair of tweezers. Thinking that this procedure was successful, Ed bandaged the area.

Sue went about her business for the next couple of days convinced that it was gone. However, every time she changed the bandage, she noticed that the site was still red and irritated. She chose to ignore it, thinking that it would get better soon. Several days later, when Sue removed the bandage to change it, the irritated site showed signs of edema and was bleeding. She immediately went to her physician and showed him the infected area. On questioning by her physician, Sue explained the events leading up to the initial symptoms. The physician, now suspicious of the presence of a parasite in the wound, made a small incision and removed the mouthpiece of the organism. The entire parasite responsible for Sue's discomfort is shown in the diagram.

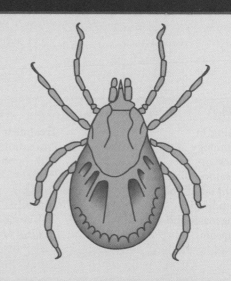

Questions and Issues for Consideration
1. Which parasite is suspected? (Objective 13-12)
2. What types of adult forms can be seen with this parasite? (Objective 13-6)
3. Name one method of prevention of infection with this parasite. (Objective 13-10)
4. Name at least two types of diseases that are notably transmitted by this organism. (Objective 13-9)

FOCUSING IN

Members of the phylum Arthropoda that affect humans as ectoparasites consist of a group of arthropods known as arachnids, including ticks, mites, spiders, and scorpions, and insects, including fleas, flies, lice, mosquitoes, and bugs. There are over four times as many species of arthropods as there are species in the remainder of the entire animal kingdom. Arthropods are of particular interest to parasitologists because they are responsible for the transmission of parasites, bacteria, viruses, and rickettsial organisms, as well as directly causing disease in humans. This chapter introduces the reader to what some might consider the most commonly encountered arthropods of interest that relate to human parasitology. It is important to note that the organization and structure of this chapter vary somewhat from that of the other parasite chapters.

MORPHOLOGY AND LIFE CYCLE NOTES

At some time in their life cycle, every arthropod shows each of the following three distinguishing characteristics: (1) pairs of jointed appendages;

(2) a **chitinized exoskeleton** (defined as a structure on the outside of an arthropod body composed of an insoluble polysaccharide that provides support for corresponding internal organs); and (3) a system of blood-containing spaces present on the body of an arthropod referred to as a **hemocele**. Other general arthropod characteristics include bilateral symmetry; often, more than one life stage is involved in human interaction. The specific morphologic forms and life cycle phases vary among the arthropods discussed in this chapter and are covered on an individual basis.

LABORATORY DIAGNOSIS

Although **ectoparasites** (parasites established in or on the exterior of the body) can be examined directly, it may be helpful to immerse them completely in 70% ethanol as a preservative. Flying insects may require inactivation with chloroform or ether before immersion in alcohol. This alcohol solution will maintain the morphology and color until examined. Samples may also be placed in 5% formalin or sterile saline solution. Some arthropods may discolor after a few days in formalin and sterile saline will not prevent eventual decomposition. Berlese's medium can be used as a permanent method to kill and fix specimens.

Although most of the arthropods in this chapter are directly visible, some stages are extremely small and microscopic examination is necessary to discern specific features. Arthropods may be diagnosed by placing them on a glass slide and examining them under the microscope or dissecting microscope. The distinguishing arthropod morphology characteristics necessary for identification are usually readily recognized on examination.

The laboratory diagnostic techniques described here basically apply to the identification of all the arthropods in this chapter, thus eliminating the need for individual laboratory diagnosis section discussions. Readers may refer back to this section for laboratory diagnosis information.

> ### Quick Quiz! 13-1
>
> All arthropods possess a hemocele at some point in their life cycle. (Objective 13-6)
> A. True
> B. False
> C. Unable to determine

ARTHROPOD-HUMAN RELATIONSHIPS

Arthropods may affect humans in various ways. They may take up residence as temporary or permanent occupants of their human host or they may cause the disease themselves. Arthropods may also transmit disease as mechanical transfer agents, such as house flies or cockroaches transmitting bacteria that cause enteric diseases (e.g., typhoid, cholera). Some arthropods are an actual part of the parasite's life cycle and are involved in direct transmission via blood meals or excrement contamination of bite wounds (e.g., ticks, mosquitoes, kissing bugs). Other arthropods such as lice or mites cause disease directly through living and growing in or on the skin or hair of their host (**infestation**). Finally, some arthropods affect humans by injecting venom during a bite (e.g., spiders, scorpions).

PATHOGENESIS AND CLINICAL SYMPTOMS

There are two mechanisms through which arthropods may cause clinical symptoms to occur. Patients who have been bitten by or infested with arthropods may exhibit symptoms related solely to the bite itself or the presence of these arthropods. In addition to these symptoms, patients who contract a disease from the arthropod will also present with symptoms relating to the invasion of the specific pathogenic microorganism transferred by the arthropod to the human. Because the clinical symptoms for each parasite studied have been noted in earlier chapters, only those symptoms associated with the arthropod itself will be discussed in this chapter.

Quick Quiz! 13-2

Arthropods that live in or on human skin are referred to as which of the following? (Objective 13-1)
A. Larvae
B. Pronotal ctenidia
C. Ectoparasites
D. Pupae

TREATMENT

Topical lotions or ointments are available for the treatment of arthropod bites. Treatment of ectoparasite infestations requires the removal of the arthropod from the skin. Additional treatment regimens are also required for patients who contract a disease from an arthropod. As with clinical symptoms, specific treatments for parasitic infections have been discussed elsewhere in this text and will not be repeated in this chapter. The treatment of arthropod bites and infestations will, however, be briefly discussed and individually noted in this chapter.

PREVENTION AND CONTROL

Complete eradication of arthropods is almost impossible. It is essential to know the geographic distribution and life cycles of the arthropod, and the disease it carries, as well as their environmental reservoirs and the diseases that these may transmit. Some arthropods can transmit the microorganism they carry to their offspring, a process known as **vertical transmission**, creating a permanent reservoir in the environment and making the disease more difficult to contain. Although chemical sprays and insecticides are available, they are often not financially feasible or physically possible to distribute over vast areas. In addition, many species of arthropods have adapted to commonly used chemicals, becoming resistant and surviving after chemical spray contact. There is also concern that chemical sprays and insecticides may harm the environment. Other potential control measures include the destruction of arthropod breeding grounds, increasing natural predators, and the

use of protective clothing and arthropod repellents, when appropriate, to prevent exposure.

Quick Quiz! 13-3

Vertical transmission occurs when an arthropod does which of the following? (Objective 13-1)
A. Bites a unsuspecting human
B. Ingests human blood
C. Passes infective agents to offspring
D. Comes in contact with insecticides

ARTHROPOD CLASSIFICATION

The phylum Arthropoda contains five classes of medically significant arthropods (Fig. 13-1). Although members of each of these arthropod classes are shown in this figure, only the most common organisms will be discussed in this chapter—those belonging to the class Arachnida (e.g., ticks, mites, spiders, scorpions) and class Insecta (e.g., fleas, flies, lice, mosquitoes, bugs). An in-depth study of all the arthropods is beyond the scope of this text. Readers interested in arthropods other than those described here are encouraged to review the Bibliography located at the end of this text (Appendix E).

Ticks

Morphology

Adult ticks, like all arachnids, characteristically have four pairs of legs, two pairs of mouth parts, and no antennae (Fig. 13-2; Table 13-1). Ticks are of the order Ixodida, which contains the family Ixodidae (hard body) and the family Argasidae (soft body) ticks. Both types of ticks are somewhat oval in shape. The head, thorax, and abdominal regions are meshed together and appear as a single structure. Ticks have four pairs of legs and lack antennae and a head region. Sexes are separate.

There are two major morphologic differences between hard and soft ticks. Both types of ticks have an anterior **capitulum**, an umbrella term referring to the mouthparts of ticks and mites. This

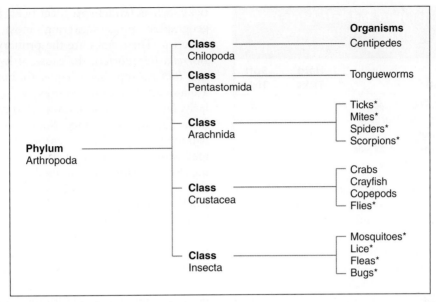

	Class	Organisms
	Class Chilopoda	Centipedes
	Class Pentastomida	Tongueworms
	Class Arachnida	Ticks* Mites* Spiders* Scorpions*
Phylum Arthropoda	Class Crustacea	Crabs Crayfish Copepods Flies*
	Class Insecta	Mosquitoes* Lice* Fleas* Bugs*

*Discussed in chapter.

FIGURE 13-1 Arthropod classification.

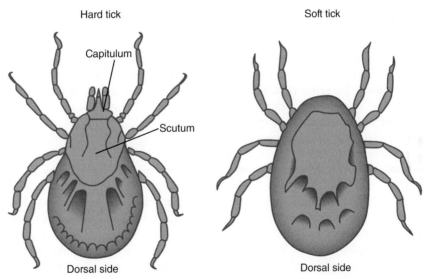

Hard tick

Capitulum

Scutum

Dorsal side

Soft tick

Dorsal side

FIGURE 13-2 Comparison of adult hard and soft ticks.

structure is visible on the dorsal side of hard ticks, but it is invisible on the dorsal side of soft ticks because of its ventral positioning. Located posterior to the capitulum on hard ticks is a dorsal hard shield known as a **scutum**. Soft ticks lack this structure and have, instead, a leathery outer surface. The typical tick ranges in size from 6 to 8 mm long.

Life Cycle Notes

Ticks are ectoparasites whose life cycles contain four morphologic stages—eggs, **larvae** (defined as juvenile stage), **nymphs** (defined as a developmental stage that resembles that of an adult), and adults of separate sexes. The life cycle typical

TABLE 13-1	Hard and Soft Adult Ticks: Typical Features at a Glance	
Characteristic	**Hard Ticks**	**Soft Ticks**
Fused spherical body (head, thorax, abdomen together)	X	X
Four pairs of legs	X	X
Visible capitulum on dorsal side	X	
Capitulum on ventral side		X
Scutum	X	

ranges from 1 to 2 years, depending on the hatch season. Ticks can also pass many microorganisms to their offspring, resulting in a renewable source of the infectious agent. The tick eggs develop and hatch on the ground. Motile larvae emerge from the eggs and migrate to sites such as blades of grass and twigs. The larvae eagerly jump onto the first viable host that passes by. Once on the host, the larvae feed via a blood meal for a few days, fall off the host and back to the ground, and molt into nymphs. These eight-legged nymphs once again migrate to potential host-passing sites and wait for another host. After attaching to a second host, the nymphs repeat the same process that they underwent in their larval stage. After falling onto the ground the second time, the nymphs molt and transform into adult ticks. It is interesting to note here that a tick completes a blood meal by making a cut into the host epidermis using a toothed structure near their mouth called a hypstome. The blood obtained during this process does not clot due to the presence of an anticoagulant in the tick's salivary gland. As the tick feeds, its body expands. Hard ticks—in particular, members of the Ixodidae family—only feed once as adults. Adult soft ticks, however, feed repeatedly. Following mating, eggs are deposited on the ground and the cycle repeats itself.

Epidemiology and Geography

Ticks are found throughout the world, including the United States and Mexico. In addition to select parasites, hard ticks are responsible for transmitting bacterial, viral, and rickettsial diseases. Hard ticks such as *Ixodes* spp. (deer ticks) have a wide geographic range covering most of North America. These ticks are the primary vector for *Borrelia burgdorferi*, the cause of Lyme disease, and *Babesia* spp. (see Chapter 6), both of which are noted for being found in New England. Similarly, *Dermacentor* spp. (dog ticks) can be found from the eastern United States to the Rocky Mountain range. *Dermacentor* ticks are associated with a number of rickettsial diseases, including Rocky Mountain spotted fever. Although concentrated in the southern states east of the Rocky Mountains, *Amblyomma americanum* (lone star tick) can also be found in the Mid-Atlantic states. *Amblyomma* ticks are the vector for human ehrlichiosis. Soft ticks belong to the genus *Ornithodorus* are primarily responsible for transmitting *Borrelia* spp., which causes relapsing fever. Different species of *Ornithodorus* are found in different geographic ranges within the United States and Canada. The *Borrelia* spp. that these ticks transmit are usually given the same species name as the tick; for example, *Ornithodoros hermsi* is found primarily in the northwestern United States and Canada and transmits *Borrelia hermsii*, whereas *Ornithodoros turicata* is the primary soft tick species found in the southwestern and midwestern states.

Clinical Symptoms

Patients infected with ticks often exhibit skin reactions to the bite site, including inflammatory infiltration of tissues, edema, local hyperemia, and hemorrhage. Additional potentially severe tissue reactions and secondary infections may occur when the mouth parts of a tick remain in the skin after attempting to remove the entire tick. Tick paralysis may occur when the salivary secretions of certain tick species (*Dermacentor*) are introduced into the host. A toxemia results and, if the tick is not readily removed, death may result.

Treatment

The recommended therapy for tick infestation consists of removal of the tick. This may be accomplished by placing a few drops of ether or chloroform on the head of a tick and pulling the tick straight out of the skin, grasping the anterior portion with forceps. It is important to remove the entire tick. Mouth parts left behind may be the source of severe tissue reactions and secondary infection.

Prevention and Control

Total tick eradication is difficult, but there are several measures that can be taken to decrease the chance of becoming infected. The avoidance of entering tick-infested areas is advisable but, if one must be in such areas, protective clothing and tick repellents are essential. A prophylactic vaccination has been developed to help protect individuals from deadly rickettsial infections transmitted by ticks. Because transfer of the infectious agents from tick bites may take hours to days, ticks should be carefully removed as soon as possible to interfere with disease transfer.

 Quick Quiz! 13-4

The morphologic form in the tick life cycle that most closely resembles an adult is which of the following? (Objective 13-1)

A. Cysts
B. Eggs
C. Larvae
D. Nymphs

 Quick Quiz! 13-5

Ixodes ticks (deer ticks) can be found throughout the United States. Those in the New England area may be responsible for transmitting which of the following diseases? (Objectives 13-7 and 13-8)

1. Malaria
2. Babesia
3. Trypanosomiasis
4. Lyme disease
    A. 1, 2, and 3 are correct
    B. 1 and 3 are correct
    C. 2 and 4 are correct
    D. Only 4 is correct
    E. None are correct

 Quick Quiz! 13-6

The presence of which of these tick anatomic parts in human skin is known to be responsible for severe tissue reactions and secondary infections? (Objective 13-9)

A. Legs
B. Mouthparts
C. Antennae
D. Wings

Mites

Morphology

Mites are extremely small, but still visible to the naked eye (Figs. 13-3 to 13-5; Table 13-2). Regardless of species, they range from 0.1 to 0.4 mm in size and are oval in shape. Microscopic examination is required to confirm their identification in a specimen.

Life Cycle Notes

Adult mites that infest humans (or other animals) burrow into the skin, hair follicles, or sebaceous glands of hosts and set up residence. They lay their eggs in the burrow, which eventually hatch

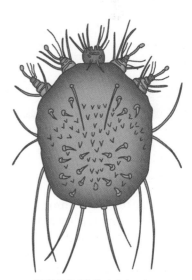

FIGURE 13-3 Adult mite.

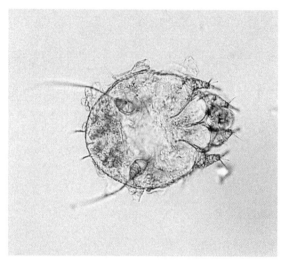

FIGURE 13-4 Adult *Sarcoptes scabiei* (itch mite); (fresh preparation, saline suspension, ×200).

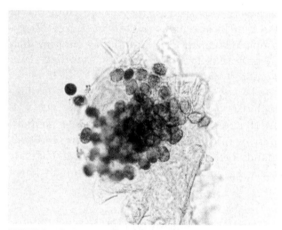

FIGURE 13-5 *Sarcoptes scabiei* (itch mite) eggs (fresh preparation, saline suspension, ×200).

TABLE 13-2	Adult Mites: Typical Features at a Glance
Parameter	**Description**
Size	0.1-0.4 mm
Shape	Oval

and mature from the larval through the nymph stage and to adult forms, all within the tunnels made by the original adult mite. Newly developed mites can then begin new burrows and continue the spread of the infestation. The life cycle takes approximately 2 weeks from egg to adult stage. Transfer from one person to another usually requires prolonged close contact, such as with household members or sexual partners, but it may also spread rapidly in overcrowded conditions such as in institutional care facilities, homeless shelters, hospitals, and refugee camps.

Epidemiology and Geography

Mites are ubiquitous in the environment, with a worldwide distribution. Mites have two different ways of affecting human hosts. Some mites cause disease directly by infesting their host and causing reactions within the skin. *Sarcoptes scabiei*, the human itch or mange mite, which causes the highly transmissible disease scabies, and *Demodex folliculorum*, the hair follicle mite, work in this way. Other mites can be carriers of rickettsial or viral diseases, transferring disease through their bite. *Trombicula akamushi*, found in Japan and the Far East, is the mite that carries scrub typhus, and *Liponyssus bacoti* (rat mite) may be a carrier of endemic typhus, rickettsial pox, and Q fever. In addition free-living mites such as house mites, *Dermatophagoides* spp., may be the cause of allergic respiratory reactions in some individuals throughout the world.

Clinical Symptoms

In many cases in which the mites do not establish long-term residency in the host, there may be little if any reaction to their presence; however, they may eventually show signs and symptoms of the microorganism that was transmitted through the mite. For itch mites, initial symptoms are minimal but, after the infestation spreads, pimple-like lesions appear on the skin where a burrow exists and intense itching begins. This is most typical for the scabies mite, *S. scabiei*. While these mites are infesting the host, there is an accumulation of fecal material and other secretions in the burrows, which generally causes a severe local pruritis and sometimes hair loss in the area of infestation.

Treatment

There are several prescription creams and lotions that can be used to treat mite infestations. It is also important to clean and disinfect clothing, bedding, and towels thoroughly by washing in hot water and drying in a hot clothes dryer.

Prevention and Control

Prevention and control are usually a concern after the fact. Because mites are ubiquitous, it is almost impossible to prevent contact unless there is an individual who is known to be infested. The focus is to prevent the spread to unaffected individuals and to prevent reinfestation of the initial case. This includes making sure that all clothing, bedding, and towels are washed in hot water and dried in a hot clothes dryer. If clothes cannot be washed right away, placing them in a plastic bag will prevent mites from spreading and finding another meal source. They will die within a few weeks without feeding, but this method should not be relied on to prevent their spread.

Quick Quiz! 13-7

The typically mite evolves from eggs to adults in this time frame. (Objective 13-6)

A. 2 days
B. 2 weeks
C. 2 months
D. 2 years

Quick Quiz! 13-8

Which of the following genera contain the organisms responsible for the disease scabies caused by the itch mite? (Objective 13-8 and 13-11)

A. *Sarcoptes* spp.
B. *Pediculus* spp.
C. *Ornithodorus* spp.
D. *Dermatophagoides* spp.

Quick Quiz! 13-9

The best way to remove mites from infected clothing and linens is to do which of the following? (Objective 13-10)

A. Wash in cold water; fluff dry.
B. Wash in warm water; fluff dry.
C. Wash in warm water; dry at medium heat.
D. Wash in hot water; dry at high heat.

Spiders

Morphology

Most people easily recognize the typical spider morphology (Fig. 13-6; Table 13-3). Spiders are found worldwide but only a few inflict damage through a venomous bite. The three species that may be found in the United States include the black widow (*Latrodectus mactans*), brown recluse (*Loxosceles reclusa*), and hobo (*Tegenaria agrestis*) spiders. The black widow spider is so-named because it is the female with the venomous bite who may kill the male after mating. Both male and female black widow spiders have a shiny black surface. The female is larger than the male and has the diagnostic red hourglass shape on the underside of her abdomen. Their webs are described as atypical or chaotic because

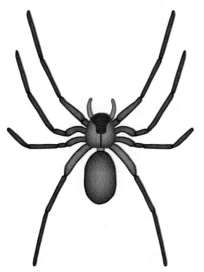

FIGURE 13-6 Adult spider.

TABLE 13-3	Adult Spiders: Typical Features at a Glance
Parameter	**Description**
Black widow spiders	Males and females have shiny black surface
	Females larger than males
	Females have diagnostic red hourglass shape on underside
	Males and females spin atypical or chaotic webs
	Males and females most active at night
Brown recluse spiders	Exhibit reclusive behavior
	Often hide in clothing or bedding
	Only bite when threatened
	Have trademark brown violin shape seen on the cephalothorax
Hobo spiders	Have muted, nondistinct, brown earth color
	Spin distinctive funnel-shaped web

there is no particular pattern or design. These spiders tend to be more active at night, with the female hanging upside down in her web, making the hourglass readily visible. Brown recluse spiders are so-named because of their reclusive behavior. They tend to hide in clothing or bedding and bite only when threatened. In addition, the trademark brown violin shape can be seen on the cephalothorax (i.e., the fused head and thorax section of the body). Hobo spiders belong to a class of spiders that creates a distinctive funnel-shaped web. These spiders have a muted, nondistinct brown earth color.

Life Cycle notes

The life cycle of spiders is less complicated than that of mites or ticks. After mating, the female spider generates an egg sack from which as many as 200 new spiders may hatch as miniature versions of the adults. As they mature, they increase in size to the adult level.

Epidemiology and Geography

Human interaction with the arachnids in this section is through a venomous bite and subsequent wound and reaction to the venom. These spiders are by nature not aggressive but will bite when provoked or disturbed. The black widow spider is found throughout the United States, with different species names for variants found in different geographic regions. The brown recluse spider is primarily found in the central United States, with high populations in Oklahoma, Arkansas, and Missouri. The hobo spider is a resident of the Pacific Northwest and western Canada.

Clinical Symptoms

All these spiders can cause a very painful bite, with a secondary reaction to the venom that is simultaneously injected. The black widow spider is considered the most venomous spider in North America but its bite rarely causes a fatality because so little venom is injected. A severe stabbing pain at the bite site may be followed by spreading of the pain, eventually creating nausea, fever, severe abdominal cramping, and excessive sweating. The brown recluse spider bite may produce a necrotizing wound; the size of the wound depends on the amount of venom that was injected, the body site location, and the immune status of the individual. Most severe reactions are in children or those with a compromised immune system. Approximately 50% of hobo spider bites do not inject venom. Cutaneous necrosis that resembles that seen in brown recluse bites has been known to result from that of a hobo spider. In some instances, the healing process takes years. Occasionally the condition from such bites worsens and evolves into systemic symptoms. For those cases in which venom is injected, the reaction usually remains localized, with a blister developing over 24 hours. This blister eventual ulcerates and healing scabs form in approximately 3 weeks.

Treatment

To treat a bite by a black widow spider, antivenin can be given to those with compromised immune systems, underlying heart conditions, or other health problems and to older adults. A hospital stay may also be required to monitor heart conditions. Antivenin for the bite of the brown recluse spider is not readily available and treatment primarily consists of palliative care, pain management, and general wound care until the site heals. Occasionally, surgical intervention may be needed for débridement of necrotic tissue. Bites by the hobo spider usually only require simple wound care to prevent secondary bacterial infections.

Prevention and Control

Prevention of venomous spider bites is a matter of minimizing places where they can hide and breed, as well as exercising caution when dealing with potential exposure locations (e.g., wood piles). Pesticides can be used around dwellings but are not always effective. Sealing holes in exterior walls where plumbing pipes and electrical wires enter a home is essential for preventing their access to inside living spaces. Minimizing clutter outside but adjacent to the home will minimize their tendency to build webs close by.

Quick Quiz! 13-10

Which type of spider is noted for its tendency to remain out of plain sight? (Objective 13-5)
A. Brown recluse
B. Hobo
C. Black widow

Quick Quiz! 13-11

The most venomous spider in North America is which of the following? (Objective 13-5)
A. Brown recluse
B. Hobo
C. Black widow

Quick Quiz! 13-12

Antivenin is a possible treatment for older adults who have encountered which of these spider(s)? (Objective 13-10)
A. Brown recluse
B. Hobo
C. Black widow
D. More than one: _____ (specify)

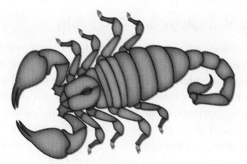

FIGURE 13-7 Adult scorpion.

TABLE 13-4	Adult Scorpions: Typical Features at a Glance
Parameter	**Description**
Body	Combined cephalothorax and elongated abdominal section that ends in up-curved tail
	Final segment in tail contains stinger and venom sac
Legs	Four pairs; first set is enlarged, with clawlike pincers to hold prey

Scorpions

Morphology

Scorpions have a distinctive body shape, with a combined cephalothorax and an elongated abdominal section that ends in an up-curved tail (Fig. 13-7; Table 13-4). Adults may reach 4 inches in length. The final segment in the tail contains a stinger and venom sac. Like all arachnids, scorpions have four pairs of legs, but their first set is enlarged, with clawlike pincers to hold prey.

Life Cycle notes

Like spiders, young scorpions are simply smaller versions of the adult. Young develop in the female's ovariuterus. After birth, the brood rides on the mother's back until the first molting, at approximately 2 weeks of age. They do not change morphology but undergo six moltings, increasing in size with each molt. The life span varies by species from 4 to 25 years.

Epidemiology and Geography

Scorpions can be found throughout the world, except for New Zealand and Antarctica, but are more prevalent in tropical and subtropical climates. Many species are found in the United States, primarily in the southern and western states. They are most common in the desert Southwest. Two species are of medical concern because their venom can have potentially lethal effects—*Hadrurus* spp. (desert hairy scorpion) and *Centruroides* spp. (bark scorpion).

Clinical Symptoms

The venom of scorpions is classified as a neurotoxin, which is used to paralyzes its prey. In addition to symptoms associated directly with the action of the toxin, some individuals may display an allergic reaction to the venom, which could lead to anaphylaxis and death. Most scorpions are not able to inject enough venom to kill a healthy adult human, but older adults, very young children and infants, and those who are immunocompromised are at risk. The sting site will become painful and swollen; there may be a tingling or numbing sensation. In the most severe cases, hypertension, pulmonary edema, and cardiac arrhythmia may result.

Treatment

Most hospital emergency rooms in desert cities in the Southwest (e.g., Phoenix, Tucson, Las Vegas) carry scorpion antivenin, which can treat at-risk patients or those displaying an intense systemic reaction. Supportive therapy, pain management, and medication to control anaphylaxis may also be needed.

Prevention and Control

Similar to prevention and control measures for spiders, prevention of a human scorpion sting is a matter of minimizing places where they can hide and breed. Pesticides can be used around dwellings but are not always effective. Sealing holes in exterior walls where plumbing pipes and electrical wires enter a home is essential for preventing their access to inside living spaces.

Quick Quiz! 13-13

Unlike the other arachnids discussed in this chapter, scorpions are equipped with a designated pair of clawlike legs used to hold their prey. (Objective 13-5)
A. True
B. False
C. Unable to determine

Quick Quiz! 13-14

With each molting, developing scorpions change morphologically and increase in size. (Objective 13-6)
A. True
B. False
C. Unable to determine

Quick Quiz! 13-15

Healthy individuals are at the greatest risk of developing serious complications following the bite of a scorpion. (Objective 13-9)
A. True
B. False
C. Unable to determine

Fleas

Morphology

Fleas range in size from 1.3 to 4 mm (Fig. 13-8; Table 13-5). Fleas are equipped with three pairs of powerful hairy legs and clawlike feet. These features, plus the fact that the rear pair of legs is extra long, allow fleas to move about quickly by jumping. Their compact segmented bodies enable them to migrate through the feathers or hairs of their hosts. The mouth parts of fleas are designed for piercing and blood sucking. The presence or absence of eyes, comblike structures located above the mouth parts (called **genal ctenidia**), and

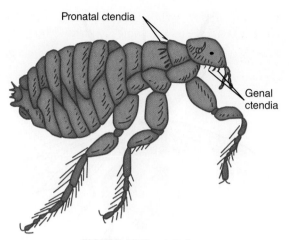

Pronatal ctendia

Genal
ctendia

FIGURE 13-8 Adult flea.

TABLE 13-5	Adult Fleas: Typical Features at a Glance
Parameter	**Description**
Size	1.3-4 mm
Mouth parts	Designed for piercing and blood sucking
Body	Compact and segmented
Legs	Three pairs; hairy with clawlike feet, back pair long for jumping

pronotal ctenidia, comblike structures located immediately behind the head and extending posteriorly on the flea's dorsal side, aid in the differentiation of the various species of fleas.

Life Cycle Notes

Flea eggs are deposited onto the ground or floor by the female adult following mating and feeding via a blood meal. Legless elongate larvae emerge following a 3- to 10-day incubation period. The actual incubation time varies, depending on environmental conditions, such as temperature and humidity. The larvae feed on organic debris. In addition, the **excrement** (feces) of adult fleas contains dried blood and serves as an additional food source for the developing larvae. Three larval phases follow. Mature third-stage larvae spin a cocoon and may remain in this **pupal** stage

for up to one year. Finally, adult fleas emerge from the cocoon and may survive for 1 year or longer. It is the adult form of the flea that is capable of serving as an ectoparasite by feeding on humans and other animals.

Epidemiology and Geography

Fleas are distributed worldwide. There are numerous species, some of which prefer tropical and subtropical regions. Fleas are responsible for transmitting the parasites *Dipylidium caninum*, *Hymenolepis nana*, and *Hymenolepis diminuta*, as well as rickettsial and bacterial diseases. For example, *Xenopsylla cheopis*, the Oriental rat flea, is the vector for *Yersinia pestis* (plague) as well as *Rickettsia typhi* (murine typhus). Between feedings, developing and adult fleas may be found on or in carpets, rugs, floors, pillows, and other household articles where dogs or cats lie. Adult fleas may reside on a variety of animals, including dogs, cats, and rodents.

Clinical Symptoms

The infestation of fleas may cause a variety of symptoms. Depending on the species, some patients with fleas remain asymptomatic, whereas others may experience intense itching, dermatitis, ulcerations, and nodular swellings at the bite site. The scratching of these itchy bites may result in secondary bacterial infection. Found in Central and South America and Africa, the chigoe flea causes a serious condition known as tungiasis. Initial contact with human hosts results in superficial tissue invasion. Human reaction to its presence in the form of inflammatory responses tyically occurs. Subsequent bacterial infection may lead to digit loss, tetanus or septicemia.

Treatment

The treatment of choice is to remove the fleas. This may be accomplished by aseptically removing them from the skin with a needle. Thorough cleaning and disinfecting of the bite site aid in preventing further discomfort to the patient.

Prevention and Control

Prevention and control measures include protecting cats and dogs from fleas. A variety of commercial products, including flea collars, powders, dips, and sprays, are available. More recently, lufenuron has been introduced, in liquid form for cats and in tablet form for dogs, as a monthly flea prevention and control medication. In addition, thorough disinfection of household articles that come into contact with dogs and cats is essential. Known flea breeding areas may be chemically treated. Fleas of rats and other rodents may be more difficult to control. Public awareness of fleas and their transmission routes, along with tips to hunters, outdoor enthusiasts, and outdoor workers, may aid in controlling the spread of fleas.

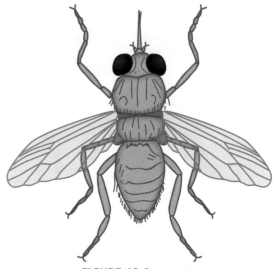

FIGURE 13-9 Adult fly.

Quick Quiz! 13-16

This distinguishing feature allows fleas to move quickly. (Objective 13-5)
A. Presence of pronotal ctenidia
B. Absence of eyes
C. Extra long rear pair of legs
D. A and C are correct

Quick Quiz! 13-17

The Oriental rat flea, *Xenopsylla cheopis*, can be involved in transmitting which of the following microorganisms? (Objective 13-8)
A. *Rickettsia typhi*
B. *Hymenolepis nana*
C. *Yersinia pestis*
D. *Plasmodium* spp.
E. A and C are correct

Quick Quiz! 13-18

The treatment of choice for flea infestations is which of the following? (Objective 13-10)
A. Topical antiflea cream
B. Prescription antiflea medication
C. Soaking infected area in hot, soapy water
D. Complete aseptic removal

TABLE 13-6	Adult Flies: Typical Features at a Glance
Parameter	**Description**
Size	1-15 mm long
Eyes	One pair
Antennae	One pair
Legs	Usually three pairs
Wings	Two pairs, one pair smaller
Body	Three separate sections—head, thorax, and segmented abdomen

Flies

Morphology

The typical fly may measure from 1 to 15 mm in length, depending on the species (Fig. 13-9; Tables 13-6). All fly species possess two pairs of wings; one pair is smaller than the other. In addition, the head, thorax, and abdomen appear as three separate sections. The abdomen is segmented, allowing for ease of movement. Flies have one pair of antennae and one pair of eyes. Three pairs of legs are the rule. The same specific features are used to speciate flies and mosquitoes (Table 13-7). A detailed discussion of each individual fly species is beyond the scope of this chapter.

TABLE 13-7	Key Features Used to Speciate Adult Flies and Adult Mosquitoes
Parameter	**Description**
Mouth parts	Presence or absence of hairs Number of segments
Antennae	Structures present for piercing of skin or sucking
Body	Size and shape as a whole Size and shape of head, thorax, and abdomen independent Color and distribution of hair
Wings	Pattern of veins

TABLE 13-8	Parasite-Transmitting Flies: Geographic Distribution and Associated Parasites	
Species	**Geographic Distribution**	**Associated Parasite**
Tsetse fly	Africa	*Trypanosoma rhodesiense* *Trypanosoma gambiense*
Sandfly	Asia, South America, Mexico, Central America, Africa, Mediterranean	*Leishmania* spp.
Black fly	Africa, Mexico, Central and South America	*Onchocerca volvulus*
Deer fly	Tropical Africa	*Loa loa*

Life Cycle Notes

Flies undergo complete transition from the developmental stage to a point at which each stage is morphologically different, a process known as **metamorphosis.** Fly larvae emerge from eggs. Fly life cycles typically contain multiple larval stages. The formation of a cocoon stage (known as a **pupa**) prior to becoming an adult is a standard occurrence in the fly life cycle. The specific life cycle of individual fly species may vary. The adult fly is capable of transmitting a variety of diseases, parasitic and bacterial, to humans through blood meals.

Epidemiology and Geography

Flies, in general, are found worldwide. Specific species of flies are more prevalent in certain regions than others. The geographic distribution of the common parasite-transmitting flies and the specific parasites involved are listed in Table 13-8.

Clinical Symptoms

Most flies affecting humans in the United States have been described as biting pests whose main function may be a concern only of sanitation. Flies can transmit various bacterial diseases

associated with enteritis caused by cross-contamination of exposed foods. They may also actively transmit specific parasites. Relatively few symptoms are associated with contact with the fly itself. An irritated and sometimes painful bite site has been described in some patients. Most of the symptoms seen are related to the parasite transmitted and not to the fly bite.

Myiasis refers to humen tissue infestation by fly larvae (often referred to as bot flies) found in Central and South America (*Dermatobia* spp.) and sub-Saharan Africa (*Cordylobia* spp.). Although primarily a problem for livestock, humans can be accidental hosts. Infection can occur after the female fly passes her eggs onto another flying insect, such as a mosquito. Accidental or opportunistic cases can occur when a female fly lands on a human host, particularly an individual with wounds or diseased tissues. The female fly takes advantage of such situations and deposits her eggs or larvae. When the mosquito bites an animal (or human) the eggs hatch and the larvae, often referred to as maggots, immediately penetrate the skin. Depending on the species of fly, the larvae (i.e., maggots) may inhabit the skin lesion for approximately 2 weeks before maturing (*Cordylobia* spp.) or 6 to 12 weeks

(*Dermatobia* spp). The skin lesion resembles a boil, with a small opening at the top. The patient may feel movement of the larval form within the lesion, which is usually pruritic and may also be painful.

Treatment

Treatment is often not necessary for a typical fly bite. Topical ointments are available to help reduce minor discomfort. Treatment for myiasis is complete excision of the lesion with treatment to prevent secondary bacterial infection.

Prevention and Control

Education regarding the fly's ability to transmit disease, wearing of protective clothing, use of screening, and use of insect repellents are essential to prevent and control the spread of disease via flies. Chemically treating fly breeding areas may also be helpful but is difficult to achieve successfully.

Quick Quiz! 13-19

Flies are identified and speciated based on which of the following characteristics? (Objective 13-5)
A. Two body sections, three pair of legs, one pair of antennae, two sets of wings
B. Three body sections, four pair of legs, one pair of antennae, two sets of wings
C. Two body sections, three pair of legs, no pair of antennae, no wings
D. Three body sections, three pair of legs, one pair of antennae, two sets of wings

Quick Quiz! 13-20

The process that flies undergo in development characterized by distinct larval stages is known as which of the following? (Objective 13-1)
A. Myiasis
B. Vertical transmission
C. Metamorphosis
D. Nymphosis

Quick Quiz! 13-21

The major symptom most often experienced by individuals who have been bitten by a fly is which of the following? (Objective 13-9)
A. Fever and chills
B. Allergic reaction
C. Irritated and painful bite site
D. Difficulty breathing

Lice

Morphology

Head and body lice (the singular form of lice is louse) are wingless ectoparasites that have three-segmented bodies consisting of a head, thorax, and abdomen (Figs. 13-10 and 13-11; Table 13-9). In general, lice are equipped with three pairs of legs with clawlike feet that extend from the thorax region. This feature allows lice to grasp body hair. A pair of antennae is located on the head of the typical louse. The louse head is narrower than the balance of its body. The mouth parts are well adapted for piercing the human skin and sucking blood. Both the head louse (*Pediculus humanus capitis*) and body louse (*Pediculus humanus humanus*) are hairless and appear long and narrow, measuring 2 to 3 mm long. The crab louse, *Phthirus pubis*, is smaller and plump, measuring up to 2 mm long, and contains hair over much of its extremities. The thorax and abdomen appear as one section.

Life Cycle Notes

Adult lice lay their eggs, also known as nits, on or very near their respective specific hosts. Head lice eggs may be found in the hair shafts of the head and neck, whereas body lice eggs are typically found in clothing fibers and occasionally on chest hairs. Pubic lice lay their eggs mainly in the pubic hair region. The young lice resemble their parents in appearance. It takes 24 to 27 days from the time the lice eggs are laid to pass through three nymph stages and transform into young adult lice. The typical adult louse lives for only 30 days.

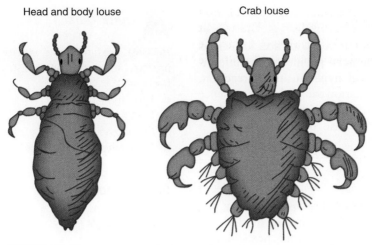

Head and body louse   Crab louse

FIGURE 13-10 Comparison of adult head and body louse with crab louse.

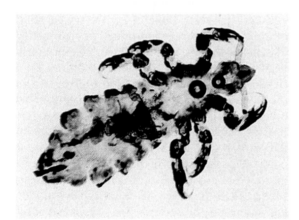

FIGURE 13-11 Adult body louse (fresh preparation, saline suspension, ×200).

TABLE 13-9	Adult Lice: Typical Features at a Glance
Parameter	**Description**
Size	Head and body lice, 2-3 mm long
	Crab lice, up to 2 mm long
Mouth parts	Adapted for piercing human skin and sucking blood
Body	Head and body lice, three segments—narrow head, thorax, abdomen
	Crab lice—plump; thorax and abdomen appear as one section
Legs	Three pairs extending from thorax with clawlike feet
Antennae	One pair
Hair	Head and body lice—absent
	Crab lice—present on extremities

Because they are sensitive to environmental changes, lice spend most of their lives feeding, via blood meals, on their respective hosts.

Epidemiology and Geography

Found worldwide, particularly in areas of poor personal and general hygiene, lice are most commonly transferred directly from person to person. Outbreaks among schoolchildren are known to occur when they share combs, scarves and hats. Further children, particularly those in day care, may bring the infestation home creating the opportunity for the lice to spread to family members. Lice have the ability to migrate from one host to another, with only slight person-to-person body contact. Crab lice are primarily transmitted through close personal contract, expecially during sexual intercourse. Infected clothing or other personal articles also serve as sources of possible head, body, and crab lice infections. In addition to being considered a nuisance in their own right, lice are capable of transmitting bacterial and rickettsial infections to humans (see Table 13-13).

Clinical Symptoms

Symptoms of an infestation with lice, known as **pediculosis**, include itchy papules at the infestation site and a local hypersensitivity reaction, followed by inflammation caused by the presence of lice saliva and fecal excretions. Secondary bacterial infections may also occur, resulting in a mangelike lesion.

Treatment

Successful treatment of lice must destroy the eggs and adults. The lice treatment of choice is the direct application of benzene hexachloride lotion.

Prevention and Control

Lice prevention and control measures include proper personal and general hygiene practices and prompt treatment of known lice infestations. In addition, the complete and thorough cleaning of all articles with which an infected person might have come into contact is essential for preventing further lice infestations.

Quick Quiz! 13-22

This type of louse is characterized by hair extremities. (Objective 13-5)
A. Head louse
B. Body louse
C. Crab louse
D. Foot louse

Quick Quiz! 13-23

The typical life span for adult lice is which of the following? (Objective 13-6)
A. 18 days
B. 24 days
C. 27 days
D. 30 days

Quick Quiz! 13-24

To treat lice infections successfully, which morphologic forms are necessary to destroy? (Objective 13-10)
A. Eggs and larvae
B. Eggs and adults
C. Larvae and adults
D. Eggs, larvae, and adults

Mosquitoes

Morphology

More than 3000 documented species of mosquitoes are known to exist (Fig. 13-12; Tables 13-10 and 13-11; also see Table 13-7). The typical adult mosquito has a three-segmented body consisting of a head, thorax, and abdomen. The roundish head is connected to the elongate thorax by a slender neck. The abdomen is also elongated in shape and is comprised of 10 segments of its own. Only eight of the abdominal segments are usually visible. Each of the single pair of antennae is long and has three segments. The three pairs of legs extend from the thorax region. Mosquitoes have two pairs of wings; one pair is smaller than the other. Mosquitoes vary in size, depending on the species. The *Anopheles* mosquito, for example, generally measures 6 to 8 mm long. The key characteristics used to differentiate the mosquito species, which are the same as those for identifying flies, are listed in Table 13-7. A detailed discussion of all mosquito species is beyond the scope of this chapter. A brief introduction to the mosquito, in general terms, is the focus of this section.

Life Cycle Notes

Adult mosquitoes lay their eggs in water or on a moist substance that eventually accumulates water. Young larvae hatch out of the eggs after an incubation period that varies with the individual species. Maturation transitions through four larval forms, resulting in the pupal form. The

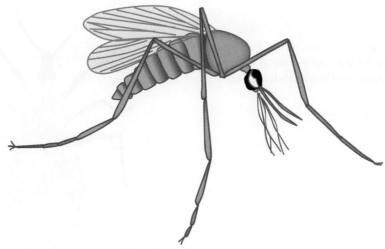

FIGURE 13-12 Adult mosquito.

TABLE 13-10	Adult Mosquitoes: Typical Features at a Glance
Parameter	**Description**
Body	Three segmented body consisting of head, thorax and abdomen
Head	Roundish in shape
Neck	Slender; connects head and thorax
Thorax	Elongate
Abdomen	Elongate, comprised of ten segments
Antennae	One pair: each is long, with three segments
Legs	Three pairs, extending from thorax region
Wings	Two pairs, one smaller than the other

TABLE 13-11	Parasite-Transmitting Geographic Distribution and Associated Parasites	
Genera	**Geographic Distribution**	**Associated Parasites**
Anopheles	Worldwide	*Plasmodium vivax* *Plasmodium ovale* *Plasmodium malariae* *Plasmodium falciparum*
Culex, Aedes, Anopheles	Worldwide, particularly the tropics, subtropics	*Wuchereria bancrofti*
Anopheles, Mansonia, Armigeres, Aedes	Parts of Asia and the South Pacific	*Brugia malayi*

pupa matures further and eventually an adult mosquito emerges. Adult mosquitoes are ecto-parasites that feed on humans via blood meals.

Epidemiology and Geography

Mosquitoes are found worldwide and are considered to be the most important group of pathogenic microorganism transmitters. In addition to carrying a number of parasites, mosquitoes are also responsible for the transmission of a variety of viruses. Areas of mosquito concentration include those in or near fresh or brackish water. The geographic distribution of the common disease-transmitting mosquitoes and specific diseases involved are listed in Table 13-11.

Clinical Symptoms

The most notable symptom of a mosquito bite is the emergence of an irritating dermatitis. Excessive scratching may also result in a secondary bacterial infection of the bite wound.

Treatment

Over-the-counter (OTC) lotions and ointments, such as calamine or Benadryl lotion, are available to relieve the itching associated with mosquito bites.

Prevention and Control

Mosquito prevention measures include the avoidance of areas of known mosquito concentration. When this is not possible, the use of insect repellents, wearing protective clothing, and using screens are recommended. The use of insecticide sprays over endemic areas may prove helpful in eradicating the mosquitoes, but this is not always financially and/or physically feasible. Further, elimination of areas of standing water and swampy areas have the potential of limiting mosquito breeding grounds and thus may decrease their population.

Quick Quiz! 13-25

The three segments of a mosquito are which of the following? (Objective 13-5)
A. Head, thorax, and abdomen
B. Thorax, abdomen, and pelvis
C. Head, neck, and thorax
D. Thorax, neck, and pelvis

Quick Quiz! 13-26

Which of the following mosquitoes are responsible for transmitting *Plasmodium* spp. parasites? (Objective 13-8)
A. *Culex* spp.
B. *Anopheles* spp.
C. *Aedes* spp.
D. *Armigeres* spp.

Quick Quiz! 13-27

For the mosquito life cycle to continue, these arthropods must lay their eggs in or near which of the following? (Objective 13-6)
A. Sand
B. Water
C. Rocks
D. Grass

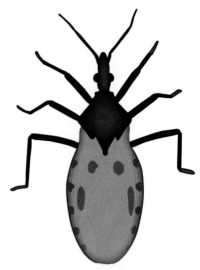

FIGURE 13-13 Adult triatomid bug.

TABLE 13-12	Adult Bugs: Typical Features at a Glance
Parameter	**Description**
Appearance	Varies; bedbugs have a reddish brown outer shell
Size	Varies; bedbugs may be up to 5 mm, whereas triatomid bugs are usually up to 4 cm in length
Legs	Three pairs; triatomid bugs and select cockroaches have fully developed wings in the adult stage
Wings	At some point in the life cycle; some wings may be vestigial

Bugs

Morphology

Because they belong to the Class Insecta, all bugs have three pairs of legs and typically have wings during certain stages of development, although some wings may be vestigial (i.e., not fully developed; Fig. 13-13; Table 13-12). Bedbugs are approximately 5 mm in length, with a reddish brown outer shell. Triatomid bugs are significantly larger, with adults up to 4 cm in length. The Triatomid bugs also have fully developed wings in the adult stage. Similarly, some species of cockroaches may have fully developed wings in the adult stage.

Life Cycle Notes

Most bugs go through a series of growth stages, with approximately six moltings from nymph to adult. Adult stages may or may not have fully developed wings.

Epidemiology and Geography

Cockroaches (order Blattaria) are primarily linked to human disease as mechanical carriers of filth. They are potential carriers of fecal pathogens since they are frequently known to move from sewers to food preparation areas. Cockroaches are found throughout the world. Organisms of the order Hemiptera are also called the true bugs, including bedbugs (e.g., *Cimex lectularius*) and the triatomid bugs that are a concern for human health management. Bedbugs can be found in tropical and subtropical climates around the world. Their migration with humans is primarily that of a pest, but they have been known to produce small red marks or hemorrhagic lesions. The presence of these marks or lesions is dependent on the individual's sensitivity to the bedbug's saliva. They live in bedding and clothing, coming out at night to take a blood meal. Triatomid bugs, on the other hand, are responsible for transmitting the parasite *Trypanosoma cruzi*, the cause of Chagas' disease. The triatomid bugs are sometimes called kissing bugs because of their tendency to bite sleeping victims on the face, especially around the mouth. The bugs discussed here transmit disease while taking a meal through defecation, which in turn may result in infection of the wound with bacteria or *T. cruzi*.

Clinical Symptoms

The most notable symptom of a bug bite is an irritating dermatitis at the bite location. Excessive scratching may also result in a secondary bacterial infection of the bite wound. Cockroaches do not directly cause symptoms. Triatomid bug bites may cause similar dermatitis reactions in their victims. *T cruzi* and the symptoms of Chagas' disease are discussed in Chapter 5.

Treatment

OTC lotions and ointments, such as calamine and Benadryl lotion, are available to relieve the itching associated with bug bites. Other bactericidal ointments may be needed for those with secondary bacterial infections.

Prevention and Control

Because these bugs exist in the environment and in human dwellings, it is almost impossible to eliminate exposure. At best, we can minimize the potential for exposure to cockroaches and bedbugs through relevant hygiene practices. Eliminating garbage and increased sanitation will minimize materials that attract cockroaches to an area. Similarly, vigilant surveillance for the presence of bedbugs and subsequent treatment and removal will minimize their spread in a residence. Treatment with pesticides in endemic areas of South America can minimize the occurrence of triatomid bugs in tribal dwellings but will not eliminate it entirely.

Quick Quiz! 13-28

Which of the following features are found in all bugs at some point during their development? (Objective 13-5)
A. Three pairs of legs and wings
B. Wings and rudimentary mouth
C. Three pairs of legs and webbed feet
D. Rudimentary mouth and webbed feet

Quick Quiz! 13-29

The most notable symptom humans experience as a result of encounters with bugs is which of the following? (Objective 13-9)
A. Breathing difficulties
B. Nausea and vomiting
C. Diarrhea and abdominal cramping
D. Intense itching at bite site

Quick Quiz! 13-30

How do cockroaches affect the health of humans? (Objectives 13-6 and 13-8)
A. They transmit diseases during a blood meal on the human host.
B. They are capable of vertical transmission of rickettsial diseases.
C. They carry and transmit diseases by mechanical transfer to uncovered food.
D. None of the above.

LOOKING BACK

Each of the arthropods discussed in this chapter is responsible for transmitting one or more parasites, as summarized in Table 13-13. In addition, each arthropod may also be the source of human infestation independent of its parasite-transmitting capabilities. In addition, each arthropod may also be the source of human infestation or illness independent of its parasite-transmitting capabilities. Thus, accurate identification of these arthropods is crucial to treat, prevent, and control infections.

Proper identification of the arthropods described in this chapter requires careful inspection of the head, thorax, and abdominal regions. Although these organisms are visible to the naked eye, microscopic examination may be helpful to confirm the identification and for speciation. Comparison drawings of the arthropods discussed are shown at the end of this chapter. These will serve as a visual summary of the arthropods' key features.

TEST YOUR KNOWLEDGE!

13-1. List the three essential characteristics common to all arthropods. (Objective 13-2)

13-2. Match the scientific name (column A) of each of the following arthropods with its common name (column B). (Objective 13-11)

Column A	Column B
___ A. *Centruroides* spp.	1. Body louse
___ B. Triatomid spp.	2. Mosquito
___ C. *Latrodectus mactans*	3. Bot fly
___ D. *Dermatobia* spp.	4. Soft tick
___ E. *Ornithodorus* spp.	5. Flea (Oriental tat)
___ F. *Xenopsylla cheopis*	6. Bark scorpion
___ G. *Pediculus humanus humanus*	7. Itch mite
___ H. *Ixodes* spp.	8. Black widow spider
___ I. *Anopheles* spp.	9. Kissing bug
___ J. *Sarcoptes scabiei*	10. Hard tick

13-3. Match each of the following arthropods (column A) with its geographic location or range (column B). Answer may be used more than once. (Objective 13-7)

Column A	Column B
___ A. *Centruroides* spp.	1. Africa
___ B. Triatomid bug	2. Central America
___ C. Hobo spider	3. South America
___ D. Tsetse fly	4. Middle East
___ E. *Dermacentor* tick	5. Desert Southwest, United States
___ F. Fleas	6. North America
___ G. *Pediculus humanus humanus*	7. Pacific Northwest, United States
___ H. *Ixodes* tick	8. East of the Rocky Mountains
___ I. *Anopheles* mosquito	9. Japan and/or Far East
___ J. *Trombicula akamushi* mite	10. Worldwide

13-4. Match each of the following arthropods (Column A) with its taxonomic class

TABLE 13-13	Select Arthropods and Associated Infectious Diseases or Reactions	
Arthropods	**Associated Organisms**	**Other Effects**
Ticks	*Anaplasma* *Arboviruses* *Babesia microti* *Borrelia burgdorferi* (Lyme disease) *Borrelia* spp. (relapsing fever) *Ehrlichia* *Francisella* *Rickettsia* spp. *Flavivirus* (tickborne encephalitis)	Secondary bite wound infections Tick paralysis (toxin reaction)
Mites	St. Louis encephalitis Western equine encephalitis *Rickettsia* spp.	Scabies
Spiders	None	Venom reaction
Scorpions	None	Venom reaction
Fleas	*Dipylidium caninum* *Hymenolepis nana* *Hymenolepis diminuta* *Yersinia pestis* *Rickettsia typhi* (murine typhus) *Francisella*	Bite reaction
Flies	*Trypanosoma rhodesiense* *Trypanosoma gambiense* *Leishmania* spp. *Onchocerca volvulus* *Loa loa* *Bartonella* (Oroya fever)	Sanitation issues (e.g., dysentery, cholera, typhoid fever, polio)
Lice	*Borrelia* (relapsing fever) *Bartonella* (trench fever) *Rickettsia prowazekii* (typhus)	Pruritis reaction to infestation
Mosquitoes	*Plasmodium* spp. *Wuchereria bancrofti* *Brugia malayi* Arboviruses Flaviviruses (dengue fever, yellow fever) Togaviruses (encephalitis)	Bite reaction
Bugs	*Trypanosoma cruzi*	Bite wound reactions Sanitation issues (e.g., dysentery, cholera, typhoid fever, polio)

(Column B). Answer may be used more be than once. (Objective 13-3)

Column A

___ A. Scorpions
___ B. Bugs
___ C. Tongue worms
___ D. Mosquitoes
___ E. Copepods

Column B

1. Crustacea
2. Chilopoda
3. Insecta
4. Pentastomida
5. Arachnida

Column A

___ F. Flies
___ G. Lice
___ H. Centipedes
___ I. Mites
___ J. Fleas

Column B

13-5. Which life cycle stage(s) of *Ixodes* ticks is most likely to transmit diseases such as Lyme disease, and why? (Objective 13-6)

13-6. Define scutum and describe how it is used in the identification of arthropods. (Objective 13-1)

13-7. Define the following key terms: (Objective 13-1)
   A. Hemocele
   B. Vertical transmission
   C. Capitulum

13-8. A physician's office calls for instructions on how to prepare a nonflying bug for laboratory examination. Which of the following is the proper method for submission of this specimen? (Objective 13-4)
   A. Ask them to place the specimen in a dry, properly labeled container and send within 2 days to the laboratory.
   B. Ask them to place the specimen in a properly labeled container with enough 70% ethanol to immerse the sample completely and send the sample to the laboratory as soon as possible.
   C. Tell them to place the sample in a small amount of gauze, place it in an envelope, and mail to the laboratory.
   D. Tell them to place the sample in a properly labeled container with enough 5% formalin to immerse the sample completely and send the sample to the laboratory as soon as possible.
   E. Two of the above are acceptable methods of specimen handling and submission for ectoparasite identification: _____ (specify)

13-9. Dermonecrotic cellulitis resulting in the progressive loss of surrounding tissue is typically associated with bites from which of the following arachnids? (Objective 13-9)
   A. Brown recluse spider
   B. Black widow spider
   C. Desert hairy scorpion
   D. Bark scorpion

13-10. An arthropod that was found on a patient in a public health clinic was sent to the laboratory for identification. The characteristics included six legs, the front pair with clawlike shapes, and a large, oval-shaped abdomen. This arthropod most likely belongs to which of the following groups? (Objective 13-5 and 13-13)
   A. Mites
   B. Lice
   C. Ticks
   D. Fleas

CASE STUDY 13-2   UNDER THE MICROSCOPE

Jared is a registered nurse at a long-term care facility. Several new residents have been admitted in the past 2 weeks and he has been assigned to perform their initial health screenings and interviews. Other than the need for intermediate-level assistance care because of the infirmities of age, most of the patients appeared relatively healthy.

One patient who is also at the beginning stages of dementia has obviously not been properly cared for in the recent past; his hygiene levels are poor. This may in part be caused by the onset of dementia and the fact that he lived alone for the past 2 years. However, Jared also notices that the patient seems restless and has a hard time sitting still or in one place for very long. A physical examination reveals appropriate indices for a person of this age but there seem to be a number of red papules on the abdomen, around the waistline. There is no fever; the heart rate, blood pressure, and respirations are normal. Further questioning reveals that the patient has been scratching this area intensely.

Questions and Issues for Consideration
1. Which ectoparasite might be involved in this case? (Objective 13-9 and 13-12)
2. What samples should be collected and how should they be processed for transporting to the laboratory? (Objective 13-4)
3. How is this ectoparasite transmitted from person to person? (Objective 13-6)
4. What type of treatment is involved and what type of isolation, if any, should be in place? (Objective 13-10)

COMPARISON DRAWINGS
Common Adult Arthropods

FIGURE 13-2. Hard and soft ticks

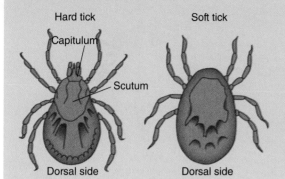

Hard tick   Soft tick

Capitulum

Scutum

Dorsal side   Dorsal side

FIGURE 13-3. Mite

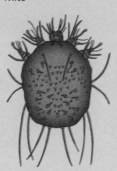

FIGURE 13-6. Spider

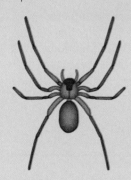

FIGURE 13-7. Scorpion

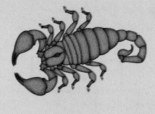

FIGURE 13-8. Flea

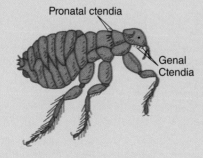

Pronatal ctendia

Genal
Ctendia

FIGURE 13-9. Fly

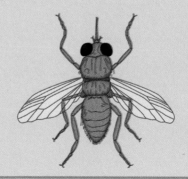

Continued

COMPARISON DRAWINGS
Common Adult Arthropods—cont'd

FIGURE 13-10. Head, body, and crab lice

Head and body louse   Crab louse

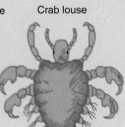

FIGURE 13-12. Mosquito

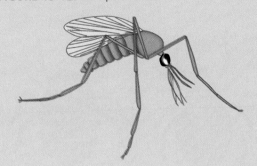

FIGURE 13-13. Triatomid bug

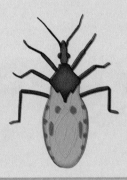

Glossary

acanthopedia Spine-like pseudopods present on the trophozoites of *Acanthamoeba* species.

accidental or incidental host (*pl.*, hosts) Host other than the normal host that is harboring a parasite.

accolé Refers to the location of parasites, specifically select species of *Plasmodium*, that assume a crescent-shaped mass at the outer edge of a red blood cell; also known as *appliqué*.

aestivoautumnal malaria Infections with *P. falciparum* that occur in the warmer months of late summer and early autumn.

amastigote (*pl.*, amastigotes) Oval, nonflagellated morphologic form found in some of the *hemoflagellate* life cycles; also known as an L.D. (Leishman-Donovan) body and leishmanial form.

ameba (*pl.*, amebas) Common name for a motile class of Protozoa (scientific name, Sarcodina) equipped with pseudopods for the purpose of locomotion; some use a different spelling (amoeba, amoebae).

amebiasis Infection with amebas.

amebic Pertaining to the amebas.

amebic colitis Any intestinal amebic infection exhibiting symptoms.

amebic dysentery Any intestinal amebic infection characterized by blood and mucus in the stool.

amebic infection Invasion of amebic parasites into the body.

anaphylactic shock Allergic response producing large amounts of histamine and other chemical mediators caused by exposure to a foreign substance; may produce fatal results; also known as anaphylaxis.

anergic Describes a patient who is unable to mount an adequate immune response.

Animalia Kingdom of animals that includes the arthropods.

appliqué Refers to the location of parasites, specifically select species of *Plasmodium*, that assume a crescent-shaped mass at the outer edge of a red blood cell; also known as *accolé*.

arthropod (*pl.*, arthropods) Organism that has a hard exoskeleton and paired jointed legs, such as an insect.

artifact (*pl.*, artifacts) A microscopic structure or form that resembles a parasite; may also be referred to as a confuser or pseudoparasite.

arthralgia (*pl.*, arthralgias) Joint pain.

autoreinfection Reinfecting oneself. For example, this process may occur in the pinworm life cycle in which the deposited eggs in the perianal region are ingested via hand-to-mouth contamination.

axoneme (*pl.*, axonemes) Intracellular portion of flagellum; the internal cytoskeletal structure that supports flagella.

axostyle Rodlike support structure found in some flagellates.

Baghdad boil (*pl.*, Baghdad boils) A common name for an infection with *Leishmania tropica*; it is a cutaneous form of leishmaniasis presenting with pus-containing ulcers.

bay sore A common name for a cutaneous form of infection caused by *Leishmania Mexicana*.

benign tertian malaria The disease caused by infection with *Plasmodium vivax* or *Plasmodium ovale*; characterized by a 10- to 17-day incubation period postexposure. The vague symptoms present mimic those generally seen in cases of the flu, including nausea, vomiting, headache, muscle pains, and photophobia. Infected patients usually experience bouts of fever and chills (known as *paroxysms*) every 48 hours.

black water fever A name for the disease caused by *Plasmodium falciparum* that develops following a relatively short incubation period of 7 to 10 days. Daily episodes of chills and fever, as well as severe diarrhea, nausea, and vomiting, rapidly develop, followed by cyclic paroxysms, which occur every 36 to 48 hours. A fulminating disease results and the intestinal symptoms (nausea, vomiting, diarrhea) mimic those seen in malignant infections—the other name for this form of malaria is ***malignant tertian malaria***. As the disease progresses, kidney involvement occurs—hence, the name black water fever.

blepharoplast Basal body structure in hemoflagellates from which an axoneme arises.

bradyzoites (*pl.*, bradyzoites) Slowly multiplying trophozoite stage of *Toxoplasma gondii*.

brood capsule (*pl.*, brood capsules) Structure inside a daughter cyst that houses developing scolices.

buccal capsule Oral cavity of adult roundworms; also known as the *buccal cavity*.

buccal cavity Oral cavity of adult roundworms; also known as the *buccal capsule*.

Calabar swelling Swelling of subcutaneous tissues that is transient in nature; occurs with infections of the filarial parasite *Loa loa*.

capitulum Umbrella term referring to the mouth parts of ticks and mites.

cardiomegaly An enlargement of the heart.

carrier (*pl.*, carriers) Parasite-harboring host that is not exhibiting any clinical symptoms but is capable of shedding the parasite and infecting others.

cercaria (*pl.*, cercarie) Final stage of fluke development occurring in the first intermediate host (snail); possesses a body and a tail, which allow the organism to become mobile.

cestoda Referring to the cestodes (tapeworms).

cestode (*pl.*, cestodes) Alternate name for members in the class of helminths known as Cestoda; common name is *tapeworm*. In this group of parasites, each adult worm consists of a flat, ribbon-like, segmented body that resembles a tape measure.

Chagas' disease A common name for the disease caused by *Trypanosoma cruzi*.

chagoma Primary lesion at the site of *Trypanosoma cruzi* infection; it is an acute inflammatory response that results in blocking of the lymphatics and production of erythema.

chancre Local inflammation leading to painful ulceration at the site of an insect bite.

chiclero ulcer A form of cutaneous leishmaniasis caused by *Leishmania mexicana*; it is commonly found in Belize, Guatemala, and the Yucatan peninsula in areas in which chicle sap is harvested for use in making chewing gum.

chitin Nitrogen-containing polysaccharide coating; also referred to as a *shell*; commonly seen on *Ascaris* eggs.

chitinized exoskeleton Structure on the outside of the arthropod body composed of an insoluble polysaccharide providing support for internal organs.

chromatoid bar (*pl.*, bars) Rod-shaped structures in the cytoplasm of some amebic cysts that contain condensed RNA material.

cilia Hairlike projections present on *Balantidium coli* trophozoites that function as the means of locomotion.

ciliate (*pl.*, ciliates) Common name for a parasite that moves by means of cilia (scientific name, class Kinetofragminophorea).

coccidia Group of protozoal parasites in which asexual replication occurs outside a human host and sexual replication occurs inside a human host.

commensal Relating to commensalism; the association between two different organisms in which one benefits and has a neutral effect on the other.

commensalism Association of two different species of organisms that is beneficial to one member and neutral to the other.

concentrated iodine wet preparation (*pl.*, preparations) Slide made by placing a drop of Lugol's or D'Antoni's iodine on a glass slide (a 3- × 2-inch size is suggested) and mixing with a small portion of specimen after a debris removal process using a wooden applicator stick or another mixing tool. The resulting slide should be thin enough for newspaper print to be read through the smear. A 22-mm^2 cover slip is placed on the slide and the preparation is examined microscopically in a systematic fashion.

concentrated saline wet preparation (*pl.*, preparations) Slide made by placing a drop of 0.85% saline on a glass slide (a 3- × 2-inch size is suggested) and mixing with a small portion of specimen after a debris removal process using a wooden applicator stick or another mixing tool. The resulting slide should be thin enough for newspaper print to be read through the smear. A 22-mm^2 cover slip is placed on the slide and the preparation is examined microscopically in a systematic fashion.

concentration technique (*pl.*, techniques) Process that provides the ability to detect small numbers of parasites that might not be detected using a direct wet preparation. It is carried out by performing a debris removal process that forces parasites present to congregate (concentrate) together through several centrifugation steps. Wet preparations, preferably saline and iodine, are then made from the concentrated specimen for microscopic examination.

concentrate wet preparation (*pl.*, preparations) Slide made by mixing a small portion of specimen with saline or iodine after a debris removal process and subsequent examination of the resultant mixture under the microscope.

confuser (*pl.*, confusers) A microscopic structure or form that resembles a parasite; may also be referred to as an artifact or a pseudoparasite.

congenital transmission Passage of disease from mother to unborn child.

copepod (*pl.*, copepods) Water flea that resides in freshwater sources such as streams and wells; also known as *Cyclops* spp. Serves as the intermediate host in the life cycle of select *helminths* such as *Dracunculus*.

copulation Sexual union or mating of certain helminths, including the nematodes.

copulatory bursa Umbrella-like structure at the posterior end of adult male nematodes that aids in copulation.

coracidium Ciliated larval stage of *Diphyllobothrium latum*; consists of a hexacanth embryo that develops from the egg stage and hatches when the egg is exposed to fresh water.

corticated Presence of an outer, mammillated albuminous coating; commonly seen on *Ascaris* eggs.

costa Rodlike structure located at the base of the undulating membrane, between the undulating membrane and the body of certain flagellate trophozoites, thus connecting the two structures. It may also aid in supporting the undulating membrane.

cutaneous An infection localized in the capillaries of the skin.

cuticle Surface covering present on adult nematodes; provides protection against destruction by human stomach acid.

cyst (*pl.*, cysts) Amebic stage characterized by a thick cell wall that allows for survival of the organism in the environment and its subsequent transmission into an uninfected host.

cysticercoid larval stage Scolex surrounded by a bladder-like cyst that contains little or no fluid that emerges from the larvae of certain tapeworm species, such as *Hymenolepis nana*.

cysticercosis Human tissue infection contracted by ingestion of *Taenia solium* eggs that have been passed in human feces.

cysticercus larva Scolex surrounded by a bladder-like cyst that is thin-walled and filled with fluid. It emerges from the larvae of certain tapeworms, such as *Taenia* spp.; also known as a bladder worm.

cytostome Rudimentary mouth.

daughter cyst (*pl.*, daughter cysts) Miniaturized hydatid cyst complete with cyst wall, layers of germinal tissue, and fluid-filled bladder; contains numerous scolices.

decorticated Absence of an outer, mammillated, albuminous coating.

definitive host (*pl.*, hosts) Host in which the adult and/or sexual phase of a parasite occurs.

developing trophozoite (*pl.*, trophozoites) Consists of a number of stages of malarial development emerging from the ring form, characterized by an increased presence of parasites that take up more space within the red blood cell. Remnants of the ring may be visible.

diagnostic stage Stage in the parasitic life cycle that can be identified by examining appropriate specimens from the host.

Digenea A name for the class of parasites that includes the *flukes*.

dioecious Refers to parasites that reproduce via separate sexes.

direct wet mount (*pl.*, mounts) A slide made by mixing a small portion of unfixed stool with saline or iodine and subsequent examination of the resultant mixture under the microscope to detect the presence of motile protozoan trophozoites; also known as a *direct wet preparation*.

direct wet preparation (*pl.*, preparations) A slide made by mixing a small portion of unfixed stool with saline or iodine and subsequent examination of the resultant mixture under the microscope to detect the presence of motile protozoan trophozoites; also known as a *direct wet mount*.

distomiasis General term for (human) infection with flukes.

direct iodine wet preparation (*pl.*, preparations) Slide made by placing a drop of Lugol's or D'Antoni's iodine on a glass slide (a 3- × 2-inch size is suggested) and mixing with a small portion of unfixed stool, using a wooden applicator stick or another mixing tool. The resulting slide should be thin enough for newspaper print to be read through the smear. A 22-mm² cover slip is placed on the slide and the preparation is examined microscopically in a systematic fashion.

direct saline wet preparation (*pl.*, preparations) Slide made by placing a drop of 0.85% saline on a glass slide (a 3- × 2-inch size is suggested) and mixing with a small portion of unfixed stool using a wooden applicator stick or another mixing tool. The resulting slide should be thin enough for newspaper print to be read through the smear. A 22-mm² cover slip is placed on the slide and the preparation is examined microscopically in a systematic fashion.

disease Destructive process having characteristic symptoms.

distomiasis Name for the pulmonary condition caused by infection with *Paragonimus westermani*.

diurnal Occurring during the daytime hours.

dum dum fever A common name for the visceral leishmaniasis caused by *Leishmania donovani*.

ectoparasite (*pl.*, ectoparasites) Parasite that is established in or on the exterior surface of its host.

edema Localized swelling of tissues, most often seen in the joints.

egg (*pl.*, eggs) Female sex cell (gamete) after fertilization. Synonyms include oocyst, ovum, and zygote.

elephantiasis Enlargement of the skin and subcutaneous tissue caused by the presence of some filariae (e.g., *Wuchereria bancrofti*), which obstruct the circulation of the lymphatic tissues. Affected areas include the breast, leg, and scrotum.

embryonated Fertilized.

embryophore Shell of certain intestinal tapeworm eggs, such as those of *Taenia* spp.

encystation Transformation of a trophozoite stage into a cyst stage.

endoparasite Parasite that is established inside the body.

epidemiology Study of the factors that determine the distribution and frequency of an infectious process or disease in a particular location.

epimastigote (*pl.*, epimastigotes) Long, spindle-shaped, hemoflagellate morphologic form equipped with a free flagellum and an undulating membrane that extends over half of the body length. It is found in the vectors responsible for transmitting *Trypanosoma* spp.

erythematous Refers to a localized reddening of the skin.

erythrocytic cycle Asexual cycle of *Plasmodium* that occurs in human red blood cells (RBCs).

espundia Another name for an infection caused by the presence of *Leishmania braziliensis*, the principle cause of mucocutaneous disease in Central and South America, particularly in Brazil.

excrement Waste matter of the body—for example, feces.

excystation Transformation of a cyst stage into a trophozoite stage.

exoerythrocytic cycle Asexual cycle of *Plasmodium* that occurs in human liver cells.

extraintestinal Refers to when parasites migrate and/or take up residence outside the intestines.

facultative parasite Parasite that is able to exist independently of its host.

filaria (*pl.*, filariae) A blood or issue roundworm that requires an arthropod intermediate host or vector for transmission; belongs to the order Filariata, superfamily Filarioidea.

filarial Pertaining to the group of parasites that belong to the filariae.

filariform larva (*pl.*, larvae) Infective nonfeeding larvae.

fixative (*pl.*, fixatives) A substance that preserves the morphology of protozoa and prevents further development of certain helminth eggs and larvae.

flagellate (*pl.*, flagellates) Protozoan parasite that moves by means of flagella; scientific name, phylum Mastigophora.

flagellum (*pl.*, flagella) Tail-like extension of the cytoplasm, which provide a means of motility and perhaps aids in obtaining food; movement of the flagellum is whiplike in nature.

fluke (*pl.*, flukes) Common name for a *trematode*.

forest yaws Another name for the infection caused by the presence of *Leishmania guyanensis*, the principle cause of leishmaniasis in the Guianas, parts of Brazil and Venezuela; also known as pian bois.

gametogony Phase in the life cycle of certain parasites, such as malaria, in which macrogametocytes and microgametocytes are formed.

gametocyte (*pl.*, gametocytes) Sex cells (males are called microgametocytes and females are known as macrogametocytes) that are capable of sexual reproduction.

genal ctenidia Comblike structures located just above the mouth parts of some fleas.

genital primordium Precursor to the reproductive system consisting of a clump of cells in an ovoid formation. It is present in the rhabditiform larvae of hookworm and *Strongyloides*.

glomerulonephritis Inflammation of the filtering mechanisms in the nephrons of the kidney called glomeruli.

glycogen mass A cytoplasmic area without defined borders that is believed to represent stored food and is also usually visible in young cysts. As the cyst matures, the glycogen mass usually disappears, a process that likely represents usage of the stored food.

gravid Pregnant.

helminth (*pl.*, helminthes, helminths) A generic term for multicellular worms that includes the roundworms (nematodes), tapeworms (cestodes), and flukes (trematodes).

hemocele System of blood-containing spaces present in the body of arthropods.

hemoflagellate (*pl.*, hemoflagellates) Flagellates that are found in blood and tissue.

hemoglobinuria Presence of hemoglobin in the urine

hemozoin A remnant of the parasite feeding on RBC hemoglobin that is visible as a brown pigment.

hepatosplenomegaly Enlargement of the liver and spleen.

hermaphroditic Parasites capable of self-fertilization. Each tapeworm segment contains both male and female reproductive organs.

hexacanth embryo Motile first larval stage of some tapeworms. Armed with six small hooks, known as *hooklets*—hence, the name hexacanth; also known as an onchosphere.

hooklet (*pl.*, hooklets) A small hook located in a hexacanth embryo that is believed to function in piercing the intestinal wall of the infected host.

host (*pl.*, hosts) Species of animal or plant that harbors a parasite.

hydatid cyst Larval stage of *Echinococcus granulosus*; made up of a fluid-filled bladder surrounded by a cyst wall and laminated layers of germinal tissue. The inner germinal layer gives rise to daughter cysts and scolices.

hydatid sand Components found in the fluid of older *Echinococcus granulosus* cysts; consists of daughter cysts, free scolices, hooklets, and miscellaneous nondescript material.

hypnozoite (*pl.*, hypnozoites) Dormant liver cells infected with *Plasmodium vivax* or *Plasmodium ovale*. These cells may remain dormant for months to years and, when reactivated, may cause relapsing malarial infections.

immature schizont (*pl.*, schizonts) Beginning stage of the developed asexual sporozoa trophozoite (i.e., *Plasmodium* spp.); characterized by the early stages of merozoite formation.

infection Invasion of parasites (except arthropods) into the body. Strict use of this term does not imply a disease process.

infective stage Stage in the parasitic life cycle that is capable of invading a definitive host.

infestation Invasion of arthropods in or on the skin or hair of a host.

intermediate host (*pl.*, hosts) Host in which the larval or asexual phase of a parasite occurs.

ischemia Insufficient blood supply in body tissues caused by blockage of the capillaries and blood sinuses.

kala-azar Another name for the most severe form of visceral leishmaniasis caused by members of the *Leishmania donovani* complex.

karyosome (karyosomal chromatin) Small mass of chromatin located within the nucleus of certain protozoan parasites; also known as karyosomal chromatin or endosome.

Katayama fever A systemic hypersensitivity reaction to the presence of a schistosomulae migrating through tissue. The rapid onset of fever, nausea, myalgia, malaise, fatigue, cough, diarrhea, and eosinophilia occurs 1 to 2 months after exposure.

Kerandel's sign A delayed sensation to pain often associated with trypanosomal infections.

Kernig's sign Diagnostic sign for meningitis. The patient is unable to straighten his or her leg fully when the hip is flexed at 90 degrees because of hamstring stiffness.

kinetoplast Umbrella term often used to refer to the blepharoplast and small parabasal body.

larva (*pl.*, larvae) Juvenile stage of a worm. Singular, larva.

larval Pertaining to larvae.

leishmaniasis General and collective name for the diseases caused by any organisms of the genus *Leishmania*.

lymphadenopathy Enlargement of the lymph nodes.

macrogametocyte (*pl.*, macrogametocytes) Female sex cell that occurs in the malarial life cycle.

macronucleus Large, often kidney-bean shaped nucleus found in *Balantidium coli*. The macronucleus shape may vary.

malaria, malarial Name for the disease caused by infection with *Plasmodium* spp.; pertaining to *malaria*.

malarial malaria Name for the form of malaria caused by *plasmodium malarial*.

malignant tertian malaria Disease caused by *Plasmodium falciparum* that develops following a relatively short incubation period of 7 to 10 days. Daily episodes of chills and fever, as well as severe diarrhea, nausea, and vomiting, rapidly develop, followed by cyclic *paroxysms*, which occur every 36 to 48 hours. A fulminating disease results and the intestinal symptoms (nausea, vomiting, diarrhea) mimic those seen in malignant infections—hence, the name malignant tertian malaria. It is also known as *black water fever*.

mature schizont (*pl.*, schizonts) Fully developed stage of the asexual sporozoa trophozoite (i.e., *Plasmodium* spp.) characterized by the presence of mature merozoites.

Maurer's dot (*pl.*, dots) A dark-red staining, irregular to comma-shaped dot located in the cytoplasm of red blood cells infected with *Plasmodium falciparum*; also known as *Maurer's clefts*. Maurer's dots tend to have a more bluish tint after Giemsa staining than Schüffner's dots.

median body (*pl.*, median bodies) Slightly rodlike-shaped structure (resembling a comma) located in the posterior portion of *Giardia intestinalis* trophozoites and cysts. Although they are believed to be associated with energy or metabolism, or with supporting the organism's posterior end, their exact function is unclear.

megacolon Enlargement of the colon seen in infections caused by the presence of *Trypanosoma cruzi*.

megaesophagus Enlargement of the esophagus seen in infections caused by the presence of *Trypanosoma cruzi*.

merozoite (*pl.*, merozoites) Contents of the fully developed stage of the asexual Sporozoa trophozoite (i.e., *Plasmodium* spp., the mature schizont) produced in both the liver cells and RBCs and capable of initiating infection in previously healthy red blood cells.

metacercaria (*pl.*, metacerariae) Encysted form of the fluke life cycle; occurs on water plants or in the second intermediate host, such as fish, crabs, or crayfish. It is the infective stage for humans.

metamorphosis Transition of one developmental stage into another. In the case of the arthropods, the nymphs resemble the adults morphologically in incomplete (simple) metamorphosis. In complete metamorphosis, the developmental stages (larvae and pupa) do not morphologically resemble the adults.

Metazoa Subkingdom that consists of multicellular organisms, including parasitic worms.

microfilaria (*pl.*, microfilariae) The embryonic stage of a filarial parasite. Adult female filarial worms lay live microfilariae; there is no known egg stage.

microgametocyte (*pl.*, microgametocytes) Male sex cell that occurs in the malarial life cycle.

micron (*pl.*, microns) Measuring unit of parasites; also known as a micrometer; one thousandth (10^{-3}) of a millimeter or one millionth (10^{-6}) of a meter. Microns are abbreviated as μ or μm.

micronucleus Small dotlike nucleus found in *Balantidium coli*; often difficult to see, even in stained preparations.

miracidium First-stage larva of flukes that emerge from the egg in fresh water, equipped with cilia, which aid in movement. This is the infective stage for the first intermediate host (snail).

mode of transmission (*pl.*, modes of transmission) The means whereby a parasite gains entry into an unsuspecting host.

Montenegro skin test A test similar to that of the tuberculin skin test used for screening large populations at risk for contracting *Leishmania* spp. infections.

mucocutaneous Refers to disease that causes lesions of the skin and mucous membranes, specifically in the oral and nasal mucosa regions of the body.

mutualism Association of two different species of organisms that is beneficial to both members.

myalgia (*pl.*, myalgias) Muscle pain.

myiasis (*pl.*, myiases) Condition resulting after a female fly passes her eggs onto another flying insect, such as a mosquito. These eggs are transmitted onto human skin during a mosquito blood meal and subsequently hatch. The eggs evolve into larvae known as maggots and immediately penetrate the host's skin, often causing a pruritic and painful skin lesion.

myocarditis Inflammation of the cardiac muscles (inflammation of the heart).

nagana A form of trypanosomiasis often found in cattle.

Nematoda Referring to the Nematodes (roundworms).

nematode (*pl.*, nematodes) Alternate name of members in the class of helminths known as **Nematoda**; common name, intestinal *roundworms*. Adults may possess a variety of anterior structures and appear round when seen in cross section.

nocturnal Occurring during the nighttime hours.

nymph (*pl.*, nymphs) Developmental stage of certain arthropods that morphologically resemble the adult.

O&P (ova and parasites) The traditional method for parasite examination in which O stands for ova and P stands for parasites; consists of direct macroscopic and microscopic analysis and microscopic examination after a debris removal process is performed.

obligatory parasite Parasite that is unable to survive outside its host.

occult Not apparent, hidden, concealed.

ocular micrometer Specially designed ocular device equipped with a measuring scale designed to measure parasites and other structures under a microscope.

onchosphere Motile, first larval stage of some tapeworms; armed with six small hooks, known as *hooklets*, and also known as a *hexacanth embryo*.

oocyst (*pl.*, oocysts) Encysted form of a zygote that in *Plasmodium* develops in the stomach of the *Anopheles* mosquito; characterized by the presence of mature sporozoites.

ookinete (*pl.*, ookinetes) Fertilized cell; the product of the union of a male and female sex cell, also known as a *zygote*.

operculum Caplike structure or lid present on select tapeworm and fluke eggs.

Oriental sore Common reference for the cutaneous leishmaniasis caused by the hemoflagellates that comprise *Leishmania tropica* complex.

parasite (*pl.*, parasites) Organism that gains its nourishment from and lives in or on another organism.

parasitemia (*pl.*, parasitemias) Parasitic infection of the blood.

parasitic Relating to or characteristic of a parasite; disease caused by the presence of parasites.

parasitic life cycle Route that a parasite follows from any one stage in its development throughout its life, back to the stage where the route began.

parasitology Study of parasites.

parasitism Symbiotic relationship of two different species of organisms in which one member benefits at the other member's expense.

paroxysm (*pl.*, paroxysms) Chills and fever syndrome associated with malaria. Chills occur in response to schizont development followed by a fever. which corresponds to the release of merozoites and toxic waste by-products from infected red blood cells.

parthenogenic Formation of a new organism without fertilization. It occurs in the life cycle of *Strongyloides* in which the adult male does not participate in reproduction; its ultimate fate is unknown. The parasitic female is thus responsible for this process.

pathogenic Refers to an agent (parasite) that has demonstrated the ability to cause disease.

pathogenicity Ability to cause an infectious disease; may also be referred to as the ability to produce tissue changes.

pediculosis Lice infestation.

periodicity Recurring regularly during a specific time period.

peripheral chromatin Chromatin portion of the nucleus that surrounds the karyosome. It may be evenly or unevenly distributed when present.

permanent stained smear (*pl.*, smears) A microscope slide that contains a fixed sample fixed in a preservative such as polyvinyl alcohol (PVA) that has been allowed to dry and subsequently stained.

pian bois Another name for the infection caused by *Leishmania guyanensis*, the principle cause of mucocutaneous leishmaniasis in the Guianas, parts of Brazil and Venezuela; also known as forest yaws.

Platyhelminthes Phylum of organisms known as platyhelminths that are commonly known as the flatworms; contains the tapeworms as well as the *flukes*.

pleurocercoid Precursor larval stage of *Diphyllobothrium latum* that develops following the ingestion of the first known larval stage, a *procercoid*, by a freshwater fish (the second of two intermediate hosts in the life cycle); the infective stage for humans.

preparation (*pl.*, preparations) The result of one placing a portion of sample for parasite study onto a microscope slide with or without adding iodine or saline and adding a coverslip, when appropriate, for subsequent microscopic examination; often referred to using the abbreviation *prep(s)*.

procercoid First known larval stage of *Diphyllobothrium latum* that develops following the ingestion of the coracidium by a copepod, the first of two intermediate hosts in the life cycle.

proglottid (*pl.*, proglottids) Individual segment of a tapeworm. Each mature proglottid contains both male and female reproductive organs.

promastigote (*pl.*, promastigotes) Long, slender hemoflagellate morphologic form containing a free flagellum. It is found mainly in the vector responsible for transmitting *Leishmania* spp.

pronotal ctenidia Comblike structures located immediately behind the head and extending posteriorly on the dorsal surface of some fleas.

protozoa Subkingdom that consists of single-celled eukaryotic animals.

protozoal, protozoan Pertaining to members of the subkingdom Protozoa.

pruritis Intense itching.

pseudopod (*pl.*, pseudopods) An extension of the cytoplasm of the ameba that aids the organism in motility; literal translation is "false feet." The presence of this feature classifies a parasite as an ameba. It has been suggested that pseudopods may also assist the parasite in gathering food as it moves.

pupa/pupal (*pl.*, pupae) The enclosed resting stage of select arthropods; also known as a cocoon stage.

quartan malaria, malarial malaria Form of malaria caused by infection with *Plasmodium malariae* characterized by an 18- to 40-day incubation period postexposure, followed by the onset of flulike symptoms. Infected patients usually experience bouts of fever and chills (known as *paroxysms*) every 72 hours.

recrudescence Rupture of malarial infected RBCs and the subsequent clinical symptoms following an initial infection in which neither chemotherapy nor the body's immune system has eliminated the parasite.

red water fever Condition caused by *Babesia* that severely affected the cattle industry; also known as Texas cattle fever.

redia (*pl.*, rediae) Intermediate larval stage of the flukes (may be a second or third, depending on species). Development occurs inside the sporocyst, which is located in the snail host. Each redia has the capability to produce numerous cercariae.

reservoir host (*pl.*, hosts) Host that harbors a parasite that is also parasitic for humans, and from which humans may become infected.

retroinfection In pinworm-specific terms, a process that may occur when hatched pinworm larvae migrate back into the body via the rectum and mature into adults.

rhabditiform larva (*pl.*, larvae) First-stage feeding larvae that are noninfective.

rigor Shivering or trembling caused by chills.

ring form (*pl.*, forms) Earliest morphologic form of malarial parasites after infecting a previously healthy RBC; also known as an early trophozoite. It is characterized by the presence of a ring-like structure in the erythrocyte.

Romaña's sign Conjunctivitis and unilateral edema of the face and eyelids resulting from infection with *Trypanosoma cruzi*.

rostellum Fleshy extension of the scolex of some tapeworms; may or may not be armed with hooks, which aid suckers in intestinal attachment.

roundworm (*pl.*, roundworms) Common name for an intestinal *nematode*.

schistosomule Form of a schistosome that results following penetration of the cercaria into human skin and concurrent loss of the organism's tail during this process.

schizodeme analysis Restriction analysis of kinetoplast DNA.

schizogony Asexual multiplication of some parasites, including malarial organisms. The process consists of multiple nuclear divisions followed by cytoplasmic division.

schizont (*pl.*, schizonts) Morphologic form, most notably found in the *Plasmodium* spp. life cycle, responsible for the development and maturing of a merozoite, a morphologic form critical to the survival and continued replication of the parasites in a human host.

Schüffner's dot (*pl.*, dots) Tiny granule visible in the cytoplasm of red blood cells infected with *Plasmodium vivax* or *Plasmodium ovale* that appears red with Giemsa stain; also known as eosinophilic stippling.

scolex (*pl.*, scolices) Anterior end of a tapeworm.

scutum Dorsal surface shield of hard ticks. The scutum of females covers part of the dorsal surface, whereas that of the males covers the entire dorsal surface.

sheath Delicate membrane that surrounds the microfilariae; also known as an egg membrane because when present, it is visible at birth. The sheath extends past the anterior and posterior ends and may be retained or lost by the microfilaria, depending on the species.

somnolence Excessive sleepiness.

sparganosis Human condition that results from the accidental ingestion of the procercoid larval stage of *Diphyllobothrium latum*.

sparganum Condition that occurs after a tapeworm migrates and invades subcutaneous tissue, often described as white, wrinkled, and ribbon-shaped; may occur with infections of *Diphyllobothrium latum*, known as *sparganosis*.

sporoblast (*pl.*, sporoblasts) Roundish immature sac within the oocyst consisting of developing sporozoites.

sporocyst (*pl.*, sporocysts) Roundish mature sac (pertaining to sporozoa) within the oocyst containing fully developed, sausage-shaped sporozoites; or saclike structure (pertaining to flukes) serving as the larval form of flukes that is formed in the snail and that emerges from the miracidium.

sporogony Process of spore and sporozoite production via sexual reproduction.

Sporozoa Motile class of Protozoa that has no apparent organelles for locomotion.

sporozoite (*pl.*, sporozoites) Infective stage of malaria developed in the mosquito vector and transmitted via a blood meal to an unsuspecting human.

stippling Fine speckled dots within a blood cell, visible when treated with a basic stain.

strobila General term used to denote the entire tapeworm body.

subperiodic Term that describes when the timing of an occurrence, such as the presence of *microfilariae* in the blood, is not clear-cut.

sucker (*pl.*, suckers) A cup-shaped structure located on the scolex that aid cestodes in intestinal attachment. Each scolex typically contains four suckers.

swimmer's itch Condition (zoonosis) in which the cercariae of select animal and bird *Schistosoma* spp. penetrate human skin and cause an allergic response. The life cycle is not completed.

symbiosis Living together (association) of two organisms, each of a different species.

tachyzoite (*pl.*, tachyzoites) Rapidly multiplying trophozoite stage of *Toxoplasma gondii*.

tapeworm (*pl.*, tapeworms) Common name for a *cestode*.

tegument Outer surface of the cestodes and trematodes.

Texas cattle fever The condition caused by *Babesia* that severely affected the cattle industry; also known as *red water fever*.

tissue roundworm (*pl.*, tissue roundworms) Common name for a *filaria*.

transport host (*pl.*, hosts) A host responsible for transferring a parasite from one location to another.

Trematoda Referring to the trematodes (flukes).

trematode (*pl.*, trematodes) Alternate name of the class of helminths known as **Trematoda**; common name, *flukes*. Consists primarily of organisms that are nonsegmented, flattened, and leaf-shaped.

trophozoite (*pl.*, trophozoites) Amebic stage characterized by its ability to move, obtain food, and multiply; often abbreviated as troph or trophs.

trypanosomiasis General and collective term for the diseases caused by any of the trypanosomal hemoflagellates.

trypomastigote (*pl.*, trypomastigotes) Long and slender to stubby hemoflagellate morphologic form of *Trypanosoma* spp. that typically looks like the letter C or U on permanent stain; characterized by a full body length undulating membrane. A free flagellum may or may not be present. It is found in vectors and humans.

undulating membrane Finlike structure connected to the outer edge of some flagellates; aids in the organism's locomotion, moving in a wavelike pattern.

unembryonated Unfertilized.

unfixed Refers to specimens that do not contain added preservatives.

uta Refers to mucocutaneous leishmaniasis in the Peruvian Andes.

vector (*pl.*, vectors) Living carrier (e.g., an arthropod) responsible for transporting a parasite from an infected host to a noninfected host.

vertical transmission Process whereby some arthropods transmit the microorganism they carry to their offspring.

viscera Soft parts and internal organs of the major cavities in the body.

visceral Pertaining to the internal organs of the body, especially the liver, spleen, and lymph nodes; also may be referred to a systemic infection.

Winterbottom's sign Enlargement of the postcervical chain of lymph nodes related to trypanosomal infections.

xenodiagnosis A procedure, primarily performed in areas of the world with little, if any, means for parasite identification, in which a noninfected reduviid bug is allowed to feed on a person suspected of having Chagas' disease; feces from the bug is then examined several weeks later for the presence of trypomastigotes.

Ziemann's dot (*pl.*, dots) A fine dustlike dot that stain pale pink and is seen in the cytoplasm of heavily stained RBCs infected with *Plasmodium malariae*; also known as Ziemann's stippling.

zoonosis (*pl.*, zoonoses) Accidental human infection with a parasite whose normal host is an animal. As a result, completion of the parasite life cycle may or may not occur; also referred as a *zoonotic* occurrence.

zoonotic Parasitic disease that normally infects animals and that may also infect humans; also known as a *zoonosis*.

zygote (*pl.*, zygotes) Fertilized cell, the product of the union of a male and female sex cell; also known as an **ookinete**.

zymodeme analysis Procedure used to diagnose and identify parasitic infections that involves the study of isoenzyme patterns of an organism.

Answers to Case Studies: Under the Microscope

CHAPTER 1

Case Study 1-1: Under the Microscope

1. A parasite is an organism that gains it nourishment from and lives in or on another organism.

2. Joe most likely came into contact with parasites during his mission trip to Haiti. Increased population density, poor sanitation, marginal water sources, poor public health practices, and environmental changes are all factors that might have contributed to Joe's current condition.

3. Other populations at risk for contracting parasite infections include the following: (1) individuals in underdeveloped areas/countries; (2) refugees; (3) immigrants; (4) visitors from foreign countries; (5) immunocompromised individuals; (6) individuals living in close quarters; and (7) children attending day care centers.

4. The most likely additional symptoms of individuals with intestinal parasitic infections are fever and chills.

5. The key components of a traditional O&P study include direct macroscopic and microscopic examination and microscopic examination of the sample following a fecal debris removal process.

CHAPTER 2

Case Study 2-1: Under the Microscope

1. The most common procedure performed in the area of parasitology is the examination of a stool specimen for O&P. Based on the patient's history and symptoms, it is also advisable for the technologist to recommend that the physician order a stool screen for *Giardia* and *Cryptosporidium*.

2. Because parasites are often shed intermittently, it is recommended that three specimens be collected within 10 days. Because the patient will need to transport the specimens to the laboratory, the specimens should be collected in vials containing fixatives.

3. A macroscopic examination can be performed to detect the presence of gross abnormalities and determine the consistency and color of the sample. However, if the specimen is submitted in a fixative, this step would be eliminated. The microscopic examination of the stool would include a direct wet preparation, concentrated wet preparation, and permanently stained smear. Again, if the specimen is received in fixative, the direct wet preparation can be eliminated.

4. Stool screening methods that detect antigen in the patient's specimen are commercially available for a limited number of parasites. Because the patient's symptoms are consistent with those of *Giardia* and *Cryptosporidium* infection, it is recommended that testing begin using this protocol. These tests are highly sensitive and specific and not as technically demanding as the O&P examination. If the result of this test is negative, a complete O&P examination is recommended.

CHAPTER 3

Case Study 3-1: Under the Microscope

1. The most likely cause of the infection is the atrial ameba *Naegleria fowleri*.

2. Patients who contract *N. fowleri* resulting in colonization of the nasal passages are usually asymptomatic. However, in this case, the patient developed primary amebic meningoencephalitis (PAM). This condition occurs when the ameboid trophozoites of *N. fowleri* invade the brain, causing rapid tissue destruction.

3. *N. fowleri* has three morphologic forms—ameboid trophozoite, flagellate trophozoite, and cyst. The ameboid trophozoites of *N. fowleri* are the only form known to exist in humans. Replication of the ameboid trophozoites occurs by simple binary fission. The ameboid trophozoites transform into flagellate trophozoites in vitro after being transferred to water from a tissue or culture. The flagellate trophozoites do not divide but lose their flagella and convert back into the ameboid form, in which reproduction resumes. The cyst form is known to exist only in the external environment. It appears that the entire life cycle of *N. fowleri* occurs in the external environment; it is primarily found in warm bodies of water, including lakes, streams, ponds, and swimming pools. Humans primarily contract this ameba by swimming in contaminated water. The ameboid trophozoites enter the human body through the nasal mucosa and often migrate to the brain, causing rapid tissue destruction. Some infections may be caused by inhaling dust infected with *N. fowleri* cysts. The mechanics of how, when, and where the transition of the cysts to ameboid trophozoites occurs after the cysts have been inhaled by a human have not been described. The ameboid trophozoite is the diagnostic stage of the infection.

4. Unfortunately, medications used to treat meningitis and amebic infections are ineffective against *N. fowleri*. There is evidence, however, that prompt and aggressive treatment with amphotericin B may be of benefit to patients suffering from infections with *N. fowleri*, despite its known toxicity. In rare cases, amphotericin B in combination with rifampin or miconazole has also proved to be an effective treatment. Amphotericin B and miconazole damage the cell wall of *N. fowleri*, inhibiting the biosynthesis of ergosterol and resulting in an increased membrane permeability that causes nutrients to leak out of the cells. Rifampicin inhibits RNA synthesis in the ameba by binding to beta subunits of DNA-dependent RNA polymerase, which in turn blocks RNA transcription. A person can survive if signs are recognized early but, if not, PAM almost always results in death. The survival rate is low, so prevention and early detection are important. However, because of the numerous bodies of water that may potentially be infected, total eradication of *N. fowleri* is highly unlikely.

5. Microscopic examination of cerebrospinal fluid (CSF) is the method of choice for recovery of *N. fowleri* ameboid trophozoites (see Chapter 2).

6. The diagnosis of PAM is difficult because the infection is often confused with other bacterial or viral infections because of similarities in clinical manifestations and laboratory results. The peripheral white blood cell (WBC) count is elevated with a neutrophilia in PAM. Analysis of the spinal fluid reveals an increased pressure, resulting in a hemorrhagic specimen. There is also a high white blood cell count with a neutrophilic predominance and high red blood cell (RBC) count, as well as an elevated protein level and a low to normal glucose level in the spinal fluid. The Gram stain of the spinal fluid is negative for bacteria. A basic metabolic panel may show abnormalities such as hyponatremia associated with acquired hyperglycemia. PAM is obvious when the spinal fluid is purulent, with no bacteria present. It is best diagnosed with a wet mount examination of the spinal fluid for *N. fowleri* along with standard laboratory tests (e.g., WBC, RBC, glucose, protein, bacterial and fungal cultures) of the spinal

fluid. Further specificity for diagnosis can be achieved through molecular and immunologic methods (e.g., polymerase chain reaction [PCR], restriction fragment length polymorphism, isoelectric focusing, monoclonal antibody testing).

Case Study 3-2: Under the Microscope
1. Protozoa and, in particular, the amebas.
2. Size, position of the karyosome, arrangement of peripheral chromatin, and cytoplasmic inclusions; specific to trophozoites, the presence of pseudopods, specific to cysts, the number of nuclei.
3. Trophozoite, yes.
4. Red blood cells.
5. *Entamoeba histolytica* trophozoite. Features that substantiate this identification are size (13 μm), with a single nucleus that contains a central karyosome and evenly distributed peripheral chromatin, and the presence of RBCs (diagnostic for this organism).
6. Yes, this organism is pathogenic in the human host and is known to cause the patient's symptoms.
7. Yes, *Entamoeba histolytica* cysts (Fig. 2-2A) may also be present in a fresh stool sample. The typical cyst measures 12 to 18 μm and contains one to four nuclei. The appearance of the nuclei is identical to that in the trophozoite form, a centrally located karyosome surrounded by evenly distributed peripheral chromatin. The cytoplasm resembles ground glass and may contain chromatin bars with large blunt ends as well as a glycogen mass.

CHAPTER 4

Case Study 4-1: Under the Microscope
1. The most likely identification of the organism is *Giardia intestinalis*. *G. intestinalis* cysts are ovoid in shape, ranging in size from 8 to 17 μm long by 6 to 10 μm wide. Immature cysts contain two nuclei and two median bodies. Mature cysts can have four nuclei.
2. Bryan most likely contracted his illness by drinking unfiltered water while hiking. *G.*

intestinalis can be found in the environment, commonly in stagnant or slowly moving water such as streams, marshes, and lake shores. Campers and hikers should always carry bottled water or use a water purification method such as filtering or chemical treatment.
3. If a *G. intestinalis* infection is suspected, multiple stool samples collected on subsequent days should be submitted for routine O&P analysis.

Case Study 4-2: Under the Microscope
1. *Dientamoeba fragilis.*
2. Trichrome.
3. Chromatin granules.
4. Pseudopods.
5. None, the trophozoite is the only known form in the *Dientamoeba fragilis* life cycle.
6. The exact mode of transmission is not clear. One theory suggests that transmission of *Dientamoeba* trophozoites occurs via the eggs of select helminth parasite eggs such as those of *Enterobius vermicularis* and *Ascaris lumbricoides* (see Chapter 8).

CHAPTER 5

Case Study 5-1: Under the Microscope
1. *Leishmania donovani.*
2. Amastigote (Fig. 5-1).
3. Playing outdoors in Kenya with dogs and other animals known to be reservoir hosts for Leishmania species and increased potential of coming into contact with the sandfly vectors.
4. India, Thailand, Peoples Republic of China, Burma, East Pakistan.
5. Weight loss, anemia, emaciation, darkening of the skin.
6. Venous blood may sometimes reveal the parasites.

Case Study 5-2: Under the Microscope
1. Lymph node aspirations and peripheral blood; Giemsa staining of the preparations.
2. Trypomastigotes.

3. Winterbottom's sign and Kerandel's sign.
4. *Trypanosoma brucei gambiense*.
5. West African sleeping sickness and Gambian trypanosomiasis.
6. Humans become infected with *T. brucei gambiense* following the injection of trypomastigotes by the tsetse fly during its blood meal. The entering trypomastigotes migrate through the bloodstream and into the lymphatic system, multiplying by binary fission. The trypomastigotes are transmitted back to the tsetse fly vector when it feeds on an infected human. Once ingested by the tsetse fly, the trypomastigotes continue to multiply and eventually migrate back to the salivary gland, converting into epimastigotes along the way. Once in the salivary gland, the epimastigotes transform back into trypomastigotes, thus completing the cycle.
7. Treatments include melarsoprol, suramin, pentamidine, and eflornithine. The treatment of choice is situation-dependent and is dictated by a number of factors, including patient age and stage of disease. The toxicity level of the chosen medication must be monitored to ensure that the appropriate dose is used.

CHAPTER 6

Case Study 6-1: Under the Microscope
1. *Plasmodium falciparum*.
2. The presence of two rings in the red blood cell and a double chromatin dot seen in form A; the banana-shaped organism seen in forms B and C.
3. Form A, ring form; form B, microgametocyte; form C: macrogametocyte. The organization of chromatin in the macrogametocyte is condensed and centered in the cytoplasm, whereas that of the microgametocyte shows a diffuse pattern.
4. Only ring forms and gametocytes are typically seen in the peripheral blood with this species. Other species may show schizonts and merozoites.
5. Black water fever.
6. Bite of a mosquito.

7. Maurer's dots. Schüffner's dots are often seen with other species.

Case Study 6-2: Under the Microscope
1. Babesiosis.
2. Serologic or PCR techniques.
3. *Ixodes dammini* tick blood meal lasting 12 hours or longer.
4. Lyme disease, human granulocytic ehrlichiosis.

CHAPTER 7

Case Study 7-1: Under the Microscope
1. *Blastocystis hominis*, vacuolated form, The parasite described exactly matches the features of *Blastocystis*, which is characterized by a center fluid-filled vacuole surrounded by a cytoplasmic ring containing small nuclei.
2. False-negative results may appear if the sample containing *Blastocystis* is only examined using one or more saline wet preps. Saline (as well as water) is known to lyse the parasite, therefore making the sample appear negative.
3. *Blastocystis hominis* reproduces by sporulation or by binary fission.
4. *Blastocystis hominis* was initially considered as a yeast most likely because of its size, shape and minimal internal structures. It has since been reclassified as a Protozoa.
5. Proper treatment of fecal material, thorough hand washing, and subsequent proper handling of food and water are critical to halt the spread of *Blastocystis hominis*.

Case Study 7-2: Under the Microscope
1. *Cryptosporidium parvum*; the patient's diagnosis and the presence of oocysts that resemble yeastlike cells in the wet preparations indicate the presence of this parasite.
2. Modified acid-fast stain; these organisms are acid-fast and stain red. *Cryptosporidium* oocysts may display small, dark-staining granules.
3. Yeast; yeast are not acid-fast and thus stain blue after modified acid-fast staining.

CHAPTER 8

Case Study 8-1: Under the Microscope
1. *Trichuris trichiura* egg.
2. Whipworm.
3. Ingestion of infective eggs.
4. Trichuriasis; whipworm infection.
5. Adult worms.

Case Study 8-2: Under the Microscope
1. *Ascaris lumbricoides*. Figure A, adult pregnant female; Figure B, mature egg.
2. Large intestinal roundworm, human roundworm.
3. The life cycle of *A. lumbricoides* is relatively complex compared with the parasites presented thus far. Infection begins following the ingestion of infected eggs that contain viable larvae. Once inside the small intestine, the larvae emerge from the eggs. The larvae then complete a liver-lung migration by first entering the blood via penetration through the intestinal wall. The first stop on this journey is the liver. From there, the larvae continue the trip via the bloodstream to the second stop, the lung. Once inside the lung, the larvae burrow their way through the capillaries into the alveoli. Migration into the bronchioles then follows. From here, the larvae are transferred through coughing into the pharynx, where they are then swallowed and returned to the intestine.

   The larvae then mature, resulting in adult worms, which take up residence in the small intestine. The adults multiply and a number of the resulting undeveloped eggs (up to 250,000/day) are passed in the feces. The outside environment, specifically soil, provides the necessary conditions for the eggs to embryonate. Infective eggs may remain viable in soil, fecal matter, sewage, or water for years. The resulting embryonated eggs are the infective stage for a new host and, when consumed by a human host, initiate a new cycle.
4. The avoidance of using human feces as fertilizer, as well as exercising proper sanitation and personal hygiene practices, are critical measures for breaking the life cycle of *Ascaris*.

CHAPTER 9

Case Study 9-1: Under the Microscope
1. *Loa loa*
2. *Loa loa*, is known to inhabit areas of Africa especially the rain forest belt and as such is referred to as the African Eye Worm. It is estimated that the infection rates may be over 70% in the areas in which a large vector population exists.
3. Yes, the blood sample was drawn at the appropriate time. Samples collected between 10:15 am and 2:15 pm yield the best recovery rate of *Loa loa* microfilariae. This parasite exhibits diurnal periodicity.
4. Surgical removal is the treatment of choice for the removal of adult *Loa loa* worms. The medication of choice for the treatment of *Loa loa* is diethylcarbamazine (DEC).

Case Study 9-2: Under the Microscope
1. The organism observed in the stained blood smear in this case is that of a *Wuchereria bancrofti* microfilaria.
2. Technically, the timing of the blood collection was not optimal for the best recovery of microfilariae. *Wuchereria bancrofti* generally exhibits nocturnal periodicity. The organism can also exhibit subperiodic periodicity and can be prevalent in the late afternoon. This may explain why the organism was detected in Sir Thomas' blood even though the timing of his blood collection was not optimal.
3. The vectors responsible for parasite transmission in this case consist of *Culex, Aedes,* and *Anopheles* spp. of mosquitoes.
4. Sir Robert is exhibiting the signs and symptoms of Bancroft's filariasis or elephantiasis.
5. Prevention and control strategies that Sir Robert should have implemented on his adventure include using personal protection when entering known endemic areas, avoiding mosquito infested areas, and using mosquito netting and insect repellants.

CHAPTER 10

Case 10-1: Under the Microscope

1. *Hymenolepis nana.*
2. No intermediate host is required.
3. Adult worm develops in humans following ingestion of an egg.
4. Praziquantel.

Case 10-2: Under the Microscope

1. Proglottid.
2. A, Uterine branches; B, radial striations; C, hexacanth embryo; D, hooklets.
3. *Taenia solium.*
4. Pork tapeworm.
5. The proglottids of *T. solium* differ from *T. saginata* in that the latter has 15 to 30 uterine branches, whereas the former possesses less than 15 uterine branches. Eggs of both organisms are identical morphologically.
6. See E. Also, the rostellum of *T. solium* possess hooklets, whereas that of *T. saginata* possesses no hooklets.

CHAPTER 11

Case Study 11-1: Under the Microscope

1. *Clonorchis sinensis.* The other trematodes that cause infections from eating raw fish, metagonimiasis and heterophyiasis, live in the intestine, not the liver.
2. Human infection occurs following the ingestion of undercooked fish contaminated with encysted metacercariae. Maturation of the immature flukes takes place in the liver. The adult worms take up residence in the bile duct. Eggs are passed in bile to the intestine, where they can be identified in feces. On contact with fresh water, the miracidium emerges from each egg. Specific species of snails serve as the first intermediate host. The miracidium penetrates into the snail, where a sporocyst develops. Numerous rediae result and ultimately produce many cercariae. The cercariae emerge from the snail and enter a fish, where they encyst.
3. Clonorchiasis.

4. Appropriate strategies in a prevention plan include practicing proper sanitation procedures, especially the practice of proper human and reservoir host feces disposal, and avoiding the practice of consuming raw, undercooked, or freshly pickled freshwater fish and shrimp.

Case Study 11-2: Under the Microscope

1. Eggs of *Schistosoma haematobium.*
2. Schistosomiasis, bilharziasis.
3. Snail.
4. Penetration of cercariae through the skin that takes place when unsuspecting humans swim in contaminated fresh water.

CHAPTER 13

Case Study 13-1: Under the Microscope

1. A type of hard shell tick is the most likely suspect.
2. There are both male and female forms of ticks, as well as hard and soft shell ticks.
3. If you must enter an area where ticks are prevalent, you should wear clothing that covers as much of the body as possible. Tick repellants are also recommended.
4. Hard ticks (*Ixodes* spp.) are capable of transmitting a number of bacterial, rickettsial, and parasitic diseases.

Case Study 13-2: Under the Microscope

1. The most likely arthropod involved is the itch mite *Sarcoptes scabiei*, the cause of scabies.
2. Skin scrapings should be collected from the lesions and placed in a sterile container with 70% ethanol and 5% formalin or sterile saline, enough to cover the sample.
3. This parasite is transmitted from person to person through close contact. Members of the household or other patients in an institutional care facility are easily infected.
4. There are several prescription level topical treatments available but it is also necessary to treat the clothing, bedding, and close contacts of this patient to prevent reinfection of the patient or the spread of scabies to others in the facility (e.g., staff, patients, family members).

Answers to Quick Quiz! Questions

CHAPTER 1

1-1. C
1-2. D (A and C)
1-3. A
1-4. B
1-5. D
1-6. B
1-7. C
1-8. D
1-9. C

CHAPTER 2

2-1. C
2-2. C
2-3. D
2-4. A
2-5. A
2-6. B
2-7. B
2-8. A
2-9. A
2-10. B
2-11. A
2-12. C
2-13. A
2-14. D

CHAPTER 3

3-1. B
3-2. B
3-3. A
3-4. A
3-5. B
3-6. B
3-7. D
3-8. C
3-9. C
3-10. A
3-11. B
3-12. B
3-13. B
3-14. B
3-15. D
3-16. B
3-17. C
3-18. A
3-19. D
3-20. C
3-21. A
3-22. C
3-23. A
3-24. D
3-25. C
3-26. A
3-27. C
3-28. D
3-29. A
3-30. D

CHAPTER 4

4-1. B
4-2. C
4-3. D
4-4. D
4-5. C
4-6. A
4-7. B
4-8. B

4-9. D
4-10. A
4-11. B
4-12. D
4-13. A
4-14. A
4-15. C
4-16. B
4-17. D
4-18. A
4-19. C
4-20. C
4-21. B
4-22. A
4-23. D (A, B, C)
4-24. B
4-25. D

CHAPTER 5

5-1. B
5-2. B
5-3. A
5-4. C
5-5. B
5-6. A
5-7. D
5-8. A, B
5-9. C
5-10. C
5-11. D
5-12. C
5-13. A
5-14. B
5-15. D
5-16. D
5-17. A
5-18. C
5-19. A
5-20. B
5-21. D
5-22. B
5-23. C
5-24. D
5-25. A
5-26. C
5-27. C

CHAPTER 6

6-1. C
6-2. A
6-3. C
6-4. B
6-5. A
6-6. B
6-7. A
6-8. D
6-9. C
6-10. B
6-11. B
6-12. A
6-13. C
6-14. B
6-15. D
6-16. A
6-17. D
6-18. C
6-19. D
6-20. A
6-21. D

CHAPTER 7

7-1. C
7-2. A
7-3. B
7-4. C
7-5. D
7-6. D
7-7. A
7-8. A
7-9. A
7-10. B
7-11. A
7-12. B
7-13. B
7-14. C
7-15. B
7-16. B
7-17. A
7-18. B
7-19. A
7-20. B
7-21. B

7-22. A
7-23. D
7-24. A
7-25. D
7-26. A
7-27. C
7-28. C

CHAPTER 8

8-1. C
8-2. B
8-3. D
8-4. C
8-5. B
8-6. A
8-7. C
8-8. A
8-9. D
8-10. C
8-11. D
8-12. A
8-13. A
8-14. B
8-15. D
8-16. B
8-17. C
8-18. D
8-19. C
8-20. A
8-21. C
8-22. B
8-23. A
8-24. B

CHAPTER 9

9-1. C
9-2. B
9-3. D
9-4. A
9-5. B
9-6. D
9-7. A
9-8. D
9-9. C
9-10. D

9-11. B
9-12. A
9-13. B
9-14. C
9-15. D

CHAPTER 10

10-1. B
10-2. C
10-3. B
10-4 C
10-5. B
10-6. A
10-7. D
10-8. B
10-9. A
10-10. C
10-11. A
10-12. B
10-13. B
10-14. C
10-15. D
10-16. A
10-17. B
10-18. C
10-19. B
10-20. C
10-21. D

CHAPTER 11

11-1. B
11-2. B
11-3. A
11-4. D
11-5. C
11-6. A
11-7. C
11-8. C
11-9. D
11-10. C
11-11. B
11-12. A
11-13. C
11-14. B
11-15. A

11-16. A
11-17. D
11-18. B

CHAPTER 12

12-1. C
12-2. B
12-3. A
12-4. A
12-5. C
12-6. D
12-7. D (A, B, C)

CHAPTER 13

13-1. A
13-2. C
13-3. C
13-4. D
13-5. C
13-6. B
13-7. B

13-8. A
13-9. D
13-10. A
13-11. C
13-12. C
13-13. A
13-14. B
13-15. B
13-16. C
13-17. E
13-18. D
13-19. D
13-20. C
13-21. C
13-22. C
13-23. D
13-24. B
13-25. A
13-26. B
13-27. B
13-28. A
13-29. D
13-30. C

Answers to Test Your Knowledge
(Review Questions)

CHAPTER 1

1-1. A. 6
B. 4
C. 1
D. 9
E. 8
F. 3
G. 10
H. 5
I. 2
J. 7

1-2. Parasites are endemic in underdeveloped tropical and subtropical countries and areas around the world. Examples of these places include Guatemala, Myanmar (Burma), and Africa. Factors that contribute to their presence include the following: (1) increased population density; (2) poor sanitation; (3) marginal water sources; (4) poor public health practices; (5) environmental changes affecting vector breeding areas; and (6) habits and customs of the inhabitants.

1-3. The increasing prevalence of world travel accounts for the increased incidence of parasitic infections in nonendemic areas of the world.

1-4. Primary modes of parasitic transmission include the following: (1) ingestion of contaminated food or drink; (2) hand-to-mouth transfer; (3) insect bite; (4) entry via drilling through the skin; (5) unprotected sexual relations; (6) mouth-to-mouth contact; (7) droplet contamination; and (8) eye contact with infected swimming water.

1-5. A. Types of parasites: Endoparasites, ectoparasites, obligatory parasites and facultative parasites.
B. Types of host: Accidental or incidental hosts, definitive hosts, intermediate hosts, reservoir hosts, transport hosts, and vectors.
C. Types of parasite-host relationships: Symbiosis, commensalisms, mutualism, and parasitism; in some cases the association may become pathogenic.
Optional activity: Any reasonable informational flyer is considered acceptable. Follow your instructor's guidelines and requirements for completion; creativity is encouraged. Keep the audience in mind and use wording that the audience will understand.

1-6. Parasites have the ability to alter their makeup so that the host will not recognize its presence as being foreign will therefore not mount an immune response against it. This in turn often creates an environment that is conducive for parasite establishment.

1-7. The two common phases of a parasitic life cycle are the following: (1) occurs when the parasite is in or on the human body and: (2) occurs independently from the human body.

1-8. (1) When parasite is in or on the human body: Provides information about the method of diagnosis, symptomatology, pathology and selection of appropriate antiparasitic medication.

(2) When parasite is independent of the human body: Provides information about epidemiology, prevention, and control.

1-9. E (A, B, C, and D)

1-10. E (C and D)

1-11. The three groups of clinically significant parasites areas follows: (1) Protozoa, single-celled parasites; (2) Metazoa, multicellular worms (helminths); and Animalia, arthropods.

1-12. Possible prevention and control strategies include the following: (1) practicing good hygiene and sanitation practices; (2) protecting picnic food from flies; (3) proper handling and preparation of food; and (4) educating at-risk individuals regarding the proper use of insecticides and other chemicals.

1-13. Any reasonable informational flyer is considered acceptable; follow your instructor's guidelines and requirements for completion. Creativity is encouraged. Keep the audience in mind and use wording that the audience will understand.

1-14. Any reasonable generic life cycle is considered acceptable; the use of illustrations and key words and phrases is encouraged. Follow your instructor's guidelines and requirements for completion; creativity is encouraged. It is important that two life cycle phases (those that occur when the parasite is in or on the human body and independently from the human body) are clearly distinguished and delineated.

CHAPTER 2

2-1. B

2-2. C

2-3. B

2-4. C

2-5. True.

2-6. The purpose of the ocular micrometer is to measure objects accurately under the microscope. It must be calibrated to determine the number of microns in the units that make up the ocular scale.

2-7. It is acceptable to eliminate the direct wet prep examination on a specimen that is received in fixative. The main purpose of the direct wet prep examination is to detect the motility of trophozoites. Because fixatives kill the trophozoites, no motility will be observed.

2-8. The zinc sulfate flotation procedure does yield a cleaner microscopic preparation; however, some parasites will not be detected with this method. Large helminth eggs and eggs that have an operculum will not float and will be missed. Thus, most laboratory technicians prefer the use of the sedimentation technique because it results in a better recovery.

2-9. The specific gravity of the zinc sulfate solution must be 1.18 to 1.20 to recover the parasites in the specimen. If the specific gravity is not within this range, recovery will not be optimal.

2-10. The permanent stained smear allows the technologist to observe more detailed features of protozoa. In addition, it allows for detection of protozoan trophozoites that are not usually recovered in the concentration procedure. *Dientamoeba fragilis* is an example of a parasite that will only be detected in the stained smear because it only has a trophozoite stage.

2-11. Rapid stool screens detect antigens to specific protozoa in a stool sample. They are available for *Cryptosporidium* spp., *Giardia intestinalis*, *Entamoeba histolytica*, and *Entamoeba histolytica–Entamoeba dispar* group. These methods do not detect tapeworms; therefore, this test request is inappropriate. As tests become available in parasitology, it is important for the laboratory to provide education to medical providers about the purpose and usefulness of assays.

2-12. Parasites that reside in the small intestine can be difficult to detect from a stool specimen. Duodenal material is an alternative sample that will allow detection of parasites such as *Giardia intestinalis, Cryptosporidium* spp., *Isospora belli,* and *Strongyloides stercoralis.*

2-13. B

2-14. Thick films are prepared by placing drops of blood onto a microscope slide and spreading them in a circular fashion to the size of a dime or nickel. The slide is then air-dried and, prior to staining, the cells are ruptured by placing the slide into buffered water. An advantage is increased recovery of malaria because of the concentration of cells. A disadvantage is that is difficult to identify species because of poor morphology.

Thin films are prepared by placing a drop of blood toward the end of a microscope slide and then using the edge of another slide to spread the blood cells into a thin layer. On staining, the red blood cells are left intact for observation of intracellular malaria parasites. An advantage is the speciation of the malaria. A disadvantage is that is difficult to detect because the cells are not concentrated.

2-15. *Entamoeba histolytica, Trichomonas vaginalis, Leishmania* spp., *Trypanosoma cruzi, Toxoplasma gondii.*

2-16. A. 2
B. 5
C. 6
D. 3
E. 1
F. 4

2-17. Xenodiagnosis is a diagnostic tool that uses a reduviid bug to diagnose patients with Chagas' disease (*Trypanosoma cruzi*). An uninfected bug is allowed to feed on a patient. The insect is later tested to determine whether the parasite was transmitted from the patient to the insect.

2-18. In most cases, immunologic tests are used in parasitology as an adjunct to diagnosis. In some cases, when the infection is difficult to diagnose by demonstrating the diagnostic stage, or the technique is too invasive, more immunology testing may be necessary. See Table 2-8 for examples of antigen tests and antibody tests.

2-19. The reporting of parasitology results is a critical component of the postanalytic phase of laboratory testing. It is important to spell out the genus and species. In this situation, reporting *E. coli* instead of *Entamoeba coli* would confuse the physician because of the confusion with the bacteria *Escherichia coli.*

2-20. Quality assurance in parasitology must include the following:
Procedure manuals
Reagents and solutions
Controls
Calibration of centrifuges and ocular micrometer
Recording of temperatures
Action plans for out of control results
References
Proficiency testing of personnel

CHAPTER 3

3-1. A. 4
B. 8
C. 3
D. 1
E. 2
F. 7
G. 5
H. 6

3-2. C

3-3. Cysts.

3-4. *Entamoeba histolytica,* intestinal; *Entamoeba hartmanni,* intestinal; *Entamoeba coli,* intestinal; *Entamoeba polecki,* intestinal; *Endolimax nana,* intestinal; *Iodamoeba butschlii,* intestinal; *Entamoeba gingivalis,* atrial; *Naegleria fowleri,* atrial; *Acanthamoeba* spp., atrial.

3-5. The life cycles of all of the intestinal amebas are similar, with one exception. Amebic life cycles require two morphologic forms, the trophozoite and the cyst. Trophozoites are characteristically delicate, fragile, and motile. The most common means whereby amebas are transferred to humans is through ingestion of the infective cyst in contaminated food or water. In most cases, trophozoites are easily destroyed by the gastric juices of the stomach. Trophozoites are also very susceptible to the environment outside the host. Therefore, trophozoites are not usually transmitted to humans. Excystation occurs in the ileocecal area of the intestine. Replication only occurs in the trophozoite stage by multiplication of the nucleus via asexual binary fission. Encystation occurs in the intestine when the environment becomes unacceptable for continued trophozoite multiplication. A number of conditions solely or in combination may trigger encystation, including ameba overpopulation, pH change, food supply (too much or too little), and available oxygen (too much or too little). Contrary to trophozoites, cysts are equipped with a protective cell wall. The cell wall allows cysts to enter the outside environment with the passage of feces and remain viable for long periods of time. The ingestion of the infective cysts completes the typical intestinal amebic life cycle.

3-6. *Entamoeba gingivalis* typically lives around the gum line of the teeth in the tartar and gingival pockets of unhealthy mouths. In addition, *E. gingivalis* trophozoites have been known to inhabit the tonsillar crypts and bronchial mucus. There is no known cyst stage of *E. gingivalis.* Infections of *E. gingivalis* are contracted via mouth-to-mouth (kissing) and droplet contamination, which may be transmitted through contaminated drinking utensils.

Naegleria fowleri is the only ameba with three known morphologic forms—ameboid trophozoite, flagellate trophozoite, and cyst. The ameboid trophozoites of *N. fowleri* are the only form known to exist in humans. Replication of the ameboid trophozoites occurs by simple binary fission. The ameboid trophozoites transform into flagellate trophozoites in vitro after being transferred to water from a tissue or culture. The flagellate trophozoites do not divide but, instead, lose their flagella and convert back into the ameboid form, in which reproduction resumes. The cyst form is known to exist only in the external environment. It appears that the entire life cycle of *N. fowleri* occurs in the external environment. Humans primarily contract this ameba by swimming in contaminated water. The ameboid trophozoites enter the human body through the nasal mucosa and often migrate to the brain, causing rapid tissue destruction. Some infections may be caused by inhaling dust infected with *N. fowleri* cysts. The mechanics of how, when, and where the transition of the cysts to ameboid trophozoites occurs after the cysts have been inhaled by a human have not been described.

3-7. A

3-8. A. *Entamoeba histolytica* is the only known pathogenic intestinal ameba. Symptoms range from asymptomatic carrier state to symptomatic intestinal amebiasis (amebic colitis) to symptomatic extraintestinal amebiasis.

B. Infections with *E. coli* are usually asymptomatic.

C. Patients who contract *N. fowleri* resulting in colonization of the nasal passages are usually asymptomatic. Primary amebic meningoencephalitis (PAM) occurs when the ameboid trophozoites of *N. fowleri* invade the brain, causing rapid tissue destruction.

D. Central nervous system (CNS) infections with *Acanthamoeba* are also known as granulomatous amebic encephalitis (GAE). On occasion, *Acanthamoeba* invade other areas of the body, including the kidneys, pancreas, prostate, and uterus, and form similar granulomatous lesions. *Acanthamoeba* infections of the cornea of the eye are known as amebic keratitis.

3-9. A. True

3-10. B

3-11. 1. A

2. A

3. A

4. C

5. B, D

6. B

3-12. Amebic trophozoites and cysts may be seen in stool samples submitted for parasite study. Trophozoites are primarily recovered from stools that are of soft, liquid, or loose consistency. Formed stool specimens are more likely to contain cysts. The morphologic forms present in samples other than stool are noted on an individual basis. It is important to point out that the presence of either or both morphologic forms is diagnostic. Proper determination of organism size, using the ocular micrometer (see Chapter 2), is essential when identifying the amebas. In addition, the appearance of key nuclear features, such as the number of nuclei present and the positioning of the nuclear structures, is crucial to correctly differentiate the amebas. The presence of other amebic structures and characteristics, such as cytoplasmic inclusions and motility, also aids in the identification of the amebas. Traditional microscopic procedures include saline wet preparations, iodine wet preparations, and permanent stains. The saline wet preparation and iodine wet preparation each have an advantage supporting their use. Saline wet preparations are of value because they will often show motility of the amebic trophozoites. The internal cytoplasmic, as well as the nuclear structures, may be more readily seen with the use of iodine wet preparations. It is important to note that permanent smears of samples suspected of containing amebas must be performed to confirm parasite identification. In most cases, the key identifying features cannot be accurately distinguished without the permanent stain. The permanent stain allows for many of the otherwise refractive and invisible structures to be more clearly visible and thus easier to identify. The permanent smear procedure may, however, shrink amebic parasites, causing measurements smaller than those typically seen in wet preparations.

CHAPTER 4

4-1. A. 3

B. 4

C. 2

D. 6

E. 1

F. 5

4-2. Intestinal flagellates: *Giardia intestinalis, Chilomastix mesnili, Dientamoeba fragilis, Trichomonas hominis, Enteromonas hominis, Retortamonas intestinalis*; atrial flagellates: *Trichomonas tenax, Trichomonas vaginalis.*

4-3. Any of the flagellates may be found in the United States.

4-4. *Trichomonas vaginalis.*

4-5. The life cycle of *Trichomonas vaginalis* is relatively simple. *T. vaginalis* trophozoites reside on the mucosal surface of the vagina in infected women. The trophozoites multiply by longitudinal binary fission in the vagina, feeding on bacteria and leukocytes. In the male, the organism typically invades the prostate gland and epithelium of the urethra.

Beyond this, the life cycle in a male host is unknown.

4-6. *Enteromonas hominis* cysts are oval in shape, with a predominant cell wall. The cysts may be binucleated or quadrinucleated. The nuclei show central karyosomes but do not have peripheral chromatin.

4-7. Trophozoite and cyst stages: *Giardia intestinalis, Chilomastix mesnili, Enteromonas hominis, Retortamonas intestinalis*; trophozoite stage only: *Dientamoeba fragilis, Trichomonas hominis, Trichomonas tenax, Trichomonas vaginalis*; cyst stage only—not applicable.

4-8. *Giardia intestinalis, Dientamoeba fragilis.*

4-9. A. Axoneme—intracellular portion of the flagellum.

B. Axostyle—rodlike support structure found in some flagellates.

C. Costa—rodlike structure located at the base of the undulating membrane. It is located between the undulating membrane and the body of some flagellates, connecting the two structures. It may also aid in supporting the undulating membrane.

D. Cytosome—rudimentary mouth.

E. Median bodies—comma-shaped structures located in the posterior end of *Giardia intestinalis* trophozoites and cysts; believed to be associated with energy and metabolism or with supporting the organism's posterior end. Their exact function is unclear.

F. Undulating membrane—finlike structure connected to the outer edge of some flagellates; aids in the organism's locomotion, moving in a wave-like pattern.

4-10. *Dientamoeba fragilis* can be difficult to diagnose for two primary reasons. First, *D. fragilis* sheds irregularly and so may not be present in all stool samples of an infected individual. The parasite resides in deeper mucosal crypts in the large intestine and may shed sporadically as a result. Second, *D. fragilis* can be difficult to identify in stained stool preparations. The parasite can stain very lightly and also has few distinguishing features, so it easily blends into the background material on a stained slide. Therefore, multiple stool samples collected over several days may be necessary to diagnose *D. fragilis*.

4-11. *Giardia intestinalis, Chilomastix mesnili, Enteromonas hominis, Retortamonas intestinalis.*

4-12. *Chilomastix mesnili, Trichomonas hominis, Enteromonas hominis, Retortamonas intestinalis, Trichomonas tenax.*
Note: there is considerable controversy over the pathogenicity of *Dientamoeba fragilis.*

4-13. *Trichomonas tenax.*

CHAPTER 5

5-1. A. 4
B. 5
C. 2
D. 1
E. 3

5-2. C

5-3. D

5-4. E

5-5. B

5-6. B

5-7. A

5-8. C

5-9. B

5-10. D

5-11. A

5-12. Belize, Guatemala, the Yucatan Peninsula, the Amazon River Basin, Venezuela, Brazil, the Venezuelan Andes.

5-13. Enlargement of the postcervical lymph nodes commonly seen in infections with *Trypanosoma brucei gambiense* and occasionally in *Trypanosoma brucei rhodesiense* infections.

5-14. Cattle, sheep, wild game animals.

5-15. Complement fixation (CF), direct agglutination (DAT), and indirect immunofluorescence (IIF).

CHAPTER 6

6-1. D
6-2. C
6-3. B
6-4. B
6-5. A
6-6. C
6-7. B
6-8. B
6-9. D
6-10. A

CHAPTER 7

7-1. A. 2, 4
    B. 1, 2
    C. 2
    D. 2
    E. 2
    F. 2
7-2. Liver, lungs, pleura, mesenteric nodes, and urogenital tract.
7-3. A. Cat—*Toxoplasma gondii.*
    B. Pig—*Balantidium coli, Isospora belli, Sarcocystis* spp.
    C. Cow—*Isospora belli, Sarcocystis* spp., *Cryptosporidium* (primarily in calves).
7-4. *Isospora belli, Blastocystis hominis.*
7-5. *Pneumocystis jiroveci.*
7-6. B
7-7. C
7-8. B
7-9. D
7-10. B

CHAPTER 8

8-1. A. 3
    B. 6
    C. 4
    D. 2
    E. 1
8-2. B
8-3. C
8-4. A. 1
    B. 3

    C. 4
    D. 5
    E. 6
8-5. D
8-6. A
8-7. A. 2
    B. 4
    C. 1
    D. 5
8-8. D
8-9. A. 5
    B. 3
    C. 2
    D. 7
    E. 4
8-10. D

CHAPTER 9

9-1. B
9-2. B
9-3. A
9-4. C
9-5. D
9-6. D
9-7. B
9-8. C
9-9. A
9-10. C

CHAPTER 10

10-1. A. 3
    B. 9
    C. 7
    D. 8
    E. 10
    F. 1
    G. 2
    H. 5
    I. 6
    J. 4
10-2. A. Beef tapeworm.
    B. Dog and cat tapeworm; pumpkin seed tapeworm.
    C. Dwarf tapeworm.
    D. Fish tapeworm.

E. Pork tapeworm.

F. Hydatid tapeworm; dog tapeworm, less commonly.

G. Rat tapeworm.

10-3. Great Lakes region; parts of South America, Asia; Central Africa; Baltic region; Finland.

10-4. A. Cysticercus.

B. Cysticercoid larva (in flea).

C. Egg.

D. Plerocercoid.

E. Cysticercus.

F. Egg.

G. Cysticercoid larva (in beetle or flea).

10-5. A. Vitamin B_{12} deficiency.

B. Cyst development in various organs.

10-6. A. Stool.

B. Stool.

C. Stool.

D. Stool.

E. Stool.

F. Serum specimen for serology or biopsy.

G. Stool.

10-7. A. Four suckers and no hooks.

B. Four suckers and rows of tiny hook-like spines.

C. Four suckers and short rostellum with one row of hooks.

D. Lateral sucking grooves.

E. Four suckers with two rows of hooks.

F. Four suckers and up to 36 hooks.

G. Four suckers and rostellum with no hooks.

10-8. *Taenia saginata* proglottids have 15 to 30 lateral uterine branches, whereas *Taenia solium* has less than 15 lateral uterine branches.

10-9. *Taenia solium.*

10-10. *Diphyllobothrium latum.*

CHAPTER 11

11-1. C

11-2. B

11-3. A

11-4. D

11-5. A

11-6. B

11-7. B

11-8. C

11-9. D

11-10. 1. B

2. B

3. A

4. C

5. A

6. A

CHAPTER 12

12-1. A. 7

B. 6

C. 5

D. 2

E. 4

F. 3

G. 1

12-2. Charcot-Leyden crystals, diamond-shaped crystals, indicate that an immune response has occurred as they develop from the breakdown of eosinophils. This immune response could be caused by the presence of parasites.

12-3. C

12-4. Epithelial cells differ from amebic parasites in that epithelial cells lack the typical amebic trophozoite interior structures and appear smooth, with no inclusions.

12-5. D

12-6. Clumped, fused platelets, Giemsa stain precipitate, red cell abnormalities.

CHAPTER 13

13-1. Pairs of jointed appendages, chitinized exoskeleton, and hemocele.

13-2. A. 6

B. 9

C. 8

D. 3

E. 4
F. 5
G. 1
H. 10
I. 2
J. 7

13-3. A. 5
B. 3
C. 7
D. 1
E. 8
F. 10
G. 10
H. 6
I. 10
J. 9

13-4. A. 5
B. 3
C. 4
D. 3
E. 1
F. 3
G. 3
H. 2
I. 5
J. 3

13-5. The larval and nymph stages are more likely to transmit microorganisms such as Lyme disease because they are often overlooked as a result of their small size. It takes at least 24 hours of contact feeding to obtain a good transmission rate. Adult ticks are sufficiently large that most people see them quickly and they are removed before complete transmission can occur.

13-6. A scutum is the hard plate or shell on the dorsal surface of a hard tick, such as *Ixodes* spp.

13-7. Hemocele—a blood sac or cavity in which the blood meal is held; found in the body of blood-sucking arthropods.
Vertical transmission—some arthropod hosts are capable of transmitting their infecting microorganism to their progeny, perpetuating the environmental source of human infection (e.g., ticks).
Capitulum—the head and mouth parts of a hard shell tick.

13-8. E (B and D)

13-9. A

13-10. B

Bibliography

Abrams C: *Donor center vigilance essential to maintain safe blood supply*, King of Prussia, PA, 1992, Merion Publications.

Ashrafi K, Valero MA, Massoud J, et al: Plant-borne human contamination by fascioliasis. *Am J Trop Med Hyg* 75:295–302, 2006.

Beth Israel Deaconess Medical Center: Laboratory manual, 2004 (http://home.caregroup.org/departments/pathology/default.asp).

Bope ET, Kellerman RD, editors: *Conn's current therapy 2012*, Philadelphia, 2012, Saunders.

Bottone EJ, Madayag RM, Qureshi MN: *Acanthamoeba* keratitis: Synergy between amebic and bacterial co-contaminants in contact lens care systems as a prelude to infection. *J Clin Microbiol* 30:2447–2450, 1992.

Bracha R, Diamond S, Ackers JP, et al: Differentiations of clinical isolates of *Entamoeba histolytica* by using specific DNA probes. *J Clin Microbiol* 28:680–684, 1990.

Casey K: *Specimen processing in clinical parasitology.* Senior Research Project, 1994, St. Louis University Department of Clinical Laboratory Science.

Centers for Disease Control and Prevention (CDC): Parasites—enterobiasis (also known as pinworm infection), 2010 (http://www.cdc.gov/parasites/pinworm/treatment.html).

Centers for Disease Control and Prevention (CDC): Parasites—drancunculiasis (also known as guinea worm infection), management and treatment, 2010 (http://www.cdc.gov/parasites/guineaworm/ treatment.html).

Centers for Disease Control and Prevention (CDC): Parasites—enterobiasis (also known as pinworm infection), treatment, 2010 (http://www.cdc.gov/parasites/pinworm/treatment.html).

Centers for Disease Control and Prevention (CDC): Parasites—trichinellosis (also known as trichinosis), treatment, 2010 (http://www.cdc.gov/parasites/trichinellosis/treatment.html).

Centers for Disease Control and Prevention (CDC): parasites—trichuriasis (also known as whipworm infection), treatment, 2010 (http://www.cdc.gov/parasites/whipworm/treatment.html).

Centers for Disease Control and Prevention (CDC), Division of Parasitic Diseases and Malaria: DPDx: Laboratory identification of parasites of public concern, 2009 (http://www.dpd.cdc.gov/dpdx).

Centers for Disease Control and Prevention (CDC): Parasites—*Giardia*, biology, 2010 (http://www.cdc.gov/parasites/giardia/biology.html).

Centers for Disease Control and Prevention (CDC): Parasites—*Giardia*, treatment, 2010 (http://www.cdc.gov/parasites/giardia/treatment.html).

Chan FH, Guan MX, Mackenzie AMR: Application of indirect immunofluorescence to detection of *Dientamoeba fragilis* trophozoites in fecal specimens. *J Clin Microbiol* 31:1710–1714, 1993.

Chandler FW, Watts JC: Immunofluorescence as an adjunct to the histopathologic diagnosis of Chagas' disease. *J Clin Microbiol* 26:567–569, 1988.

Clark JK: *Giardia lamblia continues to plague water supplies*, King of Prussia, PA, 1992, Merion Publications, pp 10–11.

Current Topics: Despite intensified awareness, STDs are increasing. *ASM News* 57:10–11, 1991.

Dorland: *Dorland's pocket medical dictionary*, ed 29, Philadelphia, 2012, Saunders.

Edwards DD: Troubled waters in Milwaukee. *ASM News* 59:342–345, 1993.

Fan PC, Lin CY, Chen CC, Chung WC: Morphological description of *Taenia saginata asiatica* (Cyclophyllidea: Taeniidae) from man in Asia. *J Helminth* 69:299–303, 1995.

Fenwick A, Webster JPL: Schistosomiasis: Challenges for control, treatment and drug resistance. *Curr Opin Infect Dis* 19:577–582, 2006.

Flores BM, Garcia CA, Stamm WE, et al: Differentiation of *Naegleria fowleri* from *Acathamoeba* species by using monoclonal antibodies and flow cytometry. *J Clin Microbiol* 28:1999–2005, 1990.

Food and Drug Administration (FDA): Draft prescribing information, Alinia, 2004 (http://www.accessdata.fda.gov/drugsatfda_docs/label/2004/21497.21498s001lbl.pdf).

Food and Drug Administration (FDA): Flagyl, metronidazole, 2010 (http://www.accessdata.fda.gov/drugsatfda_docs/label/2010/012623s061lbl.pdf).

Food and Drug Administration (FDA): Highlights of prescribing information, Tindamax, 2007 (http://www.accessdata.fda.gov/drugsatfda_docs/label/2007/021618s003lbl.pdf).

Fritsche TR, Gautom RK, Seyedirashti S, et al: Occurrence of bacterial endosymbionts in *Acanthamoeba* spp. isolated from corneal and environmental specimens and contact lenses. *J Clin Microbiol* 31:1122–1126, 1993.

Garcia LS: *Diagnostic medical parasitology*, ed 5, Washington, DC, 2007, ASM Press.

Garcia LS: *Practical guide to diagnostic parasitology*, Washington, DC, 2009, ASM Press.

Garcia LS, Shimizu RY: Diagnostic parasitology: Parasitic infections and the immunocompromised host. *Lab Med* 24:205–214, 1993.

Garcia LS, Shimizu RY: Medical parasitology: Update on diagnostic techniques and laboratory safety. *Lab Med* 24:81–88, 1993.

Garcia LS, Shum AC, Bruckner DA: Evaluation of a new monoclonal antibody combination reagent for direct fluorescence detection of *Giardia* cysts and *Cryptosporidium* oocysts in human fecal specimens. *J Clin Microbiol* 30:3255–3257, 1992.

Gilbert DN, Moellering RC, Jr, Eliopoulos GM, editors: *The Sanford guide to antimicrobial therapy 2008*, ed 38, Sperryville, VA, 2008, Antimicrobial Therapy.

Gross U, Roos T, Appoldt D, et al: Improved serological diagnosis of *Toxoplasma gondii* infection by detection of immunoglobulin A (IgA) and IgM antibodies against P30 by using the immunoblot technique. *J Clin Microbiol* 30:1436–1441, 1992.

Gryseels B, Polman K, Clerinx J, Kestens L: Human schistosomiasis. *Lancet* 368:1106–1118, 2006.

Hobbs MM, Lapple DM, Lawing LF, et al: Methods for Detection of *Trichomonas vaginalis* in the Male Partners of Infected Women: Implications for Control of Trichomoniasis. *J Clin Microbial* 44:3994–3999, 2006.

John JT, Petri WA: *Markell and Voge's medical parasitology*, ed 9, St. Louis, 2006, Saunders.

Keiser J, Utzinger J: Artemisinins and synthetic trioxolanes in the treatment of helminth infections. *Curr Opin Infect Dis* 20:605–612, 2007.

Keiser J, Utzinger J: Emerging foodborne trematodiasis, 2005 (http://wwwnc.cdc.gov/eid/article/11/10/05-0614_article.htm).

Kilvington S, Larkin DF, White DG, et al: Laboratory investigation of *Acanthamoeba* keratitis. *J Clin Microbiol* 28:2722–2725, 1990.

King CH, Dickman K, Tisch DJ: Reassessment of the cost of chronic helmintic infection: A meta-analysis of disability-related outcomes in endemic schistosomiasis. *Lancet* 365:1561–1569, 2005.

Lang HK: *Gulf War mystery disease getting renewed attention*, King of Prussia, PA, 1993, Merion Publications.

Le TH, Nguyen VD, Phan BU, et al: Case report: Unusual presentation of Fasciolopsis buski in a Vietnamese child. *Trans R Soc Trop Med Hyg* 98:193–194, 2004.

Leishmaniasis: History, 2006 (http://www.stanford.edu/class/humbio103/ParaSites2006/Leishmaniasis/history.htm).

Lim JH, Kim SY, Park CM: Parasitic diseases of the biliary tract. *Am J Roentgenol* 188:1596–1603, 2007.

Linsalata L: *Incidence of intestinal parasites in the St. Louis area: A five-year analysis*. Senior Research Project, 1994, St. Louis University Department of Clinical Laboratory Science.

Lun ZR, Gasser RB, Lai DH, et al: Clonorchiasis: A key foodborne zoonosis in China. *Lancet Infect Dis* 5:31–41, 2005.

MacPherson DW, McQueen R: Cryptosporidiosis: Multi-attribute evaluation of six diagnostic methods. *J Clin Microbiol* 31:198–202, 1993.

Mahon CR, Lehman DC, Manuselis G: *Textbook of diagnostic microbiology*, ed 4, St. Louis, 2011, Saunders.

Malaria threat low. MT Today August 1993.

Malowitz R: Clinical parasitology. In Lehmann CA, editor: *Saunders manual of clinical laboratory science*, Philadelphia, pp 687–770, 1998, WB Saunders.

Mann CC: A pox on the new world, 2010 (http://www.americanheritage.com/content/pox-new-world).

Mejia E: *Parasitic infections in the St. Louis area: Prevalence from November 1988 to November 1990*. Senior Research Project, 1990, St. Louis University Department of Clinical Laboratory Science.

Moser DR, Kirchoff LV, Donelson JE: Detection of *Trypanosoma cruzi* by DNA amplification using the polymerase chain reaction. *J Clin Microbiol* 27:1477–1482, 1989.

Mountford AP: Immunological aspects of schistosomiasis. *Parasite Immunol* 27:243–246, 2005.

Murat L: *Parasitology case studies*. Senior Research Project, 1994, St. Louis University Department of Clinical Laboratory Science.

Murray PR, Rosenthal KS, Pfaller MA: *Medical microbiology*, ed 6, Philadelphia, 2009, Mosby.

Park do H, Son, HY: Images in clinical medicine. Clonorchis sinensis. *Am J Trop Med Hyg* 358:e18, 2008.

Peek R, Reedeker FR, van Good T: Direct amplification and genotyping of *Dientamoeba fragilis* from human stool specimens. *J Clin Microbiol* 42:631–635, 2004.

PCR could lead to toxoplasmosis test. *ASM News* 55:530, 1989.

Qureshi MN, Perez II AA, Madayag RM: Inhibition of *Acanthamoeba* species by *Pseudomonas aeruginosa*: Rationale for their selective exclusion in corneal ulcers and contact lens care systems. *J Clin Microbiol* 31:1908–1910, 1993.

Ruiz AG, Haque R, Rehman T, et al: A monoclonal antibody for distinction of invasive and noninvasive clinical isolates of *Entamoeba histolytica. J Clin Microbiol* 30:2807–2813, 1992.

Samuelson J, Soto RA, Reed S, et al: DNA hybridization probe for clinical diagnosis of *Entamoeba histolytica. J Clin Microbiol* 27:671–676, 1989.

Schuurman T, Lankamp P, Van Belkum A, Kooistra-Smid M, Van Zwet A: Comparison of microscopy, real-time PCR and a rapid immunoassay for the detection of *Giardia lamblia* in human stool specimens. *Clin Microbiol Infect* 13:1186–1191, 2007.

Smith LA: *Entamoeba histolytica:* The question of pathogenicity. *Clin Lab Sci* 5:334–335, 1992.

Spread of drug-resistant malaria poses threat. MT Today. August, 1993.

Steinmann P, Keiser J, Bos R, et al: Schistosomiasis and water resources development: Systematic review, meta-analysis, and estimates of people at risk. *Lancet Infect Dis* 6:411–425, 2006.

Thewjitcharoen Y, Poopitaya S: Paragonimiasis presenting with unilateral pseudochylothorax: Case report and literature review. *Scand J Infect Dis* 38:386–388, 2006.

Thielman N, Reddy E: Intestinal parasites. In Bope ET, Kellerman RD, editors: *Conn's current therapy 2012: Expert consult—online and print*, Philadelphia, 2012, Saunders, pp 538–547.

van Belkum A, Jonckheere J, Quint WGV: Genotyping *Naegleria* spp. and *Naegleria fowleri* isolates by inter-repeat polymerase chain reactions. *J Clin Microbiol* 30:2595–2598, 1992.

Vennervald B, Dunne DW: Morbidity in schistosomiasis: An update. *Curr Opin Infect Dis* 17:439–447, 2004.

Versalovic J: *Manual of clinical microbiology*, ed 10, Washington DC, 2012, ASM Press.

Weber R, Bryan RT, Juranek DD: Improved stool concentration procedure for detection of *Cryptosporidium* oocysts in fecal specimens. *J Clin Microbiol* 30:2869–2873, 1992.

Wilson M, Arrowood MJ: Diagnostic parasitology: Direct detection methods and serodiagnosis. *Lab Med* 24:145–148, 1993.

Yao A, Hammond N, Alasadi R, Nikolaidis P: Central hepatic involvement in paragonimiasis: Appearance on CT and MRI. *Am J Roentgenol* 187:W236–W237, 2006.

Zeibig EA: *Introduction to medical parasitology: Laboratory course manual*, St. Louis, 1994, Saint Louis University Department of Clinical Laboratory Science.

Zierdt CH: *Blastocystis hominis,* a protozoan parasite and intestinal pathogen of human beings. *Clin Microbiol Newslett* 5:57–59, 1983.

Page numbers followed by "f" indicate figures, "t" indicate tables, and "b" indicate boxes.

A

Acanthamoeba
  keratitis, 70b
    diagnosis, 30
  name, reference, 71b
Acanthamoeba species, 68b
  clinical symptoms, 70
  cysts, 69b
    characteristics, 69t
    cytoplasm/vacuoles, 69f
    illustration, 69f
  diagnosis, reasons, 71b
  epidemiology, 70b
  granulomatous amebic encephalitis,
    70b
  human acquisition, 71b
  identification, 70t
  infections, 72b
    prevention, 72b
  laboratory diagnosis, 69b
  life cycle notes, 69b-70b
  morphology, 68
  prevention/control, 71b
  treatment, 70b-71b
  trends, 71b
  trophozoites, 68b-69b
    acanthopodia, presence, 68f
    characteristics, 68t
Acanthamoeba spp.
  laboratory techniques, 44
  presence, 29
Acanthopodia, presence, 68f
Adult body louse, 313f
Adult bugs, features, 316t
Adult fleas, 309f
  features, 309t
Adult flies, 310f
  features, 310t
  speciation, 311t
Adult lice, features, 313t
Adult mites, 303f
  features, 304t
Adult mosquitoes
  features, 315t
  illustration, 315f
  speciation, 311t
Adult scorpion, 307f
Adult spiders, 305f
  features, 306t
Adult worms, 223-224
  nematoda form, 190

African sleeping sickness, 29
Alternative single-vial systems, 19
Amastigotes, 106-107
  characteristics, 107t
  illustration, 107f
  Leishmania spp., illustration, 107f
Amebas
  case study, 42b-43b
  classification, 45-72
  clinical symptoms, 44-45
  focus, 43-72
  form, 43
  iodine wet preparation, usage, 44
  laboratory diagnosis, 44
    techniques, alternatives, 44
  life cycle, 43-44
    notes, 43-44
  morphology, 43-44
  organism size, determination, 44
  parasite classification, 45f
  pathogenesis, 44-45
  permanent smear procedures, 44
  saline wet preparation, usage, 44
  transformation, 44b
Amebic cysts, white blood cells
  (differentiation), 287b
Amebic trophozoites
  epithelial cells, comparison, 290
  presence, 44
Ameboid trophozoites, *Naegleria
  fowleri*, 65b
Anaphylactic shock, 242
Ancylostoma duodenale, 202b
  adult female, 204f
  adult hookworm, buccal cavity,
    207b
  adults, 204b-205b
  asymptomatic hookworm infection,
    206b
  buccal capsule, 204f
  clinical symptoms, 206
  eggs, 202b-203b
    illustration, 202f
  epidemiology, 205b-206b
  filariform larvae, 204b
  hookworm
    contraction process, 207b
    disease, ancylostomiasis/
      necatoriasis, 206b
  laboratory diagnosis, 205b
  life cycle notes, 205b

Ancylostoma duodenale *(Continued)*
  morphology, 202
  prevention/control, 206b
  rhabditiform larvae, 203b-204b
  treatment, 206b
  trends, 206b-207b
Ancylostomiasis, 206b
Animal inoculation, 31
Animalia, arthropods, 10
Anopheles (malaria transmission),
    133-134
Antibody detection, 32
  endemic area, consideration,
    32b
Antigen detection, 32
Antimalarial medication,
    consideration, 143b
Antiparasitic medications, availability,
    7-8
Apicomplexan parasites, genus
    location, 152
Arthropods
  animalia, 10
  case study, 298b
  characteristics, 298-299
  classes, 300-318
  classification, 300-318
    breakdown, 301f
  clinical symptoms, 299-300
  focus, 298-318
  hemocele, presence, 299b
  humans, relationship, 299
  infectious diseases/reactions,
    319t
  laboratory diagnosis, 299
  life cycle notes, 298-299
  morphology, 298-299
  parasite classification, 11f
  pathogenesis, 299-300
  prevention/control, 300
  skin location, 300b
  treatment, 300
  vector (insect vector), parasite
    entry, 4
  vertical transmission, occurrence,
    300b
  visibility, 299
Artifacts (confusers), 9
  focus, 286-292
Ascariasis (roundworm infection),
    201b

Ascaris lumbricoides, 197b
  adult female, 200f
  adult male, 200f
  adults, 198b
    characteristics, 198t
  asymptomatic patients, 201b
  clinical symptoms, 201
  contraction, method, 201b
  corticated mature egg, 199f
  decorticated egg, 199f
  epidemiology, 201b
  fertilized eggs, 197b-198b
    characteristics, 198t
  infection, 30
  laboratory diagnosis, 198b-199b
  life cycle notes, 199b-201b
  mature egg, 199f
  morphology, 197
  outer mamilated albuminous
      coating, absence, 202b
  prevention/control, 201b
    strategies, 207b
  recovery, specimen selection, 202b
  treatment, 201b
  unfertilized eggs, 197b
    characteristics, 198t
    illustration, 198f
Asymptomatic carrier state
  Balantidium coli, 164b
  Dientamoeba fragilis, 90b
  Entamoeba histolytica, 49b
  Giardia lamblia (G. lamblia), 84b
  Trichomonas vaginalis, 99b
Asymptomatic hookworm infection,
    206b
Atypical interstitial plasma cell
    pneumonia, 184b

B

Babesia divergens, 154b
  clinical symptoms, 155b
  epidemiology, 154b-155b
  laboratory diagnosis, 154b
  laboratory diagnostic procedures,
      recommendation, 155b
  life cycle notes, 154b
  morphology, 154b
  prevention/control, 155b
  treatment, 155b
Babesia microti, 154b
  infection location, 155b
Babesia species, 152-156
  accidental human host, 153b
  classification, 154-156
  clinical symptoms, 153-154
  historical perspective, 152

Babesia species *(Continued)*
  laboratory diagnosis, 153
  life cycle notes, 152-153
  merozoite, 152b-153b
    characteristics, 152t
  morphological forms, 152-153
  morphology, 152-153
  parasite classification, 154f
  pathogenesis, 153-154
  recovery, specimen selection, 153b
  trophozoite, 152b
    characteristics, 152t
Babesia spp.
  parasite recovery, 27
  quantitation, 33
Babesiosis, 131
  severity, 155b
Babesiosis, characterization, 154b
Background material
  appearance, 25t
  parasitic structures, appearance,
      28t
Balantidiasis, 164b-165b
Balantidium coli, 162b
  asymptomatic carrier state, 164b
  clinical symptoms, 164
    comparison, 165b
  cysts, 163b-164b
    characteristics, 163t
  epidemiology, 164b
  infection, prognosis (factors),
      165b
  laboratory diagnosis, 164b
  life cycle
    comparison, 165b
    notes, 164b
  morphology, 162
  prevention/control, 165b
  stained cyst/troph, structure
      (visibility), 165b
  treatment, 165b
  trends, 165b
  trophozoite, 162b-163b
    characteristics, 163t
    illustration, 161f
Beef tapeworm infection (taeniasis),
    245b
Benign tertian malaria, 139b
Bilharziasis, 280b
Biopsy specimens, 29-30
Black water fever, 150b
  description, 151b
Blastocystis hominis, 172b
  clinical symptoms, 174
    responsibility, 174b
  epidemiology, 173b-174b

Blastocystis hominis (Continued)
  identification, screening method,
      174b
  infection, 174b
  laboratory diagnosis, 173b
  life cycle notes, 173b
  morphology, 172b-173b
  prevention/control, 174b
  quantitation, 33
  spread, prevention, 174b
  treatment, 174b
  trends, 174b
  vacuolated forms, 173b
    characteristics, 173t
    illustration, 166f, 168f
Blood, 27-29
  buffy coat slides, 29
  collection, 27-28
    timing, variation, 28
  cultures, 29
  films, smears, 134
  handling, 27-28
  Knott technique, 29
  parasites (detection), Giemsa stain
      preference (identification), 31b
  processing, 28-29
    permanent stains, usage, 28
    thick/thin smears, usage, 28
  sample, *Loa loa* recovery (timing),
      231b
  specimen collection,
      ethylenediaminetetraacetic acid
      (usage), 27-28
Blood-dwelling trematodes, 267
Body
  disease processes, 7
  infection, parasites (impact), 3
  infestation, parasites (impact), 3
  Naegleria fowleri ameboid
      trophozoites (entry), 68b
Broad fish tapeworm infection
    (diphyllobothriasis), 255b-256b
Brugia malayi, 227b
  adults, 228b
  characteristic, contrast, 229b
  clinical symptoms, 229
  epidemiology, 228b-229b
  laboratory diagnosis, 228b
  life cycle notes, 228b
  Malayan filariasis, 229b
  microfilariae, 229b
    characteristics, 228t
    illustration, 228f
    sheath/nuclei, illustration, 228f
  morphology, 227
  prevention/control, 229b

Brugia malayi (Continued)
  sample collection, timing, 229b
  treatment, 229b
  trends, 229b
Buffy coat slides, 29
Bugs, 316
  adult bugs, features, 316t
  adult triatomid bug, illustration, 316f
  clinical symptoms, 317b
  encounters, impact, 317b
  epidemiology, 317b
  features, presence, 317b
  geography, 317b
  life cycle notes, 317b
  morphology, 316b-317b
  prevention/control, 317b
  treatment, 317b

C

Cat tapeworm disease (dipylidiasis), 253b
Category names, variation, 10
Cellophane tape preparation, 27
Cercariae, 267
Cerebral paragonimiasis, 276b
Cerebrospinal fluid (CSF) specimens, 29
Cervical lymph nodes, enlargement, 121b
Cestodes
  case study, 240b
  characteristics, 241b
  classification, 242-259
  clinical symptoms, 242
  focus, 240-259
  infection, association, 242b
  internal structures, visibility, 241
  laboratory diagnosis, 241
  life cycle notes, 240-241
  morphologic forms, 240-241
    characterization, 241b
  morphology, 240-241
  parasite classification, 242f
  pathogenesis, 242
  stool, recovery, 241
Chagas' disease, 124b
  characteristics, 125b
Charcot-Leyden crystals, 288-289
  presence, clinical significance, 289b
Chiclero ulcer, presence, 113b
Chilomastix mesnili, 86b
  clinical symptoms, 88b
  cysts, 87b
    characteristics, 87t
    illustration, 87f

Chilomastix mesnili (Continued)
  epidemiology, 88b
  morphologic characteristics, 88b
  morphologic forms, liquid stool recovery, 88b
  morphology, 77-78
  prevention/control, 88b
  treatment, 88b
  trophozoites, 86
    characteristics, 86t
    illustration, 86f
Chitinized exoskeleton, 298-299
Cilia, cytoplasmic extensions, 161-185
Ciliates, 161-185
Clinical symptoms, amebas, 44-45
Clonorchiasis, 272b-273b
Clonorchis sinesis, 271b
  adults, 271b
    illustration, 269b
    recovery procedures, 273b
  asymptomatic patients, 272b
  cases, increase (determination), 273b
  clinical symptoms, 272
  eggs, 271b
    characteristics, 271t
    illustration, 272f
  epidemiology, 272b
  Heterophyes heterophyes (differentiation), 274b
  laboratory diagnosis, 271b
  life cycle notes, 271b-272b
  morphology, 271
  prevention/control, 273b
    strategy, recommendation, 273b
  quantitation, 33
  specimen, observation, 26
  treatment, 273b
Clumped platelets, 291
Cockroaches, impact, 318b
Colon biopsy material, collection, 26-27
Commensal associations, 5
Commensualism, 5
Concentrated iodine wet preparations, 23
Concentrated saline wet preparations, 23
Concentrated wet preparations, 23
Concentration methods, 22-23
  formalin-ethyl acetate sedimentation procedure, 23
  types, 23
  zinc sulfate flotation techniques, 23

Confusers (artifacts), 9
  focus, 286-292
Congenital toxoplasmosis, 180b-181b
Cryptosporidiosis, 171b
Cryptosporidium
  oocysts, 163f
    detection, 25
  spp., detection (absence), 32-33
  tests, indication, 25-26
Cryptosporidium parvum, 170b
  autoinfection, stage identification, 172b
  clinical symptoms, 171
  epidemiology, 171b
  gametocytes, 171b
  laboratory diagnosis, 171b
  life cycle notes, 171b
  morphology, 170
  oocysts, 170b
    characteristics, 170t
    illustration, 162f
  prevention/control, 172b
    recommendation, 172b
  recovery, permanent stain (selection), 172b
  schizonts, 171b
  treatment, 172b
  trends, 172b
Culture methods, 31
Cutaneous leishmaniasis
  new world cutaneous leishmaniais, 116b-117b
  old world cutaneous leishmaniasis, 118b
Cyclic paroxysms, occurrence, 134t
Cyclospora cayetanensis, 174b
  clinical symptoms, 175
    association, 176b
  diagnosis, 176b
  epidemiology, 175b
  infection, 175b
  laboratory diagnosis, 175b
  life cycle notes, 175b
  mature oocyst, characteristics, 175t
  morphology, 174
  oocysts, 174b-175b
  prevention step, 176b
  prevention/control, 175b
  trends, 175b-176b
Cyclospora genera, 161
Cysts, 43
  amebic trophozoites, presence, 44
  conversion, 43

D

Deer ticks (*Ixodes* ticks), U.S. location, 303b
Developing trophozoites, 132-133
   appearance, variation, 132-133
   Plasmodium falciparium, 147b
   Plasmodium malariae, 144b-145b
   Plasmodium ovale, 141b
   Plasmodium vivax, 136b
Diagnostic stage (parasitic life cycle), 6
Diagnostic test, completion, 34b
Dientamoeba fragilis, 88b
   asymptomatic carrier state, 90b
   clinical symptoms, 90
   cysts, 89b
   epidemiology, 89b-90b
   flagellate trophozoite, description, 90b
   life cycle notes, 89b
   morphology, 88b
   permanent stain, selection, 90b
   prevention/control, 90b
   symptomatic patients, 90b
   treatment, 90b
   trends, 90b
   trophozoites, 88b-89b
      characteristics, 89t
      illustration, 89f
Digenea, 266
Diphyllobothriasis (fish tapeworm infection), 255b-256b
Diphyllobothrium latum, 253b
   adults, characteristics, 255t
   associations, correctness, 256b
   asymptomatic patients, 255b
   clinical symptoms, 255
   eggs, 254b
      characteristics, 254t
      illustration, 254f
      uniqueness, 256b
   epidemiology, 255b
   laboratory diagnosis, 254b-255b
   life cycle notes, 255b
   morphology, 254
   prevention/control, 256b
   primary pathology, 256b
   proglottids, 254b
      illustration, 255f
   scolices, 254b
      illustration, 254f
   treatment, 256b
   trends, 256b
Dipylidiasis (dog/cat tapeworm disease), 253b

Dipylidium caninum, 251b
   adults, characteristics, 252t
   asymptomatic patients, 253b
   characteristic, 253b
   clinical symptoms, 253
   egg packets, 251b
      illustration, 252f
   eggs, characteristics, 252t
   epidemiology, 253b
   infection, diagnosis/acquisition, 253b
   laboratory diagnosis, 252b
   life cycle notes, 252b-253b
   morphology, 251
   prevention/control, 253b
      measures, 253b
   proglottids, 252b
      illustration, 252f
   scolices, 251b
   treatment, 253b
Direct fluoroscent antibody (DFA), 25
Direct iodine wet preparation, 22
Direct saline wet preparation, procedure, 22
Direct wet mount, 21-22
Direct wet preparation, 21-22
   elimination, 21
      specimen fixation, 22b
   purpose, 21-22
Disease processes/symptoms, 7
Dog tapeworm disease (dipylidiasis), 253b
Dracunculosis (Guinea worm infection), 214b
Dracunculus medinensis, 213b
   adults, 213b-214b
      characteristics, 214t
   clinical symptoms, 214
   epidemiology, 214b
   first-stage larva, 213t
   human contraction, 215b
   laboratory diagnosis, 214b
   larvae, 213b
   life cycle notes, 214b
   morphologic stages, 215b
   morphology, 213
   prevention/control, 215b
   recovery, specimen selection, 215b
   treatment, 214b-215b
   trends, 215b
Drancunculiasis (Guinea worm infection), 214b
Duodenal fluid, examination, 26
Duodenal specimens, 26
Dwarf tapeworm disease (hymenolepiasis), 251b

E

Early trophozoites (ring forms), 132
East African (Rhodesian) sleeping sickness, 122b
Echinococcosis, 258b
Echinococcus granulosus, 256b
   adults, 257b
   clinical symptoms, 258
   eggs, 256b-257b
   epidemiology, 258b
   human site, location, 259b
   hydatid cysts, 257b
      characteristics, 257t
      illustration, 257f
   infection
      diagnostic procedure, 259b
      impact, 259b
   laboratory diagnosis, 258b
   life cycle notes, 258b
   morphology, 256
   prevention/control, 259b
   treatment, 258b-259b
   trends, 259b
Echinococcus spp. (pathogen recovery), 29
Ectoparasites, 4-5
   examination, 299
   impact, 298
Eggs (nematoda form), 190
Encystation, occurrence, 43
Endemic area, consideration, 32b
Endolimax nana, 58b
   characteristics, 60b
   clinical symptoms, 60b
   cysts, 59b
      characteristics, 60t
      illustration, 59f
   epidemiology, 60b
   karyosome, appearance, 60b
   laboratory diagnosis, 59b-60b
   morphology, 58
   prevention/control, 60b
   treatment, 60b
   trophozoites, 58b-59b
      characteristics, 58t
      illustration, 59f
Endoparasite, 4-5
Entamoeba coli, 53b
   characteristics, identification, 56b
   clinical symptoms, 56b
   cysts, 54b-55b
      characteristics, 55t
      nuclei, visibility, 55f
   epidemiology, 56b

Entamoeba coli (Continued)
  laboratory diagnosis, 55b
  morphology, 53
  prevention/control, 56b
  treatment, 56b
  trends, 56b
  trophozoites, 53b-54b, 54f
    characteristics, 53t
    identification, 56b
    pseudopod, nuclear perimeter
      (irregularity), 54f
Entamoeba gingivalis, 63b
  characteristics, 64b
  clinical symptoms, 64b
  cysts, 63b
  epidemiology, 64b
  identification, 64b
  infection, 30
  laboratory diagnosis, 63b-64b
  life cycle notes, 64b
  morphology, 63
  prevention/control, 64b
  treatment, 64b
  trends, 64b
  trophozoites, 63b
    characteristics, 63t
    illustration, 63f
Entamoeba hartmanni, 51b
  characteristics, identification,
    53b
  clinical symptoms, 53b
  cysts, 52b
    characteristics, 52t
  epidemiology, 52b-53b
  laboratory diagnosis, 52b
  morphology, 51b
  prevention/control, 53b
  treatment, 53b
  trends, 53b
  trophozoites, 51b-52b
    characteristics, 52t
    contrast, 53b
Entamoeba histolytica (E. histolytica),
    45b
  antigen detection method, 25
  asymptomatic carrier state, 49b
    factors, 51b
  clinical symptoms, 49b
  cyst, 47b-48b, 47f
    characteristics, 47t
    nucleus/chromatoid bars,
      presence, 47f
  dispar cyst, 47f
  epidemiology, 48b-49b
  infection, diagnosis method
    (identification), 51b

Entamoeba histolytica (E. histolytica)
    (Continued)
  infective stage, identification,
    51b
  laboratory diagnosis, 44, 48b
  life cycle notes, 48b
  morphology, 45
  presence, 26
  prevention/control, 50b
  symptomatic extraintestinal
    amebiasis, 49b
  symptomatic intestinal amebiasis,
    49b
  treatment, 49b
  trends, 50b
  trophozoite, 45b-47b, 46f
    characteristics, 46t
    contrast, 53b
    karyosome, presence, 46f
    structures, identification, 50b
Entamoeba polecki, 56b
  characteristics, identification, 58b
  clinical symptoms, 58b
  cysts, 57b
    characteristics, 57t
    illustration, 57f
  epidemiology, 57b-58b
  infection, transmission, 58b
  laboratory diagnosis, 57b
  morphology, 56
  prevention/control, 58b
  treatment, 58b
  trophozoites, 56b-57b
    characteristics, 57t
    illustration, 56f
Enterobius vermicularis (pinworm),
    192b
  adult female, example, 193f
  adults, 192b-193b
    characteristics, 193t
  clinical symptoms, 194
  contraction, identification, 194b
  eggs, 192f
    characteristics, 192t
    detection, 27
    morphology, 192b
  epidemiology, 194b
  laboratory diagnosis, 193b
  life cycle notes, 193b-194b
  morphologic forms, recovery,
    194b
  morphology, 192
  prevention/control, 194b
  recovery, specimen (selection),
    194b
  treatment, 194b

Enteromonas hominis, 92b
  clinical symptoms, 93b
  cysts, 93b
    characteristics, 93t
    illustration, 93f
    nuclei, position, 94b
  epidemiology, 93b
  laboratory diagnosis, 93b
  morphology, 92
  prevention/control, 94b
  treatment, 93b
    indication, 94b
  trophozoites, 92b-93b
    characteristics, 92t
    illustration, 92f
Enterotest
  simplicity, 26
  usage, identification, 27b
Enzyme immunoassay (EIA), 25
Epidemiology, 3-4
Epimastigotes, 107-108
  characteristics, 108t
  illustration, 108f
Epithelial cells, 290
  amebic trophozoites, comparison,
    290
  parasites, confusion, 290b
Erythrocyte structural abnormalities,
    135
Erythrocytic cycle, 133
Ethylenediaminetetraacetic acid
    (EDTA), usage, 27-28
Eyes
  Loa loa morphologic form,
    extraction, 231b
  specimens, 30

F

Facultative parasite, 4-5
Fascioliasis (sheep liver rot),
    270b
Fasciolopsiasis, 270b
Fasciolopsis
  determination, contrast,
    271b
  eggs, caplike structure, 271b
Fasciolopsis buski, 269b
  adult, 269f
  eggs
    characteristics, 269t
    illustration, 269f
  organ infection, 271b
Fasciolopsis hepatica, 269b
  adults, 269b-270b
    illustration, 270f
  clinical symptoms, 270

Fasciolopsis hepatica (Continued)
   eggs
      characteristics, 269t
      illustration, 269f
   epidemiology, 270b
   laboratory diagnosis, 270b
   life cycle notes, 270b
   morphology, 269
   prevention/control, 271b
   treatment, 270b-271b
Fecal specimens
   parasite testing, considerations, 17
   SAF-preserved fecal samples, usage,
      25
Filariae
   case study, 223b
   classification, 225-233
   clinical symptoms, 224-225
      variation, 224-225
   focus, 223-236
   laboratory diagnosis, 224
   life cycle
      comparison, 224
      notes, 223-224
   morphologic forms, 223-224
   morphology, 223-224
   parasites
      classification, 225f
      symptoms, display, 225b
   pathogenesis, 224-225
Filarial organisms, 233-236
Filariform larvae, 204b
   characteristics, 204t
Fish tapeworm infection
      (diphyllobothriasis), 255b-256b
Fixatives, 18
   alternative single-vial systems, 19
   formalin, 18-19
   modified polyvinyl alcohol, 19
   polyvinyl alcohol, 19
   purpose, identification, 19b
   selection, 18
   sodium acetate formalin (SAF), 19
Flagellates
   case study, 78b
   characteristics, 79
   classification, 80-100
   clinical symptoms, 80
   iodine wet preparations, usage,
      79
   laboratory diagnosis, 79
   life cycles, 79
      amebas, comparison, 79
      notes, 78-79
      trophozoite/cyst morphologic
         forms, possession, 79b

Flagellates *(Continued)*
   morphologic structure, invisibility,
      79b
   morphology, 78-79
   movement, accomplishment, 78-79
   nuclear characteristics, 79
   parasite classification, 80f
   pathogenesis, 80
   recovery, 80
   saline wet preparations, usage, 79
   structures (flagella), 78-79
Fleas, 308
   adult flea, 309f
   clinical symptoms, 309b
   epidemiology/geography, 309b
   infestations, treatment, 310b
   life cycle notes, 309b
   microorganism, transmission,
      310b
   morphology, 308b-309b
   movement, 310b
   prevention/control, 310b
   treatment, 309b
Flies, 310
   adult flies, 310f
      features, 310t
      speciation, 311t
   clinical symptoms, 311b-312b
   development, larval stages, 312b
   epidemiology, 311b
   geography, 311b
   identification, 312b
   life cycle notes, 311b
   morphology, 310b
   parasite-transmitting flies,
      geographic distribution,
      311t
   prevention/control, 312b
   speciation, 312b
   symptoms, 312b
   treatment, 312b
Formalin, 18-19
   advantages/disadvantages, 18
   sodium acetate formalin (SAF),
      19
   usage, health hazard, 18-19
Formalin-ethyl acetate sedimentation
      procedure, 23
Fungal elements, 290
Fused platelets, 291

G

Gametocytes
   Cryptosporidium parvum, 171b
   ingestion, 133-134
Genital secretions, 30

Giardia lamblia (G. lamblia),
      80b-81b
   antigen detection method, 25
   asymptomatic carrier state, 84b
   clinical symptoms, 84b
   contraction, risk, 86b
   cysts, 82b-83b
      characteristics, 83t
      illustration, 82f
   epidemiology, 83b-84b
   giardiasis (traveler's diarrhea), 84b
   infection, 86b
   laboratory diagnosis, 83b
   life cycle notes, 83b
   median bodies, presence, 85b
   morphology, 81
   prevention/control, 84b-85b
   tests, indication, 25-26
   treatment, 84b
   trends, 85b
   trophozoites, 81b-82b
      characteristics, 81t
      illustration, 81f
      mucosa, attachment, 85b
      observation, 26
      red-staining nuclei, 81f-82f
Giardiasis (traveler's diarrhea), 84b
Giemsa stains
   detection preference, 31b
   parasitic structures, appearance,
      28t
   precipitate, visibility, 291
   usage, preference, 28
Giemsa-stained peripheral blood
      films, usage, 134
Global travel, impact, 4
Granulomatous amebic encephalitis
      (GAE), 70b
Guinea worm infection
      (dracunculosis/drancunculiasis),
      214b

H

Hard adult ticks
   comparison, 301f
   features, 302t
Helminth eggs
   plant material, differentiation, 290b
   quantitation, 33
Helminth larvae
   plant hair, resemblance, 289
   vegetable spirals, comparison, 288
Helminths
   morphologic forms, detection, 16
Helminths, parasite classification, 10f
Hemocele, presence, 299b

Hemoflagellates
  amastigotes, 106-107
  case study, 106b
  classification, 110
  clinical symptoms, 110b
  epimastigotes, 107-108
  focus, 106-126
  general morphology, 108-110
  infections, symptoms (range), 110b
  laboratory diagnosis, 109b
  life cycle notes, 106-110
  morphologic form, external
      flagellum (absence), 109b
  morphology, 106-110
  parasite classification, 110f
  pathogenesis, 110b
  promastigotes, 107
  stool sample presence, 110b
Hermaphroditic tapeworms, 241
Heterophyes heterophyes, 273b
  adults, 274b
  asymptomatic patients, 274b
  Clonorchis sinesis differentiation,
      274b
  eggs, characteristics, 273t
  epidemiology, 274b
  laboratory diagnosis, 274b
  life cycle notes, 274b
  prevention/control, 274b
  recovery, specimen selection, 275b
  treatment, 274b
    selection, 275b
Heterophyiasis, 274b
Hexacanth embryo (onchosphere),
      240-241
Homosexual population, parasitic
      infection (increase), 4
Hooklets, 240-241
Hookworms, 202-216
  adults, characteristics, 205t
  disease, ancylostomiasis/
      necatoriasis, 206b
  eggs, characteristics, 203t
  filariform larvae
    characteristics, 204t
    illustration, 204f
  rhabditiform larva
    characteristics, 203t
    illustration, 203f
Host, parasite (entry/infection), 4
  symbiosis, 5
Humans
  Acanthamoeba species
    acquisition, 71b
    identification, 70t
  arthropods, relationship, 299

Humans (*Continued*)
  Babesia species, accidental host,
      153b
  bugs, encounters (impact), 317b
  Dracunculus medinensis
      (contraction), 215b
  Echinococcus granulosus site,
      location, 259b
  Fasciolopsis buski (organ infection),
      271b
  health, cockroaches (impact),
      318b
  Hymenolepis diminuta (infective
      stage), 249b
  Paragonimus westermani
      (transmission route), 277b
  Toxoplasma gondii infection,
      initiation, 182b
Hydatid cysts, 258b
Hydatid disease, 258b
Hydatidosis, 258b
Hymenolepiasis
  dwarf tapeworm disease,
      251b
  rat tapeworm disease, 248b
Hymenolepis diminuta, 247b
  adult, characteristics, 248t
  asymptomatic patients, 248b
  clinical symptoms, 248
  eggs, 247b
    characteristics, 247t, 249b
    illustration, 247f
  epidemiology, 248b
  infective stage, 249b
  laboratory diagnosis, 248b
  life cycle notes, 248b
  morphology, 247
  prevention/control, 248b-249b
    measures, 249b
  proglottids, 247b-248b
    illustration, 248f
  scolices, 247b
    illustration, 247f
  treatment, 248b
Hymenolepis diminuta egg,
      differentiation, 251b
Hymenolepis nana, 249b
  adults, characteristics, 250t
  asymptomatic patients, 251b
  clinical symptoms, 251
  eggs, 249b-250b
    characteristics, 250t
    differentiation, 251b
    illustration, 249f
  epidemiology, 250b-251b
  laboratory diagnosis, 250b

Hymenolepis nana (*Continued*)
  life cycle
    characteristic, differentiation,
        251b
    notes, 250b
  morphology, 249
  nonapplications, 251b
  proglottids, 250b
  scolices, 250b
    illustration, 250f
  treatment, 251b
Hypnozoites, 133

I

Immature schizonts, 133
  Plasmodium falciparium, 147b
  Plasmodium malariae, 145b
  Plasmodium ovale, 141b
  Plasmodium vivax, 136b
Immunoassays, list, 33t
Immunocompromised patients,
      toxoplasmosis (impact), 181b
Immunologic testing, 31-32
Immunologic tests
  methods, 32
  variety, 32
Infant infections, 99b
Infection, parasites (impact), 3
Infective stage (parasitic life cycle), 6
Infestation, parasites (impact), 3
Insect vector (arthropod vector),
      parasite entry, 4
Intestinal amebas
  asymptomatic patients, 44-45
  life cycle, 43-44
  prevalence, 45b
Intestinal cestodes, impact, 242
Intestinal flagellates
  life cycle, amebas (comparison), 79
  pathogenic characteristic, 80
Intestinal specimens, 26-27
Intestinal tract, encysted metacercaria
      (impact), 267
Intracellular parasites
      (demonstration), specimen
      selection, 31b
Iodamoeba bütschlii, 60b
  clinical symptoms, 62b
  cysts, 60b-61b
    characteristics, 61t
    identification, 62b
    illustration, 62f
  epidemiology, 62b
  laboratory diagnosis, 61b-62b
  morphology, 60
  prevention/control, 62b

Iodamoeba bütschlii (Continued)
transmission, occurrence, 63b
treatment, 62b
trends, 62b
trophozoites, 60b
characteristics, 61t
Iodine wet preparation, usage, 44
Iron hematoxylin, 24
stain
protozoan structures/background
material, appearance, 25t
usage, 24
Isospora belli, 165b
asymptomatic patients, 167b
clinical symptoms, 167
epidemiology, 167b
identification, sample processing,
168b
infection
contraction, likelihood, 168b
initiation, stage identification,
168b
laboratory diagnosis, 166b
life cycle notes, 167b
morphology, 165
oocysts, 165b-166b
characteristics, 166t
illustration, 162f
recovery, 32-33
prevention/control, 167b-168b
specimen, observation, 26
treatment, 167b
Isosporiasis, 167b
Itch mite, cause, 305b
Ixodes ticks (deer ticks), U.S.
location, 303b

K

Kalazar, description, 116b
Knott technique, 29

L

Laboratory diagnosis, 8-9
amebas, 44
Laboratory diagnostic techniques, 9b
Laboratory techniques, 27-31
Larvae, nematoda form, 190
Leishmania braziliensis complex,
111b
chiclero ulcer, organism (impact),
113b
clinical symptoms, 112
epidemiology, 112b
list, 112t
laboratory diagnosis, 111b-112b
methods, usage, 113b
life cycle notes, 112b

Leishmania braziliensis complex
(Continued)
mucocutaneous leishmaniasis,
112b-113b
treatment, avoidance, 113b
prevention/control, 113b
treatment, 113b
Leishmania donovani (parasite
recovery), 27
Leishmania donovani complex, 113b
clinical symptoms, 114
common name, 115b
epidemiology, 114b
list, 114t
kalazar, description, 116b
laboratory diagnosis, 113b-114b
life cycle notes, 114b
prevention/control, 115b
transmission, vector (responsibility),
115b
treatment, 115b
trends, 115b
visceral leishmaniasis, 114b-115b
Leishmania mexicana complex, 116b
clinical symptoms, 116
disease, impact, 117b
epidemiology, 116b
list, 116t
laboratory diagnosis, 116b
life cycle notes, 116b
new world cutaneous leishmaniasis,
116b-117b
prevention/control, 117b
recovery, specimen (usage), 117b
reservoir host, 117b
treatment, 117b
Leishmania spp.
amastigotes, 107f
demonstration, specimen selection,
31b
NNN medium, usage, 29
Leishmania tropica complex,
117b-118b
clinical symptoms, 118
list, 119t
epidemiology, 118b
list, 118t
geographic regions, 119b
laboratory diagnosis, 117b-118b
life cycle notes, 118b
morphologic form, 119b
old world cutaneous leishmaniasis,
118b
prevention/control, 119b
specimen, recovery, 119b
treatment, 119b
trends, 119b

Leishmaniasis
diseases/conditions, 111t
historical perspective,
110-119
new world cutaneous leishmaniasis,
116b-117b
old world cutaneous leishmaniasis,
118b
Lice, 312
adult body louse, 313f
adult lice
features, 313t
life span, 314b
clinical symptoms, 314b
comparison, 313f
epidemiology, 313b
geography, 313b
hair extremities, characterization,
314b
infections, treatment, 314b
life cycle notes, 312b-313b
morphology, 312b
prevention/control, 314b
treatment, 314b
Life cycle notes, amebas,
43-44
Life larvae, 223-224
Liquid stool, trophozoites (presence),
17
Loa loa, 229b
adults, 230b
blood sample recovery, timing,
231b
clinical symptoms, 230
epidemiology, 230b
laboratory diagnosis, 230b
life cycle notes, 230b
microfilariae, 229b-230b
characteristics, 230t
illustration, 230f
morphologic form, extraction,
231b
morphology, 229
prevention/control, 231b
treatment, 231b
Loiasis, 230b

M

Macrogametocytes, 133
characteristics, 133
Plasmodium falciparium,
147b-149b
Plasmodium malariae, 145b
Plasmodium ovale, 141b
Plasmodium vivax, 138b
Macrophages, size (variation),
287

Malaria, 131
 antimalarial medication,
   consideration, 143b
 benign tertian malaria, 139b
 blood collection, timing, 134
 classification, 135-152
 clinical symptoms, 135
 description, 132
 developing trophozoites, 132-133
 endemic consideration, 132
 erythrocyte structural
   abnormalities, 135
 gametocytes, ingestion, 133-134
 Giemsa-stained peripheral blood
   films, usage, 134
 historical accounts, 130
 historical perspective, 132
 immature schizonts, 133
 laboratory diagnosis, 134-135
 life cycle notes, 132-134
 macrogametocytes, 133
 malignant tertian malaria, 150b
 mature schizonts, 133
 microgametocytes, 133
 morphology, 132-134
 parasite, transmission, 133-134
 pathogenesis, 135
 phylum, identification, 135-152
 polymerase chain reaction (PCR)
   techniques, 134-135
 ring forms (early trophozoites),
   132
 serologic tests, 134-135
 symptoms, 135
 thick blood smears,
   recommendations/
   identification, 31b
 transmission
   Anopheles (impact), 133
   modes, 133-134
Malarial malaria, 146b
Malayan filariasis, 229b
Malignant tertian malaria, 150b
Mansonella ozzardi, 233b
 adults, 233b-234b
 clinical symptoms, 234b
 epidemiology, 234b
 laboratory diagnosis, 234b
 life cycle notes, 234b
 locations, 235b
 microfilariae, 233b
   characteristics, 233t
   illustration, 234f
 morphology, 233
 prevention/control, 234b
 sheath, presence, 234b
 treatment, 234b

Mansonella perstans, 235b
 adults, 235b
 clinical symptoms, 235b-236b
 epidemiology, 235b
 laboratory diagnosis, 235b
 life cycle notes, 235b
 microfilariae, 235b
   characteristics, 235t
   illustration, 235f
 morphology, 235
 prevention/control, 236b
 recovery, sample selection, 236b
 specimen identification, timing,
   236b
 treatment, 236b
Mature oocysts
 Cyclospora cayetanensis, 175t
 Sarcocystis species, 168b
Mature schizonts, 133
 Plasmodium falciparium, 147b
 Plasmodium malariae, 145b
 Plasmodium ovale, 141b
 Plasmodium vivax, 137b
Membrane flow cartridge techniques,
   25
Mercury-based PVA, alternatives, 19
Merozoites, 133
 Babesia species, 152b-153b
 formation, 133
Metacercaria, 267
Metagonimiasis, 274b
Metagonimus yokogawai, 273b
 adults, 274b
 asymptomatic patients, 274b
 eggs, 273b-274b
   characteristics, 273t
 epidemiology, 274b
 laboratory diagnosis, 274b
 life cycle notes, 274b
 morphology, 273
 prevention/control, 274b
 recovery, specimen selection, 275b
 treatment, 274b
   selection, 275b
Metazoa, 9
 helminths, multicellular worms, 10
Microfilariae, 223-224
 Brugia malayi, 227b
 Loa loa, 229b-230b
 recovery, periodicity, 224b
 transparent membrane, term
   (usage), 224b
 Wuchereria bancroftia, 225b-226b
Microgametocytes, 133
 characteristics, 133
 Plasmodium falciparium, 147b
 Plasmodium malariae, 145b

Microgametocytes (Continued)
 Plasmodium ovale, 141b
 Plasmodium vivax, 137b
Microns, measurement unit, 21
Microscope
 considerations, 21
 objective, calibration, 21
 performing, 21
Microsporidia, 176b
 clinical symptoms, 177
 epidemiology, 177b
 laboratory diagnosis, 176b-177b
 life cycle
   infective/diagnostic stages, 177b
   notes, 177b
 morphology, 176
 species identification, laboratory
   technique, 177b
 spores, 176b
   characteristics, 176t
   protozoan spores, contrast, 177b
 treatment, 177b
 trends, 177b
Microsporidia genera, 161
Microsporidia, appearance, 25t
Microsporidial infection, 177b
Miracidium, 267
Mites, 303
 adult mites, 303f
   features, 304t
 clinical symptoms, 304b
 eggs, evolution, 305b
 epidemiology, 304b
 geography, 304b
 itch mite, cause, 305b
 life cycle notes, 303b-304b
 morphology, 303b
 prevention/control, 305b
 removal process, 305b
 treatment, 305b
Mode of transmission, 4
Modified acid-fast stain, protozoan
   structures/yeast/background
   material (appearance), 25t
Modified polyvinyl alcohol, 19
Modified trichrome stain,
   microsporidia (appearance),
   25t
Molecular techniques, list, 33t
Monocytes, size (variation), 287
Mononuclear WBCs, size (variation),
   287
Morphology
 amebas, 43-44
 Entamoeba hartmanni, 51b
 Entamoeba histolytica, 45
 trophozoites, 45b-47b

Mosquitoes, 314
  adult mosquito, 315f
    features, 315t
  clinical symptoms, 315b
  epidemiology, 315b
  geography, 315b
  life cycle
    continuation, 316b
    notes, 314b-315b
  morphology, 314b
  parasite-transmitting mosquitoes,
    geographic distribution, 315t
  Plasmodium spp. parasite
    transmission, 316b
  prevention/control, 316b
  segments, 316b
  treatment, 316b
Mouth scrapings, 30-31
Mucocutaneous leishmaniasis,
  112b-113b
Multicellular worms, 10
Mutualism, 5

N

Naegleria fowleri, 65b
  ameboid trophozoites, 65b
    body entry, 68b
    characteristics, 65t
    illustration, 65f
  asymptomatic clinical symptoms,
    66b
  clinical symptoms, 66
  contraction method, 67b
  cysts, 65b
    illustration, 66f
  epidemiology, 66b
  flagellate forms, 65b
    illustration, 65f
  laboratory diagnosis, 45
  life cycle notes, 66b
  morphologic forms, 67b
  morphology, 65b
  presence, 29
  prevention/control, 67b
    measures, 68b
  primary amebic
    meningoencephalitis (PAM),
    66b
  recovery, specimen selection, 67b
  treatment, 67b
  trends, 67b
Nasal discharge, 30-31
Necator americanus, 202b
  adult male, 204f
  buccal capsule, 204f
Necatoriasis, 206b

Nematoda, morphologic forms, 190
Nematodes
  case study, 189b
  classification, 191-202
  clinical symptoms, 191
  focus, 190-216
  infections, likelihood, 191b
  laboratory diagnosis, 190
    accomplishment, 190
  life cycles, 190
    intestinal tract, involvement, 191
    notes, 190
  morphology, 190
  parasite classification, 191f
  pathogenesis, 191
  recovery, 190b
  worms, development (juvenile
    stage), 190b
New world cutaneous leishmaniasis,
  116b-117b
Nonpathogenic flagellates,
  importance, 80b
Novy-MacNeal-Nicolle (NNN)
  medium, usage, 29
Nucleic acid tests, development, 32

O

Objectives, calibration, 21
Obligatory parasite, 4-5
Ocular micrometer
  calibration, 21f
  usage, 21
Old world cutaneous leishmaniasis,
  118b
Onchocerca volvulus, 231b
  adults, 232b
  clinical symptoms, 232
  epidemiology, 232b
  laboratory diagnosis, 232b
  life cycle notes, 232b
  microfilariae, 231b-232b
    characteristics, 232t
    illustration, 231f
    sheath, absence (illustration),
      231f
  morphologic characteristic,
    contrast, 233b
  morphology, 231
  prevention/control, 233b
  recovery, specimen selection, 233b
  treatment, 233b
Onchocerciasis (river blindness), 232b
Onchosphere (hexacanth embryo),
  240-241
Oocyst, 133-134
Ookinete, 133-134

Operculum, 266-267
Organ-dwelling flukes, discussion,
  268-277
Organ-dwelling parasites,
  presentation, 268-277
Organ-dwelling trematodes, 267
Oriental rat flea, microorganism
  transmission, 310b
Ova and parasite (O&P)
  assay, procedure elimination, 21-22
  collection protocol, stool sample
    collection number
    (identification), 17b
  concentration methods, types, 23
  direct wet preparation, elimination,
    21
  fixatives, selection, 18
  procedure, results, 32-33
  testing, stains (usage), 24
Ova and parasite (O&P) examination
  concentration methods, 22-23
  permanent stained smear,
    preparation/examination,
    23-24
  procedures, 25
  stool, usage, 16-25

P

Paragonimiasis, 276b
  cerebral paragonimiasis, 276b
Paragonimus westermani, 275b
  adults, 275b
    illustration, 276f
  clinical symptoms, 276
  differentiation, 277b
  eggs, 275b
    characteristics, 275t
    complications, 277b
    illustration, 275f
  epidemiology, 276b
  human transmission route, 277b
  infection, 30
  laboratory diagnosis, 276b
  life cycle notes, 276b
  morphology, 275
  prevention/control, 276b
  treatment, 276b
Parasite classification, 9-11
  amebas, 45f
  arthropods, 11f
  Babesia species, 154f
  cestodes, 242f
  filariae, 225f
  flagellates, 80f
  helminths, 10f
  hemoflagellates, 110f

Parasite classification *(Continued)*
  nematodes, 191f
  Plasmodium species, 136f
  protozoa, 10f
  systems, variations, 10
  trematodes, 268f
Parasite-host relationships, 4-5
  host, function (identification), 5b
  parasites, types, 4-5
  terms, association, 5t
Parasite-transmitting flies, geographic
    distribution, 311t
Parasite-transmitting mosquitoes,
    geographic distribution, 315t
Parasites
  category names, variation, 10
  detection (interference),
      medications/substances
      (impact), 17
  diagnostic stages, microscopic
      detection, 21
  discoveries, impact, 3b
  eradication, problems, 8
  examination, stool (usage), 16-25
  heaviness, 23
  laboratory diagnostic techniques,
      9b
  laboratory identification, success, 16
  life cycle, information
      (identification), 7b
  major groups, identification, 11b
  nomenclature, 9-11
  populations, risk, 4b
  prevention/control, 8
    measures, identification, 8b
    strategies, 8b
  quantitation, identification, 34b
  recovery techniques, availability,
      8-9
  samples, microscopic examination,
      9
  scientific genus names, variation,
      9-10
  scientific names, 9
  structures, appearance, 28t
  transmission, modes, 4b
  treatment options, 7b
Parasitic disease
  clinical manifestations, knowledge
      (importance), 16
  diagnosis, 31-32
  immunoassays, 33t
  impact, 7
  molecular techniques, 33t
  processes, symptoms (association),
      7b

Parasitic infections
  global travel, increase (impact), 4
  population risk, identification, 4b
  treatment, 7-8
    therapies, identification, 8b
Parasitic life cycles, 6-7
  diagnostic stage, 6
  illustration, 6f
  infective stage, 6
  phases, 6-7
Parasitic stages, detection, 23b
Parasitic, concept, 3
Parasitism, 5
Parasitology
  case study, 2b
  focus, 3-11
  historical perspective, 3
  quality assurance, 33-34
Paroxysm, definition, 135b
Pathogenesis, amebas, 44-45
Pathogenic associations, 5
Permanent smear procedures, 44
Permanent stained smear, preparation/
    examination, 23-24
Permanent stains, 23-25
  usage, 28
Persistent urethritis, 99b
Persistent vaginitis, 99b
Pinworm *(Enterobius vermicularis)*
    eggs, detection, 27
Plant hair, 289
Plant material, 289-290
  helminth eggs, differentiation, 290b
  size/comparison, 289-290
Plasmodium falciparum, 147b
  black water fever, 150b
    description, 151b
  characteristics, 147t
  clinical symptoms, 150
  composition, 149f
  developing trophozoites, 147b
  epidemiology, 150b
  immature schizonts, 147b
  laboratory diagnosis, 149b-150b
  life cycle notes, 150b
  macrogametocytes, 147b-149b
  malignant tertian malaria, 150b
  mature schizonts, 147b
  microgametocytes, 147b
  morphologic characteristics, 149b
  morphological forms, 148f
  morphology, 147b
  prevention/control, 150b-151b
  red blood cells, invasion age,
      151b
  ring forms, 147b

Plasmodium falciparum (Continued)
  treatment, 150b
  trends, 151b
  U.S. location, 151b
Plasmodium malariae, 143b
  characteristics, 145t
  clinical symptoms, 146
  developing trophozoites,
      144b-145b
  epidemiology, 146b
  immature schizonts, 145b
  laboratory diagnosis, 145b-146b
  life cycle notes, 146b
  macrogametocytes, 145b
  malarial malaria, 146b
  mature schizonts, 145b
  microgametocytes, 145b
  morphologic characteristics, 145b
  morphologic features, identification,
      146b
  morphologic forms, 144f
    absence, 146b
  morphology, 143b
  prevention/control, 146b
    avoidance, 146b
  quartan malaria, 146b
  ring forms, 143b-144b
  treatment, 146b
Plasmodium ovale, 141b
  antimalarial medication,
      consideration, 143b
  characteristics, 141t
  clinical symptoms, 143
  developing trophozoites, 141b
  epidemiology, 143b
  immature schizonts, 141b
  laboratory diagnosis, 141b-142b
  life cycle notes, 143b
  macrogametocytes, 141b
  mature schizonts, 141b
  microgametocytes, 141b
  morphological characteristics, 141b
  morphological forms, 142f
    selection, 143b
  morphology, 141b
  prevention/control, 143b
  ring forms, 141b
  suspicion, geographic regions, 143b
  treatment, 143b
Plasmodium species, 132-152
  blood collection, timing, 135b
  classification, 135-152
  clinical symptoms, 135
  cyclic paroxysms, occurrence, 134t
  developing trophozoites, 132-133
    appearance, 132-133

Plasmodium species *(Continued)*
erythrocyte structural
abnormalities, 135
Giemsa-stained peripheral blood
films, usage, 134
historical accounts, 132
historical perspective, 132
immature schizonts, 133
infective stage, 134b
laboratory diagnosis, 134-135
life cycle notes, 132-134
macrogametocytes, 133
mature schizonts, 133
microgametocytes, 133
morphology, 132-134
parasite classification, 136f
pathogenesis, 135
ring forms (early trophozoites), 132
Plasmodium spp.
parasites
recovery, 27
transmission, mosquitoes
(identification), 316b
quantitation, 33
Plasmodium vivax, 136b
benign tertian malaria, 139b
characteristics, 136t
composition, 138f
developing trophozoites, 136b
epidemiology, 139b
immature schizonts, 136b
incubation period, 140b
invasion, 140b
laboratory diagnosis, 139b
life cycle notes, 139b
macrogametocytes, 138b
mature schizonts, 137b
microgametocytes, 137b
morphologic characteristics,
138b-139b
usefulness, 140b
morphologic forms, 137f
morphology, 136b
prevention/control, 140b
ring forms, 136b
treatment, 139b-140b
trends, 140b
Pneumocystis jiroveci, 182b
clinical symptoms, 184
contraction, risk, 184b
cysts, 183b
characteristics, 183t
illustration, 173f
diagnosis method, 184b
epidemiology, 183b-184b
laboratory diagnosis, 183b
life cycle notes, 183b

Pneumocystis jiroveci (Continued)
morphology, 182b
multiple forms, 170f
Pneumocystis carinii, 182b
prevention/control, 184b
spread, medium, 184b
treatment, 184b
trophozoites, 182b-183b
characteristics, 183t
Pneumocystosis, 184b
Pollen grains, 287
Polymerase chain reaction (PCR)
techniques, 134-135
Polymorphonuclear white blood cells,
287
Polyvinyl alcohol (PVA), 19
advantages/disadvantages, 19
mercury-based PVA, alternatives,
19
modified polyvinyl alcohol, 19
Pork tapeworm infection (taeniasis),
245b
Preparations (preps), 21
Prevention/control, 8
Acanthamoeba species, 71b
Ancylostoma duodenale, 206b
Arthropods, 300
Ascaris lumbricoides, 201b
Babesia divergens, 155b
Balantidium coli, 165b
Blastocystis hominis, 174b
Brugia malayi, 229b
bugs, 317b
Chilomastix mesnili, 88b
Clonorchis sinesis, 273b
Cryptosporidium parvum, 172b
Cyclospora cayetanensis, 175b
Dientamoeba fragilis, 90b
Diphyllobothrium latum, 256b
Dipylidium caninum, 253b
Dracunculus medinensis, 215b
Echinococcus granulosus, 259b
Endolimax nana, 60b
Entamoeba coli, 56b
Entamoeba gingivalis, 64b
Entamoeba hartmanni, 53b
Entamoeba histolytica, 50b
Entamoeba polecki, 58b
Enterobius vermicularis (pinworm),
194b
Enteromonas hominis, 94b
Fasciolopsis hepatica, 271b
fleas, 310b
flies, 312b
Giardia lamblia (G. lamblia),
84b-85b
Heterophyes heterophyes, 274b

Prevention/control *(Continued)*
Hymenolepis diminuta, 248b-249b
Iodamoeba bütschlii, 62b
Isospora belli, 167b-168b
Leishmania braziliensis complex,
113b
Leishmania donovani complex,
115b
Leishmania mexicana complex,
117b
Leishmania tropica complex, 119b
lice, 314b
Loa loa, 231b
Mansonella ozzardi, 234b
Mansonella perstans, 236b
Metagonimus yokogawai, 274b
mites, 305b
mosquitoes, 316b
Naegleria fowleri, 67b
Onchocerca volvulus, 233b
Paragonimus westermani, 276b
Plasmodium falciparium,
150b-151b
Plasmodium malariae, 146b
Plasmodium ovale, 143b
Plasmodium vivax, 140b
Pneumocystis jiroveci, 184b
Retortamonas intestinalis, 95b
Sarcocystis species, 169b
Schistosoma haematobium,
280b-281b
spiders, 307b
strategies, 8b
Taenia solium, 246b
ticks, 303b
Toxoplasma gondii, 181b
Trichomonas hominis, 92b
Trichomonas tenax, 97b
Trichomonas vaginalis, 99b
Trichuris trichiura, 197b
Trypanosoma brucei gambiense,
121b
Trypanosoma cruzi, 124b
Trypanosoma rangeli, 126b
Wuchereria bancrofti, 227b
Primary amebic meningoencephalitis
(PAM), 66b
Proglottids
Diphyllobothrium latum, 254b
Dipylidium caninum, 252b
Hymenolepis diminuta, 247b-248b
Hymenolepsis nana, 250b
presence, 241
Taenia solium, 243b-244b
Promastigotes, 107
characteristics, 107t
illustration, 107f

Protozoa
case study, 160b
classification, 161-185
cysts
presence, confirmation, 23-24
starch cells, differentiation, 291b
examination, 9
focus, 161-185
genera, discussion, 161
morphologic forms, detection, 16
parasite classification, 10f
parasites, comparison, 162b
single-celled parasites, 10
spores, Microsporidia spores
(contrast), 177b
structures, appearance, 24t-25t
Pseudopods, 43
Pulmonary distomiasis, 276b

Q

Quality control, results (reporting),
32-34
Quantitation, indication/importance,
33
Quartan malaria, 146b

R

Rat tapeworm disease
(hymenolepiasis), 248b
Recrudescence, 133
Red blood cells (RBCs)
erythrocytic cycle, 133
invasion age, 151b
rupture, 134
Red cell abnormalities, 291-292
Retortamonas intestinalis, 94b
clinical symptoms, 95b
contraction method, 96b
cysts, 94b-95b
characteristics, 95t
illustration, 95f
epidemiology, 95b
identification technique, 95b
laboratory diagnosis, 95b
morphology, 94
prevention/control, 95b
treatment, 95b
trophozoites, 94b
characteristics, 94t
illustration, 94f
Rhabditiform larvae, 203b-204b
Ring forms (early trophozoites), 132
River blindness (onchocerciasis),
232b
Rostellum, 241
Roundworm infection (ascariasis),
201b

S

Saline wet preparation, usage, 44
Saline/iodine, unfixed stool (mixture),
21-22
Sarcocystis infection, 169b
Sarcocystis species, 168b
clinical symptoms, 169
epidemiology, 169b
genus, comparison, 170b
infection process, 170b
laboratory diagnosis, 168b-169b
life cycle notes, 169b
mature oocysts, 168b
morphologic forms, appearance,
170b
morphology, 168
prevention/control, 169b
treatment, 169b
Sarcocystis spp.
mature oocyst, characteristics, 169t
oocyst, 162f
Sarcoptes scabiei
adult, itch mite, 304f
eggs, 304f
Schistosoma haematobium, 277b
adults, 278b
asymptomatic patients, 280b
clinical symptoms, 280
detection, urine (usage), 30
eggs, 277b-278b
illustration, 279f
epidemiology, 279b
laboratory diagnosis, 278b
life cycle notes, 278b
morphology, 277
prevention/control, 280b-281b
treatment, 280b
trends, 281b
Schistosoma japonicum, 277b
eggs, illustration, 279f
recovery, specimen (selection), 281b
Schistosoma mansoni, 277b
eggs, illustration, 278f
Schistosoma presence, impact, 281b
Schistosoma species, 277-282
adults, location, 281b
eggs, characteristics, 278t
Schistosoma spp., quantitation, 33
Schistosomes, copula, 280f
Schistosomiasis, 280b
Schizonts
Cryptosporidium parvum, 171b
immature schizonts, 133
mature schizonts, 133
Scientific genus names, variation,
9-10

Scolex (scolices)
Dipylidium caninum, 251b
Hymenolepsis nana, 250b
presence, 241
Taenia solium, 243b
Scorpions, 307
adult scorpion, 307f
features, 307t
attack, complications
(development), 308b
clinical symptoms, 308b
epidemiology, 308b
geography, 308b
legs, usage (determination), 308b
life cycle notes, 307b
molting, changes, 308b
morphology, 307b
prevention/control, 308b
treatment, 308b
Serologic tests, usage, 134-135
Sheath, 223-224
term, usage, 224b
Sheep liver rot (fascioliasis), 270b
Sigmoidoscopy specimens, 26-27
Single-celled parasites, 10
Skin snips, 31
Sleeping sickness
East African (Rhodesian) sleeping
sickness, 122b
trypanosomal parasites, impact,
122b
West African (Gambian) sleeping
sickness, 120b-121b
Sodium acetate formalin (SAF), 19
SAF-preserved fecal samples, usage,
25
usage, 24
Soft adult ticks
comparison, 301f
features, 302t
Specimens, 27-31
collection
case study, 15b
focus, 15-34
container, labeling, 17
fixation, SAF (usage), 24
parasites, presence (examination), 8
preservation, impact, 3
processing, 8-9
focus, 15-34
submission types, identification, 9b
Spiders, 305
adult spiders, 305f
features, 306t
antivenom, treatment, 307b
clinical symptoms, 306b
epidemiology, 306b

Spiders *(Continued)*
  geography, 306b
  hiding, tendency, 307b
  life cycle notes, 306b
  morphology, 305b-306b
  prevention/control, 307b
  treatment, 306b-307b
  venomousness, U.S. location, 307b
Sporocyst, 267
Sporozoa
  case study, 131b
  focus, 131-156
  life history, 132
Sporozoites, 133
Sputum, 30
Stains
  disadvantages, 25
  permanent stains, 23-25
  precipitates, 291
  sample, 24
  specialization, 25
  usage, types, 24
Starch cells, 290-291
  protozoan cyst, differentiation, 291b
Starch granules, 290-291
Sterile fluid specimens, 29
Stool specimens
  collection, 16-17
    fixatives, purpose (identification), 19b
    method, 17
  color, 20
    importance, 20
  consistency, 20
    parasite indication, 20
  container, labeling, 17
  cysts, presence, 44
  gross abnormalities, 20
  hemoflagellates, 110b
  laboratory procedures, 18t
  liquid specimens, trophozoites (presence), 17
  macroscopic abnormalities, 20
  macroscopic examination, 20
    characteristics, identification, 20b
  microscope considerations, 21
  microscope examination procedures, identification, 21b
  microscopic examination, 21-25
    descriptive terms, 20t
  ocular micrometer, usage, 21
  parasite testing, considerations, 17
  preservation, fixatives (usage), 18-19
  preservatives, 18t

Stool specimens *(Continued)*
  processing, 20-25
  samples, collection number (identification), 17b
  screening methods, 25-26
    advantage, identification, 26b
  submission, parasite study, 79
  transport, 16-17
  trophozoites, presence, 44
  urine, noncontamination, 17
Strongyloides stercoralis, 207b
  adult female, 209b
    characteristics, 209t
  asymptomatic patients, 210b
  clinical symptoms, 210
  diagnostic stage, appearance, 210b
  eggs, 207b-208b
    characteristics, 207t
    illustration, 207f
  epidemiology, 209b-210b
  filariform larvae, 208b
    characteristics, 209t
    illustration, 208f
  hyperinfection, 30
  laboratory diagnosis, 209b
  life cycle
    comparison, 210b
    notes, 209b
  morphology, 207
  rhabditiform larvae, 208b
    characteristics, 208t
    illustration, 208f
  specimen, observation, 26
  treatment, 210b
Strongyloidiasis (threadworm infection), 210b
Subtropical countries, parasitic infections, 3-4
Suckers, 241
Swamp fever, 280b
Symbiosis, result, 5
Symptomatic bancroftian filariasis, 226b-227b
Symptomatic extraintestinal amebiasis, *Entamoeba histolytica*, 49b
Symptomatic intestinal amebiasis, *Entamoeba histolytica*, 49b

T

Taenia colium cysticercus larvae, pathogen recovery, 29
Taenia saginata, 242b
  infection, differentiation, 246b
  proglottid, 245f

Taenia solium, 242b
  asymptomatic patients, 245b
  clinical symptoms, 245
  eggs, 242b-243b
    characteristics, 243t
    illustration, 243f
  epidemiology, 245b
  infection, differentiation, 246b
  laboratory diagnosis, 244b
  life cycle notes, 245b
  morphology, 242
  prevention/control, 246b
  proglottids, 243b-244b
    illustration, 245f
  scolices, 243b
    illustrations, 244f
  treatment, 245b-246b
  trends, 246b
Taenia spp.
  adult, characteristics, 244t
  intestinal infection, development process, 246b
  intestinal infection, treatment, 246b
Taeniasis (beef/pork tapeworm infection), 245b
Tegument, 240-241
Thick blood smears, recommendation/ identification, 31b
Thick smears, usage, 28
Thin smears, usage, 28
Threadworm infection (strongyloidiasis), 210b
Ticks, 300
  anatomic parts, presence (impact), 303b
  clinical symptoms, 302b
  comparison, 301f
  epidemiology, 302b
  features, 302t
  life cycle
    morphologic form, comparison, 303b
    notes, 301b-302b
  morphology, 300b-301b
  prevention/control, 303b
  treatment, 302b-303b
  U.S. location, 303b
Tissue specimens, 29-30
Toxoplasma gondii, 177b
  asymptomatic patients, 180b
  bradyzoites, 178b
    characteristics, 178t
    illustration, 170f
  clinical symptoms, 180
  congenital toxoplasmosis, 180b-181b

Toxoplasma gondii (Continued)
  demonstration, specimen selection, 31b
  epidemiology, 179b-180b
  geographic area, 182b
  human infection, initiation, 182b
  laboratory diagnosis, 178b-179b
  life cycle
    morphologic forms, 182b
    notes, 179b
  morphology, 178b
  oocysts, 178b
  pathogen recovery, 29
  prevention/control, 181b
  tachyzoites, 178b
    characteristics, 178t
    illustration, 170f
  treatment, 181b
  trends, 181b-182b
Toxoplasmosis
  cerebral toxoplasmosis, 181b
  congenital toxoplasmosis, 180b-181b
  general symptoms, 180b
  impact, 181b
Transmission, mode, 4
Transport carriers (vectors), 3
Traveler's diarrhea (giardiasis), 84b
Treatment, 7-8
  options, 7b
  therapies, identification, 8b
Trematodes
  case study, 266b
  categorization, life cycles (impact), 267
  classification, 268-277
  clinical symptoms, 268
  focus, 266-282
  infections, species-dependent symptoms, 268b
  intermediate host, 267b
  laboratory diagnosis, 267-268
  life cycle notes, 266-267
  morphologic forms, 266-267
  morphology, 266-267
  parasite classification, 268f
  pathogenesis, 268
  Platyhelminthes (phylum), 268
  recovery, clinical samples, 268b
  Schistosoma genus, impact, 267
  Trematoda class, 266
Trichinella spiralis, 210b
  adults, 211b-212b
    characteristics, 211t
  clinical symptoms, 212
    association, 210b

Trichinella spiralis (Continued)
  diagnostic stage, 213b
  encysted larva, 211b
    characteristics, 211t
    illustration, 211f
  epidemiology, 212b
  identification, specimen selection, 213b
  laboratory diagnosis, 212b
  life cycle notes, 212b
  morphology, 211
  prevention/control, 213b
  treatment, 213b
Trichinellosis, 212b
Trichinosis, 212b
  acquisition method, 213b
Trichomonas hominis, 91b
  clinical symptoms, 92b
  cysts, 91b
  epidemiology, 91b-92b
  laboratory diagnosis, 91b
  morphology, 91
  prevention/control, 92b
  specimen, selection, 92b
  transmission method, 92b
  treatment, 92b
  tropohozoites, 91b
    characteristics, 91t
    illustration, 91f
Trichomonas tenax, 96b
  clinical symptoms, 97b
  cysts, 96b
  epidemiology, 97b
  laboratory diagnosis, 96b-97b
  life cycle notes, 97b
  membrane, extension, 97b
  morphology, 96
  prevention/control, 97b
  recovery, specimen selection, 97b
  treatment, 97b
  trophozoites, 96b
    characteristics, 96t
    illustration, 96f
Trichomonas vaginalis, 97b
  asymptomatic carrier state, 99b
  clinical symptoms, 99
  cysts, 98b
    morphologic form, existence, 100b
  epidemiology, 99b
  infant infections, 99b
    body areas, impact, 100b
  infection, symptomatic vaginitis (result), 100b
  laboratory diagnosis, 98b
  life cycle notes, 99b

Trichomonas vaginalis (Continued)
  morphology, 97
  persistent urethritis, 99b
  persistent vaginitis, 99b
  prevention/control, 99b
  specimens. recovery, 100b
  treatment, 99b
  trends, 100b
  trophozoites, 97b
    characteristics, 98t
    illustration, 98f
    structure, extension, 100b
Trichrome stain, background material (appearance), 24t
Trichuriasis (whipworm infection), 196b-197b
Trichuris trichiura, 195b
  adult male, example, 196f
  adults, 195b
    characteristics, 195t
  asymptomatic patients, 196b
  childhood infection, 197b
  clinical symptoms, 196
  eggs, 195b
    characteristics, 195t
    characterization, 197b
    illustration, 195f
  epidemiology, 196b
  infection, 196b-197b
  laboratory diagnosis, 195b-196b
  life cycle notes, 196b
  morphology, 195
  prevention/control, 197b
  quantitation, 33
  recovery, laboratory diagnostic technique, 197b
  treatment, 197b
Trophozoites, 43
  Babesia species, 152b
  Balantidium coli, 162b-163b
  cyst conversion, 43
  delicacy/fragility, 43
  developing trophozoites, 132-133
  early trophozoites (ring forms), 132
  Entamoeba coli, 53b-54b
  Entamoeba gingivalis, 63b
  Entamoeba hartmanni, 51b-52b
  Entamoeba polecki, 56b-57b
  Giardia lamblia, 81b-82b
  Iodamoeba bütschlii, 60b
  morphology, 45b-47b
  motility, demonstration, 21-22
  Pneumocystis jiroveci, 182b-183b
  presence, confirmation, 23-24
Tropical countries, parasitic infections, 3-4

Trypanosoma brucei gambiense, 120b
  animal reservoir hosts, presence/ absence, 121b
  cervical lymph nodes, enlargement, 121b
  clinical symptoms, 120
  epidemiology, 120b
  laboratory diagnosis, 120b
  life cycle notes, 120b
  prevention/control, 121b
  treatment, 121b
  trends, 121b
  West African (Gambian) sleeping sickness, 120b-121b
Trypanosoma brucei rhodesiense, 121b-122b
  clinical symptoms, 122
  diagnostic stage, 122b
  epidemiology, 122b
  laboratory diagnosis, 122b
  life cycle notes, 122b
  prevention/control, 122b
    efforts, complication, 105
  treatment, 122b
  trypanosomal parasites, impact, 122b
Trypanosoma cruzi, 123b
  C-shaped trypomastigote, blood smear, 109f
  Chagas' disease, 124b
    characteristics, 125b
  clinical symptoms, 124
  epidemiology, 123b
  laboratory diagnosis, 123b
  life cycle notes, 123b
  NNN medium, usage, 29
  prevention/control, 124b
  specimen, detection, 125b
  transmission, vector (identification), 125b
  treatment, 124b
  trends, 124b-125b
  trypomastigote, characteristics, 109f

Trypanosoma rangeli, 125b
  clinical symptoms, 125b
  diagnostic testing methods, 126b
  epidemiology, 125b
  infection, description, 126b
  laboratory diagnosis, 125b
  life cycle notes, 125b
  prevention/control, 126b
    selection, 126b
  treatment, 125b-126b
Trypanosoma spp.
  parasite recovery, 27
  trypomastigote stages, 29
Trypanosomal parasites, impact, 122b
Trypanosomiasis
  diagnostic tests, 121b
  historical perspective, 120-126
Trypomastigotes, 108
  characteristics, 109t
  illustration, 108f

U

Unfixed stool, saline/iodine (mixture), 21-22
Urethral specimens, 30
Urethritis, persistence, 99b
Urinary bladder veins, *Schistosoma* species (location), 281b
Urine secretions, 30

V

Vaginal specimens, 30
Vaginitis, persistence, 99b
Vectors (transport carriers), 3
Vegetable cells, 288
Vegetable spirals, 288
  helminth larvae, comparison, 288
    characteristics, usage, 288b
Vertical transmission, 300
  occurrence, 300b
Visceral leishmaniasis, 114b-115b

W

West African (Gambian) sleeping sickness, 120b-121b

Wheatley modification, stain usage, 24
Wheatley trichrome, 24
Whipworm infection (trichuriasis), 196b-197b
White blood cells (WBCs), 287
  amebic cysts, differentiation, 287b
  presence, 287
Wright's stain, usage (preference), 28
Wuchereria bancrofti, 225b
  adults, 226b
  asymptomatic patients, 226b
  clinical symptoms, 226
  diagnosis, specimen selection, 227b
  epidemiology, 226b
  laboratory diagnosis, 226b
  life cycle notes, 226b
  microfilariae, 225b-226b
    characteristics, 226t
  morphology, 225
  prevention/control, 227b
  preventive measure, strategy, 227b
  sheath (presence), nuclei (absence), 225f
  symptomatic bancroftian filariasis, 226b-227b
  treatment, 227b
  trends, 227b
Wuchereria bancrofti microfilaria illustration, 225f

X

Xenodiagnosis, 31
Xenopsylla cheopis (Oriental rat flea), microorganism (transmission), 310b

Y

Yeast, 289
  appearance, 25t
  characteristics, 289

Z

Zinc sulfate flotation techniques, 23